Non-Alcoholic Fatty Liver Disease: A Practical Guide

Non-Alcoholic Fatty Liver Disease: A Practical Guide

Editor: Heidi Hamlin

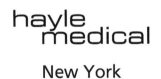

New York

Hayle Medical,
750 Third Avenue, 9th Floor,
New York, NY 10017, USA

Visit us on the World Wide Web at:
www.haylemedical.com

ISBN 978-1-64647-563-6 (Hardback)

Trademark Notice: Registered trademark of products or corporate names are used only for explanation and identification without intent to infringe.

Cataloging-in-Publication Data

Non-alcoholic fatty liver disease : a practical guide / edited by Heidi Hamlin.
    p. cm.
Includes bibliographical references and index.
ISBN 978-1-64647-563-6
1. Fatty liver. 2. Liver--Diseases. 3. Fatty liver--Treatment. 4. Fatty degeneration.
5. Hepatitis. I. Hamlin, Heidi.
RC848.F3 N66 2023
616.362--dc23

Contents

Preface

Non-alcoholic fatty liver disease (NAFLD) refers to the building up of extreme fat in the liver without any clear cause like alcohol use. NAFLD is categorized into two types that include non-alcoholic steatohepatitis (NASH), which also involves liver inflammation, and non-alcoholic fatty liver (NAFL). Non-alcoholic fatty liver is less risky when compared to NASH. Typically, it does not develop to the stage of liver cirrhosis or NASH. However, when NAFL reaches the stage of NASH, it ultimately causes severe problems including cardiovascular disease, liver failure, liver cancer and cirrhosis. The risk factors associated with NAFLD are unbalanced lifestyle, genetics, improper diet, obesity and type 2 diabetes. Liver biopsy, blood tests and imaging are some of the techniques that can be used to diagnose NAFLD. Its treatment involves weight loss which can be achieved through exercise and dietary changes. This book contains some path-breaking studies on non-alcoholic fatty liver disease. It aims to shed light on some of the unexplored aspects of this disease. This book will help new researchers by foregrounding their knowledge in this medical condition.

The information contained in this book is the result of intensive hard work done by researchers in this field. All due efforts have been made to make this book serve as a complete guiding source for students and researchers. The topics in this book have been comprehensively explained to help readers understand the growing trends in the field.

I would like to thank the entire group of writers who made sincere efforts in this book and my family who supported me in my efforts of working on this book. I take this opportunity to thank all those who have been a guiding force throughout my life.

Editor

Glutamate–Serine–Glycine Index: A Novel Potential Biomarker in Pediatric Non-Alcoholic Fatty Liver Disease

Simone Leonetti [1] , Raimund I. Herzog [2], Sonia Caprio [3], Nicola Santoro [3,4] and Domenico Tricò [1,*]

1   Department of Surgical, Medical and Molecular Pathology and Critical Care Medicine, University of Pisa, 56126 Pisa, Italy; s.leonetti@live.com
2   Department of Internal Medicine, Section of Endocrinology, Yale University School of Medicine, New Haven, CT 06510, USA; raimund.herzog@yale.edu
3   Department of Pediatrics, Yale University School of Medicine, New Haven, CT 06510, USA; sonia.caprio@yale.edu (S.C.); nicola.santoro@yale.edu (N.S.)
4   Department of Medicine and Health Sciences, "V.Tiberio" University of Molise, 86100 Campobasso, Italy
*   Correspondence: domenico.trico@unipi.it

Abstract: Preliminary evidence suggests that the glutamate–serine–glycine (GSG) index, which combines three amino acids involved in glutathione synthesis, may be used as a potential biomarker of non-alcoholic fatty liver disease (NAFLD). We investigated whether the GSG index is associated with NAFLD in youth, independent of other risk factors. Intrahepatic fat content (HFF%) and abdominal fat distribution were measured by magnetic resonance imaging (MRI) in a multiethnic cohort of obese adolescents, including Caucasians, African Americans, and Hispanics. NAFLD was defined as HFF% $\geq$ 5.5%. Plasma amino acids were measured by mass spectrometry. The GSG index was calculated as glutamate/(serine + glycine). The GSG index was higher in NAFLD patients (p = 0.03) and positively correlated with HFF% (r = 0.26, p = 0.02), alanine aminotransferase (r = 0.39, p = 0.0006), and aspartate aminotransferase (r = 0.26, p = 0.03). Adolescents with a high GSG index had a twofold higher prevalence of NAFLD than those with a low GSG index, despite similar adiposity, abdominal fat distribution, and liver insulin resistance. NAFLD prevalence remained significantly different between groups after adjustment for age, sex, race/ethnicity, and body mass index (OR 3.07, 95% confidence interval 1.09–8.61, p = 0.03). This study demonstrates the ability of the GSG index to detect NAFLD in at-risk pediatric populations with different genetically determined susceptibilities to intrahepatic fat accumulation, independent of traditional risk factors.

Keywords: amino acids; non-alcoholic fatty liver disease; pediatric obesity; insulin resistance

1. Introduction

Non-alcoholic fatty liver disease (NAFLD) has become the most common chronic liver disease worldwide, with an estimated prevalence of 40% in obese youth [1]. Therefore, there is an urgent clinical need for non-invasive, high-throughput diagnostic tools for NAFLD.

Metabolomics studies have recently identified specific amino acid patterns that may be used as potential biomarkers of liver disease [2]. Among them, Gaggini et al. [3] proposed a novel glutamate–serine–glycine (GSG) index, which combines three amino acids involved in glutathione synthesis and hepatic lipotoxicity. GSG index was found to be significantly higher in adults with biopsy-proven NAFLD compared with lean controls and was associated with liver enzymes and hepatic insulin resistance [3]. Furthermore, two preliminary reports showed that GSG index changes match longitudinal changes of surrogate markers of fatty liver after pharmacological or nutritional therapy [4,5]. These studies were limited by the lack of a control group of obese subjects without NAFLD [3,5] and of a direct quantification of liver fat content [4]. Moreover, the ability of GSG index to detect NAFLD has not been established in youths and different ethnic groups.

This study investigated whether the GSG index is associated with intrahepatic fat content in youth, independent of other risk factors.

2. Methods

2.1. Study Participants

Seventy-eight obese adolescents, including 26 (33.3%) Caucasians, 22 (28.2%) African Americans, and 29 (37.2%) Hispanics, were recruited from the Yale Pediatric NAFLD study cohort (age 13.3 ± 3.0 years, 38 boys and 40 girls, body mass index (BMI) z-score 2.31 ± 0.34), a long-term project aimed at studying metabolic and metagenomic alterations in obese youths [1,6], as previously reported [7]. All participants had a detailed medical history and a complete physical examination. Participants' ages ranged from 8–18 years and they had a BMI ≥95th percentile for age and sex. The main exclusion criteria were the use of medications known to affect liver function or amino acid metabolism; liver diseases besides NAFLD; and alcohol consumption. The study was approved by the Yale University Human Investigation Committee (HIC protocol #1104008388). All clinical investigations were conducted according to the principles expressed in the Declaration of Helsinki. Written informed parental consent and child assent were obtained from all participants.

2.2. Oral Glucose Tolerance Test

Participants were admitted to the Yale Center for Clinical Investigation (YCCI) at 8 a.m. after a 12-h overnight fast to undergo a 75 g oral glucose tolerance test (OGTT). One antecubital intravenous catheter was inserted for blood sampling after the local application of a topical anesthetic cream (Emla, Astra Zeneca, Wilmington, DE, USA). Fasting blood samples were then obtained for measurements of plasma glucose, insulin, lipid profile, amino acids, and liver enzymes. Thereafter, flavored glucose in a dose of 1.75 g per kilogram of body weight (up to a maximum of 75 g) was given orally, and arterialized venous blood samples were obtained every 30 min for 180 min for the measurement of plasma glucose and insulin.

2.3. Magnetic Resonance Imaging

Quantification of the hepatic fat fraction (HFF%) was performed by liver magnetic resonance imaging (MRI) on a Siemens Sonata 1.5 Tesla system (Erlangen, Germany) using the two-point Dixon (2PD) method as modified by Fishbein et al. [8]. NAFLD was defined as HFF% ≥ 5.5% [7]. The 2PD method was previously validated in obese adolescents against liver biopsy [1] and proton nuclear magnetic resonance (NMR) [9]. Visceral and subcutaneous fat depots were quantified by abdominal MRI [10].

2.4. Biochemical Analysis

Glucose samples were spun immediately and processed at the bedside using a YSI2700-STAT-Analyzer (Yellow Springs Instruments, Yellow Springs, OH, USA). Plasma insulin was measured by radioimmunoassay (Linco, St. Charles, MO, USA) that has <1% cross-reactivity with C-peptide and proinsulin. Plasma amino acids were measured using AbsoluteIDQ mass spectrometry-based assay kits (Biocrates Institutes, Innsbruck, Austria), as previously reported [7].

2.5. Calculations

The GSG index was calculated as glutamate/(serine + glycine) according to Gaggini et al. [3]. The hepatic insulin resistance index (HIRI) was calculated as a product of the glucose area under the curve (AUC) and insulin AUC during the first 30 min of the OGTT [11]. The Matsuda index was used to estimate whole-body insulin sensitivity (Whole-Body Insulin Sensitivity Index, WBISI) [12]. The insulinogenic index (IGI), which represents early phase insulin secretion, was calculated as the ratio of insulin at 30 min minus fasting insulin to the difference in glucose at 30 min minus fasting glucose. The disposition index (DI), which provides an integrated picture of glucose tolerance, including both insulin sensitivity and insulin secretion, was calculated as the product of the IGI and the WBISI [13].

2.6. Statistical Analysis

Group differences were analyzed using Student's *t*-test, Wilcoxon–Mann–Whitney test, or χ^2 test, as appropriate. Correlations were tested by Spearman correlation. To account for potential confounders, multivariable regression analysis was used including age, sex, BMI z-score, and race as independent variables. Odds ratios (OR) and 95% confidence intervals (95%) from logistic regression analyses are reported. A cut point of 0.36 identified the upper tertile of GSG index distribution and was used to stratify subjects in GSG-high and GSG-low. Analyses were performed using JMP Pro 14 (SAS Institutes, Cary, NC, USA) at a two-sided α level of 0.05.

3. Results

The GSG index was higher in adolescents with NAFLD (0.34 [0.28–0.51]) than without NAFLD (0.29 [0.19–0.40], $p = 0.03$) but similar in boys and girls ($p = 0.45$) and among different ethnic groups ($p = 0.40$). The GSG index correlated directly with HFF% (r = 0.26, $p = 0.02$), alanine aminotransferase (ALT; r = 0.39, $p = 0.0006$), and aspartate aminotransferase (AST; r = 0.26, $p = 0.03$). No relationships were found between GSG index and age, BMI z-score, markers of glucose control, lipid profile, visceral and subcutaneous fat, branched-chain amino acids (BCAA), and HIRI (all $p > 0.05$). The effect of GSG index on NAFLD prevalence and HFF% remained significant in multivariable models adjusted for age, sex, BMI z-score, and race ($\beta = 1.25$, $p = 0.01$ and $\beta = 1.07$, $p = 0.02$, respectively).

The two groups of GSG-high and GSG-low subjects were matched for age, sex, ethnicity, adiposity, glucose control, and cholesterol profile (Table 1). The prevalence of NAFLD and HFF% were significantly higher in adolescents with GSG-high compared with GSG-low, despite similar BMI z-score and abdominal fat distribution (Figure 1). In multivariable logistic regression analysis, the likelihood of NAFLD increased in the GSG-high group (OR 3.07, 95%CI [1.09–8.61], $p = 0.03$) independent of age, sex, BMI z-score, and race.

Table 1. Characteristics of participants stratified by glutamate–serine–glycine (GSG) index—high and low.

	GSG High (*n* = 26)	GSG Low (*n* = 52)	*p*
CLINICAL FEATURES			
Age (years)	12.7 ± 3.0	13.6 ± 3.0	0.30
Sex (M/F)	16 (62%)/10 (38%)	22 (42%)/30 (58%)	0.11
Race (Caucasian/African American/ Hispanic/Asian)	8 (31%)/4 (15%)/ 14 (54%)/0 (0%)	18 (35%)/18 (35%)/ 15 (29%)/1 (1%)	0.12
Body Mass Index (kg/m^2)	32.5 ± 6.9	34.69 ± 6.25	0.18
Body Mass Index z-score	2.29 ± 0.28	2.32 ± 0.37	0.73
Systolic blood pressure (mmHg)	115 ± 12	116 ± 9	0.66
Diastolic blood pressure (mmHg)	67 ± 8	68 ± 8	0.59
GLUCOSE METABOLISM			
Fasting glucose (mg/dL)	93 ± 7	92 ± 7	0.84
Fasting insulin (μU/mL)	27 [1.8–45]	27 [2.0–41]	0.71
2 h glucose (mg/dL)	120 ± 27	119 ± 24	0.86
Hemoglobin A1C (%)	5.52 ± 0.31	5.46 ± 0.30	0.41
HOMA-IR	6.23 [4.20–11.16]	6.51 [4.38–9.26]	0.66
Whole-Body Insulin Sensitivity Index	1.70 [0.74–2.46]	1.73 [1.11–2.39]	0.67
Hepatic Insulin Resistance Index	1611 [905–2403]	1499 [946–2018]	0.35
Insulinogenic Index	4.06 [2.43–6.50]	3.67 [2.85–5.08]	0.79
Disposition Index	5.05 [3.85–7.01]	5.88 [4.49–9.51]	0.34

Table 1. *Cont.*

	GSG High (*n* = 26)	GSG Low (*n* = 52)	*p*
LIPID PROFILE			
Total Cholesterol (mg/dL)	159 [140–179]	142 [131–169]	0.14
HDL Cholesterol (mg/dL)	40 [33–49]	46 [39–51]	0.07
LDL Cholesterol (mg/dL)	92 [76–119]	86 [72–102]	0.29
Triglycerides (mg/dL)	119 [85–140]	68 [50–106]	<0.0001
AMINO ACID PROFILE			
Glutamate (μmol/L)	147 [121–177]	73 [57–86]	<0.0001
Serine (μmol/L)	100 [88–106]	102 [87–117]	0.28
Glycine (μmol/L)	175 [149–203]	199 [180–239]	0.04
GSG index	0.50 [0.47–0.58]	0.25 [0.17–0.31]	<0.0001
BCAA (μmol/L)	413 [363–491]	423 [361–475]	0.70
ABDOMINAL FAT COMPOSITION			
Visceral (cm^2)	70.9 [48.5–90.6]	59.4 [39.6–81]	0.24
Subcutaneous (cm^2)	470.2 [356.2–680.2]	540.1 [398.8–734.1]	0.27
Visceral/Subcutaneous (%)	10.3 [8.7–14.9]	11.0 [8.2–16.7]	0.58
Visceral/Total (%)	9.4 [8.1–13.5]	10.0 [7.8–14.3]	0.67
LIVER ENZYMES			
Alanine transaminase (U/L)	24 [18–40]	17 [12–22]	0.001
Aspartate transaminase (U/L)	23 [20–32]	20 [17–25]	0.07

Data are number (percentage), mean ± SD, or median [interquartile range], as appropriate. Abbreviations: BCAA, branched-chain amino acids (i.e., isoleucine, leucine, and valine); HOMA-IR, homeostatic model assessment for insulin resistance.

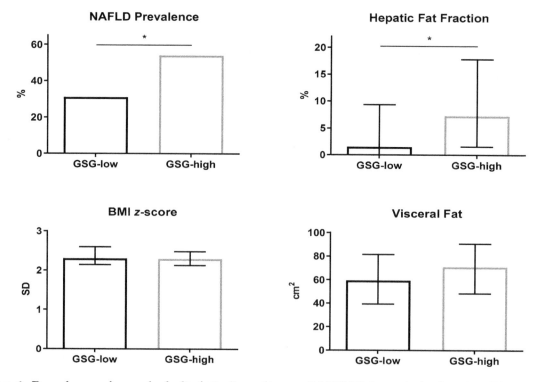

Figure 1. Prevalence of non-alcoholic fatty liver disease (NAFLD), hepatic fat fraction, BMI z-score, and visceral fat in obese adolescents with GSG-low and GSG-high. NAFLD prevalence is reported as percentage. Other data are reported as median and interquartile range. * $p < 0.05$.

4. Discussion

This study demonstrates the ability of the recently developed GSG index to detect NAFLD and its associated metabolic alterations (i.e., hypertriglyceridemia) in an at-risk population of obese adolescents. Noteworthy, by implementing an accurate MRI-based characterization of abdominal fat distribution, we observed for the first time that the relationship between GSG index and HFF% is independent of overall adiposity and visceral fat, supporting its role as a specific marker of intrahepatic fat content. This study also validates the use of the GSG index as a marker of NAFLD in pediatric populations and ethnic groups with different susceptibilities to intrahepatic fat accumulation, such as African Americans and Hispanics [1].

A recent untargeted, high-resolution metabolomics study identified several amino acid pathways dysregulated in adolescents with NAFLD, including glutamate, serine and glycine metabolism [14]. These amino acids are critical for the synthesis of glutathione, whose turnover is upregulated in NAFLD in response to oxidative stress, and of lipids associated with hepatic lipotoxicity (i.e., ceramides). Glycine and serine are consumed in these processes and are typically reduced in NAFLD [2]. Conversely, glutamate is consistently increased in NAFLD and other metabolic diseases [3]. In pathological conditions characterized by insulin resistance, such as NAFLD, obesity and metabolic syndrome, hepatic energy demands are increased due to altered mitochondrial metabolism and function [15–17]. In this context, the synthesis of liver aminotransferases is stimulated to cope with the increased need for transamination reactions [18]. Altered transaminase reactions, in turn, promote glutamate release and can justify the rise in plasma glutamate levels [19]. Furthermore, glutamate can be synthesized from proline metabolism. Higher proline concentrations have been reported in NAFLD in some [20], but not all [3], previous studies in adults. In our pediatric cohort, serum proline was similar in adolescents in the GSG-high and GSG-low group ($p = 0.72$), as well as in those with or without NAFLD ($p = 0.14$). Hence, the rise in glutamate is unlikely to be attributable to different proline concentrations. Finally, increased glutamate levels may also reflect greater dietary glutamate intake, which was not evaluated in our cohort.

The GSG index was initially associated with circulating liver enzymes and NAFLD histological severity [3], although subsequent biopsy studies do not support these findings [21]. In agreement with the earlier study, we found higher ALT and AST concentrations in the GSG-high group compared with the GSG-low group. Circulating transaminases are commonly used markers of hepatocellular damage, as they reflect the leaking of intracellular hepatocyte content into the circulation after liver injury. However, liver transaminase synthesis and release can also be enhanced in NAFLD as an adaptation to the increased metabolic demands, as mentioned above [18]. Altogether, these observations warrant further research to establish the GSG index as a reliable biomarker of NAFLD histological activity.

A marked increase in circulating branched-chain amino acids (BCAA) has been consistently reported in insulin-resistant states [22–24], including adult [3,25] and pediatric [7,14] NAFLD. Although an association between GSG index and total BCAA has been previously described [3], we could not find a significant relationship between GSG index and either single or total BCAA. This observation may be attributable to different study populations. Additionally, given that our data do not confirm the relation between GSG index and HIRI [3,4], it could be speculated that alterations in GSG index and BCAA differentially mark the distinct histological and metabolic features of NAFLD, namely inflammation/oxidative stress (for GSG index) and insulin resistance (for BCAA).

In conclusion, the GSG index represents a promising, minimally invasive biomarker for risk assessment of NAFLD in obese youths that is amenable to further validation in larger prospective cohort studies. These studies will provide an opportunity to establish whether the GSG index also correlates with NAFLD histological severity.

Author Contributions: S.L. and D.T. designed the study, analyzed the data, and wrote the first draft of the manuscript. R.I.H., S.C., and N.S. collected the data and critically revised the manuscript. All authors have read and agreed to the published version of the manuscript.

Acknowledgments: The authors are grateful to the patients and their families as well as to the Yale MS & Proteomics Resource of the WM Keck Foundation Biotechnology Resource Laboratory, the Yale Center for Clinical Investigation (YCCI) and Hospital Research Unit (HRU) personnel. This study was supported by the National Institutes of Health, National Institute of Child Health and Human Development (grants R01-HD-40787, R01-HD-28016, and K24-HD-01464, to S.C.) and National Institute of Diabetes and Digestive and Kidney Diseases (grant R01-DK-111038, to S.C.; grant R01DK114504, to N.S., grants DK045735, DK020495, and DK101984 to R.I.H.), the National Center for Research Resources (Clinical and Translational Science Award (grant UL1-RR-0249139)), the American Diabetes Association (Distinguished Clinical Scientist Award, to S.C.), and the European Foundation for the Study of Diabetes (Future Leaders Mentorship Programme for Clinical Diabetologists, to D.T.; Rising Star Fellowship, to D.T.).

References

1. Trico, D.; Caprio, S.; Umano, G.R.; Pierpont, B.; Nouws, J.; Galderisi, A.; Kim, G.; Mata, M.M.; Santoro, N. Metabolic Features of Nonalcoholic Fatty Liver (NAFL) in Obese Adolescents: Findings From a Multiethnic Cohort. *Hepatology* **2018**, *68*, 1376–1390. [CrossRef] [PubMed]

2. Trico, D.; Biancalana, E.; Solini, A. Protein and amino acids in nonalcoholic fatty liver disease. *Curr. Opin. Clin. Nutr. Metab. Care* **2020**. [CrossRef] [PubMed]

3. Gaggini, M.; Carli, F.; Rosso, C.; Buzzigoli, E.; Marietti, M.; Della Latta, V.; Ciociaro, D.; Abate, M.L.; Gambino, R.; Cassader, M.; et al. Altered amino acid concentrations in NAFLD: Impact of obesity and insulin resistance. *Hepatology* **2018**, *67*, 145–158. [CrossRef] [PubMed]

4. Gastaldelli, A.; Tripathy, D.; Gaggini, M.; Musi, N.; DeFron, O.R.A. Abstracts of 51st EASD Annual Meeting. *Diabetologia* **2015**, *58* (Suppl. S1), 1–607.

5. Khoo, J.; Koo, S.H.; Ching, J.; Soon, G.H.; Kovalik, J.P. Weight loss through lifestyle modification or liraglutide is associated with improvement of NAFLD severity and changes in amino acid concentrations. *Endocr. Abstr.* **2020**, *70*. [CrossRef]

6. Trico, D.; Koo, S.H.; Ching, J.; Soon, G.H.; Kovalik, J.P. Intestinal Glucose Absorption Is a Key Determinant of 1-Hour Postload Plasma Glucose Levels in Nondiabetic Subjects. *J. Clin. Endocrinol. Metab.* **2019**, *104*, 2131–2139. [CrossRef]

7. Goffredo, M.; Santoro, N.; Tricò, D.; Giannini, C.; D'Adamo, E.; Zhao, H.; Peng, G.; Yu, X.; Lam, T.T.; Pierpont, B.; et al. A Branched-Chain Amino Acid-Related Metabolic Signature Characterizes Obese Adolescents with Non-Alcoholic Fatty Liver Disease. *Nutrients* **2017**, *9*, 642. [CrossRef]

8. Fishbein, M.H.; Gardner, K.G.; Potter, C.J.; Schmalbrock, P.; Smith, M.A. Introduction of fast MR imaging in the assessment of hepatic steatosis. *Magn. Reson. Imaging* **1997**, *15*, 287–293. [CrossRef]

9. Cali, A.M.; De Oliveira, A.M.; Kim, H.; Chen, S.; Reyes-Mugica, M.; Escalera, S.; Dziura, J.; Taksali, S.E.; Kursawe, R.; Shaw, M.; et al. Glucose dysregulation and hepatic steatosis in obese adolescents: Is there a link? *Hepatology* **2009**, *49*, 1896–1903. [CrossRef]

10. Umano, G.R.; Shabanova, V.; Pierpont, B.; Mata, M.; Nouws, J.; Tricò, D.; Galderisi, A.; Santoro, N.; Caprio, S. A low visceral fat proportion, independent of total body fat mass, protects obese adolescent girls against fatty liver and glucose dysregulation: A longitudinal study. *Int. J. Obes. (Lond.)* **2019**, *43*, 673–682. [CrossRef]

11. Trico, D.; Galderisi, A.; Mari, A.; Polidori, D.; Galuppo, B.; Pierpont, B.; Samuels, S.; Santoro, N.; Caprio, S. Intrahepatic fat, irrespective of ethnicity, is associated with reduced endogenous insulin clearance and hepatic insulin resistance in obese youths: A cross-sectional and longitudinal study from the Yale Pediatric NAFLD cohort. *Diabetes Obes. Metab.* **2020**, *22*, 1628–1638. [CrossRef] [PubMed]

12. Matsuda, M.; DeFronzo, R.A. Insulin sensitivity indices obtained from oral glucose tolerance testing: Comparison with the euglycemic insulin clamp. *Diabetes Care* **1999**, *22*, 1462–1470. [CrossRef] [PubMed]

13. Yeckel, C.W.; Weiss, R.; Dziura, J.; Taksali, S.E.; Dufour, S.; Burgert, T.S.; Tamborlane, W.V.; Caprio, S. Validation of insulin sensitivity indices from oral glucose tolerance test parameters in obese children and adolescents. *J. Clin. Endocrinol. Metab.* **2004**, *89*, 1096–1101. [CrossRef] [PubMed]

14. Jin, R.; Banton, S.; Tran, V.T.; Konomi, J.V.; Li, S.; Jones, D.P.; Vos, M.B. Amino Acid Metabolism is Altered in Adolescents with Nonalcoholic Fatty Liver Disease-An Untargeted, High Resolution Metabolomics Study. *J. Pediatr.* **2016**, *172*, 14–19. [CrossRef] [PubMed]

15. Sunny, N.E.; Parks, E.J.; Browning, J.D.; Burgess, S.C. Excessive hepatic mitochondrial TCA cycle and gluconeogenesis in humans with nonalcoholic fatty liver disease. *Cell Metab.* **2011**, *14*, 804–810. [CrossRef]

16. Pirola, C.J.; Gianotti, T.F.; Burgueño, A.L.; Rey-Funes, M.; Loidl, C.F.; Mallardi, P.; San Martino, J.; Castaño, G.O.; Sookoian, S. Epigenetic modification of liver mitochondrial DNA is associated with histological severity of nonalcoholic fatty liver disease. *Gut* **2013**, *62*, 1356–1363. [CrossRef]

17. Sookoian, S.; Flichman, D.; Scian, R.; Rohr, C.; Dopazo, H.; Gianotti, T.F.; Martino, J.S.; Castaño, G.O.; Pirola, C.J. Mitochondrial genome architecture in non-alcoholic fatty liver disease. *J. Pathol.* **2016**, *240*, 437–449. [CrossRef]

18. Sookoian, S.; Castaño, G.O.; Scian, R.; Fernández Gianotti, T.; Dopazo, H.; Rohr, C.; Gaj, G.; San Martino, J.; Sevic, I.; Flichman, D.; et al. Serum aminotransferases in nonalcoholic fatty liver disease are a signature of liver metabolic perturbations at the amino acid and Krebs cycle level. *Am. J. Clin. Nutr.* **2016**, *103*, 422–434. [CrossRef]

19. Sookoian, S.; Pirola, C.J. Alanine and aspartate aminotransferase and glutamine-cycling pathway: Their roles in pathogenesis of metabolic syndrome. *World J. Gastroenterol.* **2012**, *18*, 3775–3781. [CrossRef]

20. Hasegawa, T.; Iino, C.; Endo, T.; Mikami, K.; Kimura, M.; Sawada, N.; Nakaji, S.; Fukuda, S. Changed Amino Acids in NAFLD and Liver Fibrosis: A Large Cross-Sectional Study without Influence of Insulin Resistance. *Nutrients* **2020**, *12*, 1450. [CrossRef]

21. Ioannou, G.N.; Nagana Gowda, G.A.; Djukovic, D.; Raftery, D. Distinguishing NASH Histological Severity Using a Multiplatform Metabolomics Approach. *Metabolites* **2020**, *10*, 168. [CrossRef] [PubMed]

22. Lynch, C.J.; Adams, S.H. Branched-chain amino acids in metabolic signalling and insulin resistance. *Nat. Rev. Endocrinol.* **2014**, *10*, 723–736. [CrossRef] [PubMed]

23. Newgard, C.B.; An, J.; Bain, J.R.; Muehlbauer, M.J.; Stevens, R.D.; Lien, L.F.; Haqq, A.M.; Shah, S.H.; Arlotto, M.; Slentz, C.A.; et al. A branched-chain amino acid-related metabolic signature that differentiates obese and lean humans and contributes to insulin resistance. *Cell Metab.* **2009**, *9*, 311–326. [CrossRef] [PubMed]

24. Trico, D.; Prinsen, H.; Giannini, C.; de Graaf, R.; Juchem, C.; Li, F.; Caprio, S.; Santoro, N.; Herzog, R.I. Elevated alpha-Hydroxybutyrate and Branched-Chain Amino Acid Levels Predict Deterioration of Glycemic Control in Adolescents. *J. Clin. Endocrinol. Metab.* **2017**, *102*, 2473–2481. [CrossRef]

25. Kalhan, S.C.; Guo, L.; Edmison, J.; Dasarathy, S.; McCullough, A.J.; Hanson, R.W.; Milburn, M. Plasma metabolomic profile in nonalcoholic fatty liver disease. *Metabolism* **2011**, *60*, 404–413. [CrossRef] [PubMed]

2

NAFLD Preclinical Models: More than a Handful, Less of a Concern?

Yvonne Oligschlaeger * and Ronit Shiri-Sverdlov

Department of Molecular Genetics, School of Nutrition and Translational Research in Metabolism (NUTRIM), Maastricht University, Universiteitssingel 50, 6229 ER, Maastricht, The Netherlands; r.sverdlov@maastrichtuniversity.nl

* Correspondence: yvonneoligschlaeger@ziggo.nl

Abstract: Non-alcoholic fatty liver disease (NAFLD) is a spectrum of liver diseases ranging from simple steatosis to non-alcoholic steatohepatitis, fibrosis, cirrhosis, and/or hepatocellular carcinoma. Due to its increasing prevalence, NAFLD is currently a major public health concern. Although a wide variety of preclinical models have contributed to better understanding the pathophysiology of NAFLD, it is not always obvious which model is best suitable for addressing a specific research question. This review provides insights into currently existing models, mainly focusing on murine models, which is of great importance to aid in the identification of novel therapeutic options for human NAFLD.

Keywords: NAFLD; mouse models; multifactorial disease; translational value

1. Introduction

Due to excess intake of fat- and/or sugar-enriched diets and a lack of exercise, overweight and obesity are currently a major and continuously growing public health concern. Strongly associated with the increasing trend in obesity is the metabolic syndrome (MetS), in which disturbed lipid homeostasis and metabolic inflammation are taking the lead. Besides type 2 diabetes (T2D) and cardiovascular diseases, MetS increases the risk of developing non-alcoholic fatty liver disease (NAFLD), the most prevalent chronic liver disease worldwide [1]. The spectrum of NAFLD ranges from benign simple steatosis [2] to steatohepatitis (NASH) and end-stage liver diseases. If steatosis is not managed in time, resident liver cells (e.g., Kupffer and hepatic stellate cells) become activated and immune cells (mainly macrophages) infiltrate the liver, a condition defined as NASH. This progressive form of NAFLD [3] can further trigger hepatocyte damage with/without fibrosis and increase the risk of cirrhosis [4] and hepatocellular carcinoma (HCC) [5]. In contrast to alcoholic liver disease- and viral hepatitis-induced HCC, NASH-related HCC is currently the most rapid growing indication for liver transplant in HCC patients [6].

Obviously, there is an urgent need for a reliable 'humanized' model that displays a liver phenotype that is identical to human disease, with macrovesicular steatosis, lobular inflammation, hepatocellular ballooning (including Mallory-Denk bodies), and fibrosis as predominant features. Subsequently, an optimal NAFLD model should have the ability to further progress to advanced fibrosis, cirrhosis, and ultimately HCC. Moreover, it should encompass MetS-related characteristics, such as obesity, disturbed lipid, glucose and insulin metabolism, as well as systemic inflammation. So far, using a wide variety of preclinical models, considerable efforts have recently been made to better understand the pathogenesis of human NAFLD and/or related clinical questions. However, none of these models resemble the complete human NAFLD spectrum, including related metabolic features that recapitulate this chronic liver disease. For instance, several models, exposed to various dietary compositions, have broadened our knowledge with regard to NAFLD progression, in particular early-onset low-grade inflammation. Alternative models (genetic or chemically-induced) provided insights into fibrotic features of human NAFLD, one of the most important predictors of human NASH progression [7]. Other models have been more suitable for testing therapeutic interventions in the context of NAFLD/NASH. Nevertheless, there are still significant unmet needs with regard to non-invasive diagnostic methods, therapeutic target identification, and drug development, which implies the need for robust preclinical models [8]. In the current Review, we will provide an update on existing preclinical NAFLD models. This Review focuses on rodents, mainly on mouse models, which are relatively low in costs and therefore allow for studying metabolic and genetic drivers of NAFLD/NASH within a considerable time frame. Moreover, these models serve as an important and well-controlled tool for preclinical drug testing in a multisystemic environment.

2. Insights into Available Preclinical Models for Non-alcoholic Fatty Liver Disease

A wide variety of dietary, genetic, chemically-induced, and/or other rodent models ([8–16]) have greatly advanced our understandings on NAFLD pathophysiology, as will be discussed in the following sections (see also Figure 1, Table 1).

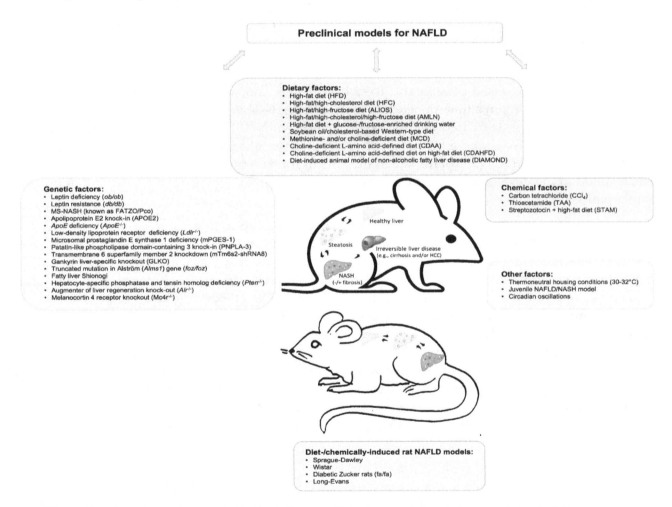

Figure 1. Brief schematic overview of existing preclinical models involving a variety of dietary, genetic, chemical, and other factors to study non-alcoholic fatty liver disease (NAFLD).

2.1. Dietary Murine Models

Diet-induced obesity is known to be the most common risk factor for NAFLD in humans [17]. The experimental NAFLD/NASH models are often based on overnutrition, a condition that can be induced by means of diets varying in macronutrient composition, amongst others.

One of the simplest ways of disturbing lipid metabolism, inducing steatosis and moderate NASH, is by the administration of a regular high-fat diet (HFD; 60% fat, 20% proteins, 20% carbohydrates) [18,19]. For instance, feeding wild-type C57BL/6 mice a HFD for 10–12 weeks resulted in phenotypic changes such as hyperlipidemia, hyperinsulinemia, and glucose intolerance [19,20]. Despite hepatic steatosis, inflammatory cell infiltration was not present until 19 weeks of HFD intake [19]. While after long-term (34–36 weeks) HFD feeding, significant increases in circulating liver enzyme levels, i.e., alanine aminotransferase (ALT) and aspartate aminotransferase (AST) were observed [19], these mice showed only minor signs of inflammation and fibrosis [21], even after prolonged administration up to 50 weeks [19]. Yet, after chronic feeding (80 weeks) of HFD, which mimics lifetime HFD consumption and enables proper design of treatment options, Velázquez et al. [17] demonstrated that mice displayed obesity and insulin resistance. In addition, these mice were shown to develop NAFLD features, including hepatic steatosis, cell injury, portal and lobular inflammation, hepatic ER stress, as well as fibrosis [17]. In line with Chen et al. [22], which showed a deterioration in NAFLD when germ-free mice were inoculated with the Firmicutes phyla, they also found increases in the Firmicutes phyla in response to prolonged HFD [17]. Though intestinal permeability was not measured in this study, these data pointed towards diet-induced gut-microbial dysbiosis [17], a well-known microbial event that has been previously observed in NAFLD patients [23]. Yet, it is unclear whether a similar but shorter dietary intervention would also provide insights into NAFLD progression [17].

In contrast to regular HFD, the atherogenic diet, composed of 1.25% cholesterol plus 0.5% cholate, resulted in increased plasma and liver lipid levels and was shown to induce NASH with hepatocellular ballooning in a time-dependent manner from 6–24 weeks [24]. Notably, the addition of a high-fat component exacerbated the histologic severity of NASH, and resulted in hepatic insulin resistance, oxidative stress, and activation of hepatic stellate cells [24]. Exposure to HFD containing 0.1–2.0% cholesterol (HFC) [25,26] for seven months in murine models, such as wild-type C57BL/6 mice, resulted in the development of obesity, hepatomegaly, hepatic steatosis, and varying degrees of steatohepatitis [27].

Due to the variability in disease onset and limited development of fibrosis, a novel so-called Amylin Liver NASH (AMLN) model was generated [28]. This model covers a high-fat/high-fructose (40%/22%) diet containing trans-fatty acids (~18%) and high-cholesterol (2%), thereby better resembling the Western-type diet and subsequent development of NASH features. Remarkably, only after 26–30 weeks of feeding an AMLN diet, wild-type C57BL/6 developed marked steatosis, moderate lobular inflammation and hepatocellular ballooning [29]. However, when obese leptin-deficient *ob/ob* mice were fed a similar AMLN diet for 12 weeks, mice displayed an accelerated and more pronounced metabolic NASH phenotype as compared to wild-type C57BL/6 [29]. Indeed, it is well-known that *ob/ob* mice, which carry a homozygous mutation in the leptin gene that protect it from binding to its receptor, are susceptible to insulin resistance and T2D, thus being predisposed to metabolic features resembling NAFLD [30]. Yet, spontaneous progression from simple steatosis to NASH and hepatic fibrosis is rather prevented in these mice [31], pointing towards the need of a second stimulus.

More recently, according to the FDA-ban on trans-fats as food additives [32], another obesogenic trans-fat-free diet substituted with saturated fat (palm oil) was explored [33]. This so-called Gubra Amylin NASH (GAN) diet has a nutrient composition and caloric density (40% high-fat, 22% high-fructose 2% high-cholesterol) similar to AMLN diet. Upon feeding *ob/ob* mice GAN diet for 16 weeks, animals displayed biopsy-confirmed liver lesions with features of fibrotic NASH. While these features were similar to AMLN-fed *ob/ob* mice, GAN-fed *ob/ob* mice showed a more pronounced weight gain and increased adiposity. In contrast, wild-type C57BL/6 mice required a prolonged feeding period (28 weeks) of GAN diet to induce consistent fibrotic NASH. However, compared to AMLN diet, GAN-fed wild-type mice had significantly greater body weight gain. Altogether, obesogenic GAN diet induces hallmarks of fibrotic NASH in both models [33], suggesting its suitability for preclinical therapeutic testing against NASH.

Administering an alternative fast-food-like nutritional regime based on high-fat/high-fructose/high-cholesterol (41%/30%/2%) was also shown to induce NASH in various genotypes [34]. These models included wild-type C57BL/6, *ob/ob* mice as well as KK-A^y [35] mice, the latter carrying a mutation in the Agouti gene that increases its susceptibility to human NAFLD-like metabolic alterations [36]. Relevantly, Abe et al. [34] showed that *ob/ob* mice under these conditions displayed more pronounced NAFLD activity score, fibrosis progression, obesity and hyperinsulinemia compared to the other models. Given that the metabolic, histologic, and transcriptomic features observed in *ob/ob* mice were similar to human NASH, this model may be further explored as a potential preclinical tool to discover novel drugs for NASH [34].

Relevantly, Henkel et al. [37] explored the impact of long-term exposure (20 weeks) with a high-caloric (43%) Western-type diet composed of soy-bean oil (high n-6-PUFA, 25g/100g) and 0.75% cholesterol. In contrast to cholesterol-free HFD [38], dietary cholesterol in soybean oil resulted in increased Kupffer cell activation and oxidative stress as well as hepatic steatosis, ballooning, inflammation and fibrosis in wild-type C57BL/6 [37], which closely resembles clinical NASH features. In line, when mice were fed an alternative high-caloric (45%) cholesterol-free HFD (composed of lard (21g/100g)/soy-bean oil (3g/100g)/5% fructose in drinking water), only mild steatosis and no signs of hepatic inflammation and fibrosis were observed [37]. Thus, in agreement with previous studies [25,26,38–40], these findings indicate that the supplementation of dietary cholesterol triggers experimental hepatic inflammation and fibrosis [37].

Other dietary variants were explored by Montandon et al. [41], comparing the high-fat atherogenic diet (60% fat plus 1.25% cholesterol and 0.5% cholic acid) versus the commonly used methionine/choline-deficient diet (MCD). In line with others [24,42], wild-type C57BL/6 mice fed a cholesterol/cholate-rich diet showed increases in hepatic cholesterol and free fatty acids, while MCD mice predominantly accumulated triglycerides in their livers [41]. Strikingly, MCD caused a reduction in liver weights, whereas atherogenic diet did not [41]. Moreover, MCD increased hepatic damage, lobular inflammation, lipogranulomas, tissue fibrosis, and liver enzymes compared to mice fed a cholesterol/cholate-rich diet. In addition, transcriptional analyses revealed a dysregulation in extracellular matrix remodeling and hepatic stellate cell activation in response to MCD, but not an atherogenic diet [41]. Altogether, these data pointed towards a more severe form of NASH in MCD mice [41], which was in line with previous studies showing that MCD triggered extensive hepatic inflammation in rats [43] and mice [44–46] within a very short time frame. To overcome the lack of severe hepatic fibrosis often observed in preclinical models, mice are commonly fed MCD [47] or a diet low in/deficient for choline (CD) [48]. Although CD exacerbated fatty liver [48], MCD resulted in rapid NASH development with severe liver fibrosis within 4–10 weeks, likely as a consequence of reduced VLDL synthesis and hepatic-β oxidation [20]. While liver inflammation and elevated circulating liver enzyme levels returned back to normal levels after switching the diet back to control within 16 weeks, fibrosis and CD68-positive macrophages remained present [47].

It is also interesting to note that leptin-resistant *db/db* mice (which carry a mutation in the leptin receptor gene [49] and lack the ability to spontaneously develop hepatic inflammation [35,50]) displayed marked hepatic inflammation and fibrosis in response to feeding an MCD diet for four weeks [45]. These data suggest that, similar to *ob/ob* mice [31,51], *db/db* mice need a second stimulus to induce NASH [45]. Nevertheless, it is noteworthy that all MCD models rather showed significant reductions in weight, concomitant loss in liver mass and cachexia, as well as low serum levels of insulin, fasting glucose, leptin and triglycerides, and a lack of insulin resistance [12,45,52]. Given that these preclinical observations are opposite to the effects seen in overweight and obese individuals with NAFLD, these data suggest that the use of MCD models as preclinical tools to represent human NAFLD is rather limited [53]. Further, though *ob/ob* and *db/db* models serve as useful preclinical tools that mimic insulin resistance as observed in humans, it should be kept in mind that these mice bear mutations that are not prevalent in obese humans or NASH patients.

Relevantly, compared to the MCD diet, mice on a choline-deficient L-amino acid-defined (CDAA) diet developed a more severe degree of NASH and fibrosis, while not having any signs of weight loss [54]. Yet, only after long-term feeding, i.e., 5–6 months with CDAA diet, wild-type C57BL/6 mice displayed increased plasma lipid levels and HOMA-IR, pointing towards the development of insulin resistance [55]. It is relevant to note that the combination of CDAA with HFD may be capable of catalysing the development of NASH [54], though humanized features of metabolic disturbances will be absent in this model [11,54].

The American lifestyle induced obesity syndrome (ALIOS) diet is also a frequently used diet, in which high fat is combined with fructose-containing drinking water [56]. Compared to high trans-fat diets without additional fructose, these mice showed increased body weight and reduced insulin sensitivity, whereas no alterations in the degree of steatosis or liver transaminase levels were observed [11,56]. Moreover, in response to ALIOS diet, some pro-fibrogenic genes were found to be increased, while fibrosis was not detectable [56]. However, when mice were additionally administered a low weekly dose of intraperitoneal carbon tetrachloride (CCl_4), these animals were shown to develop progressive stages of human fatty liver disease, ranging from simple steatosis to inflammation, fibrosis, and cancer [57]. Nevertheless, one important limitation of ALIOS is related to its dietary composition, as the amount of trans-fat per kilogram is greater than in commonly used fast foods [56].

Another promising model is the so-called diet-induced animal model of non-alcoholic fatty liver disease (DIAMOND). This model is based on wild-type C57BL/6 mice that were crossed with S129S1/svlmJ, a commonly used model to create mice with targeted mutations. After approximately four months of Western-type diet (42% kcal fat, 0.1% cholesterol, 3.1 g/L d-fructose, 18.9 g/L d-glucose), these mice have shown to recapitulate key physiological and metabolic features of human NASH [58]. However, a limitation of this dietary intervention is the high frequency of HCC development and suppression of cholesterol synthesis, which is substantially different from the human situation [12,58].

While in response to a chow diet, MS-NASH mice [59] (formerly known as FATZO/Pco mice, a cross between wild-type C57BL/6J and obesity-prone AKR/J mice [60]) spontaneously develop obesity [61], feeding these mice a Western-type fructose-supplemented diet resulted in progressive features of NAFLD/NASH [59,62]. Given the concomitant dysregulation in metabolic status, these data point towards a novel tool for studying NAFLD with high translational value.

In summary, the above-described models have provided better insights into NAFLD/NASH pathogenesis. Nevertheless, it is noteworthy that these models failed to consistently achieve the full spectrum of human NASH, thereby limiting its preclinical validity.

2.2. Genetic Murine Models

Genetic animal models are essential for unravelling the underlying mechanisms related to the progression of NAFLD. Besides obesogenic *db/db* [45] and *ob/ob* mice [31,51], other models frequently used to study the total spectrum of human NAFLD and associated complications are based on genetically-modified mice in which the murine *ApoE* gene is being substituted by the human apolipoprotein E2 (APOE2) gene, referred to as the APOE2ki model [63]. Whereas wild-type C57BL/6 mice only developed simple steatosis in response to HFD, APOE2ki mice also displayed early-stage hepatic inflammation [63]. Yet, it is important to note that the inflammatory response did not persist in these mice [63]. Therefore, it is very likely that APOE2 gene is not the main gene responsible for the development of hepatic inflammation [25,63].

Relevantly, a complete lack of the murine *ApoE* gene, i.e., *ApoE*$^{-/-}$ model [64], resulted in hyperlipidemia after feeding these mice a high-fat diet [64]. Yet, under these conditions, mice spontaneously developed atherosclerotic plaques, while lacking humanized lipoprotein profiles [64], which suggests that this model is less suitable for human NAFLD research.

Remarkably, existing knowledge on the low-density lipoprotein receptor (*Ldlr*), an important gene regulating the transport of non-modified lipids into macrophages, led to a major breakthrough in the field of NASH [25,63]. By a complete depletion of the *Ldlr*, mice fed a HFC diet for 3–12 weeks were able to resemble lifestyle-induced sustained hepatic inflammation [63]. Moreover, these mice displayed high levels of circulating LDL and low levels of HDL, thus closely mimicking the human lipoprotein profile [63]. Hence, this model is considered a physiological model to investigate early onset of NASH [25,63]. While the severity of fibrosis is rather mild, these mice have been shown to develop more fibrosis compared to regular C57BL/6 mice on a similar diet [25,63].

A more recent study investigated the relation between prostaglandin E2 and the severity of NASH, both in a clinical and preclinical context [65]. In general, prostaglandin E_2, a member of the prostaglandin family, is known to play an important role during the inflammatory processes [66,67] in diseases such as rheumatoid arthritis and osteoarthritis [68]. However, its exact role in hepatic inflammation remains unknown. Henkel et al. [65] showed that a deficiency in the expression of enzymes responsible for murine prostaglandin E2 synthesis triggered a tumor necrosis factor α (TNFα)-dependent inflammatory response in the liver, thereby increasing the severity of diet-induced murine NASH. However, given that fibrosis and genotype-specific differences in macrophage infiltration were rather absent [65], it is very likely that the timing of feeding intervention (20 weeks) was not optimal to allow for advanced-stages disease development.

Another well-known model is based on a knock-in of the Patatin-like phospholipase domain-containing 3 (PNPLA3) polymorphism [20], which was found to be present in approximately one-fifth of our population [69,70]. PNPLA3 is a functional enzyme with acyltransferase and/or lipase activity towards phospholipids and/or triglycerides and retinyl esters, respectively [71]. When mice, carrying a mutation at position 148 of the Pnpla3 gene were fed a high-sucrose diet, animals displayed increased levels of triglycerides and fatty acids, resulting in increased hepatic steatosis [72]. Nevertheless, no significant changes in hepatic inflammatory gene expression or fibrosis were observed [72]. Furthermore, in response to HFD, the development of hepatic steatosis was absent [72]. These data point towards diet as a primary trigger for PNPLA3-polymorphism-associated hepatic steatosis [72], thereby not covering the full spectrum of NAFLD.

Similarly, hepatic knockdown of transmembrane 6 superfamily member 2 (Tm6sf2), a gene responsible for regulating hepatic lipid metabolism and associated with increased susceptibility to human NAFLD [73], resulted in increased hepatic fat content and decreased VLDL secretion [74]. Though the specific role of Tm6sf2 gene is not yet known, these data point towards its contribution to NAFLD development, and hence, its translational applicability. Remarkably, a recent meta-analysis showed that rs58542926 polymorphism significantly associated with chronic liver disease in the overall population [73]. These novel data pointed towards the diagnostic ability of TM6SF2-polymorphism to identify individuals at higher risk for developing NAFLD, cirrhosis, and HCC, as well as alcohol-dependent liver disease [73].

Another recent study investigated the role of Gankyrin (Gank) [75], an oncogene frequently expressed in several types of cancer [76] and a strong driver of liver proliferation. Using mice carrying a liver-specific deletion in Gank, it was shown that feeding a HFD for 6–7 months prevented fibrosis development in Gank$^{-/-}$ mice compared to HFD-fed wild-type mice [75]. While Gank$^{-/-}$ mice showed a higher degree of hepatic steatosis compared to HFD-fed wild-type mice, it has been postulated that hepatic steatosis protects the liver from fibrosis, and therefore liver proliferation could be a trigger for hepatic fibrosis [75]. Hence, the therapeutic potential of inhibiting hepatic proliferation as a strategy against NAFLD should be further investigated.

A more recent genetically-modified model that has become popular in NAFLD research is the obese foz/foz mouse model, which carries an 11-base pair truncating mutation in the Alström gene Alms1 [12,14,77]. Alms1 is widely expressed and disrupted by mutations in a human obesity syndrome, referred to as Alstroöm syndrome [78]. When feeding a HFD within a time frame of ten months, foz/foz mice displayed features of MetS, including obesity, hyperglycemia, hyperlipidemia, and insulin resistance [77]. In addition, these mice spontaneously developed steatosis, hepatic inflammation, and fibrosis [77]. Yet, while all foz/foz models have shown to develop obesity, some develop higher NAFLD activity scores and/or fibrosis than others, implying that the severity of NASH in these mice is inconsistent [14]. Moreover, given that the exact role of *Alms1* is not yet completely understood, the translational character of this model is rather limited.

Another mouse model that spontaneously develops hepatic inflammation with rather a mild degree of fibrosis is the lean polygenetic fatty liver Shionogi (FLS) [79,80]. Remarkably, when backcrossing these mice with *ob/ob* mice, severe liver steatosis, inflammation, advanced fibrosis, and spontaneous HCC appeared to develop [81]. Nevertheless, due to its uncontrollable heterogeneity in disease onset, these models are scarcely used [82].

Other studies have used the hepatocyte-specific phosphatase and tensin homolog (PTEN)-deficient mouse model as a model for NAFLD [83,84]. PTEN, which is a phosphatase with activities towards both protein and lipids, was first discovered as a tumor suppressor protein [85]. More recently, its function as a metabolic regulator, also in the liver, has received increasing attention [85]. Indeed, PTEN-deficient mice were shown to display human-like lipid accumulation followed by liver fibrosis and HCC [83,84]. Nevertheless, these mice do not exhibit obvious human-like NASH features, such as increased circulating fatty acid levels and obesity, thereby limiting its translational potential.

In contrast, others studied the role of augmenter of liver regeneration (*Alr*) in the context of NAFLD [86]. ALR, encoded by Growth Factor ERV1 homolog of *Saccharomyces cerevisiae* (*Gfer*), is an ubiquitous and multifunctional protein [86] that plays a vital role in liver generation, via regulating Natural Killer cell function [87], as well as other liver-related functions [88], including Kupffer cell activation [89]. Though mice deficient for *Alr* were prone to develop excessive hepatic steatosis [86], hepatic lipid accumulation was reversed at 4–8 weeks. Despite reversal of steatosis, mice developed hepatic inflammation, including hepatocellular necrosis, ductal proliferation, and fibrosis, which preceded dysplasia and HCC tumor development by nearly 60% one year after birth [11,86]. Hence, this model could aid in better understanding the progression from hepatic necrosis, inflammation, and fibrosis to carcinogenesis.

Another example is the melanocortin 4 receptor knockout (*Mc4r-/-*) mouse model [90]. MC4R is a G protein-coupled receptor expressed in hypothalamic nuclei being involved in regulating food intake and body weight [90]. Whereas chow-fed *Mc4r-/-* mice were shown to develop late onset obesity, hyperphagia, and simple steatosis due to genetic mutation, feeding a HFD induced ballooning degeneration, hepatic inflammation, and pericellular fibrosis [9]. In line with these results, using MRI-based techniques, Yamada et al. [91] recently showed that *Mc4r-/-* mice fed a HFD for 20 weeks developed obesity and NASH with clear signs of moderate fibrosis. Given their ability to functionally mimic the human NASH disease state, this model holds potential for studying hepatic dysfunction during advanced stages of NASH.

Alternative genetic models to study NASH progression and (spontaneously developing) HCC are the Tsumura-Suzuki Obese Diabetes (TSOD) mice, keratin 18-, NF-κB essential modulator (NEMO)-, and methionine adenosyltransferase 1A (MAT1a)-deficient models [92]. TSOD mice spontaneously developed NAFLD-related features, including T2D, obesity, glucosuria, hyperglycemia, and hyperinsulinemia without any special treatment [93]. Keratin 18 deficiency in mice serves as a model of NASH-associated liver carcinogenesis [94]. Liver-specific deletion of *NEMO* triggered steatosis, NASH, inflammatory fibrosis and subsequently HCC [95]. *Mat1a* gene deletion in mice impaired VLDL synthesis and plasma lipid homeostasis, thereby contributing to NAFLD development [96]. Yet, these models are generally less common and therefore less well-described in literature.

2.3. Chemically-induced Murine Models

As earlier described, alternative ways to explore the progression and/or regression of liver fibrosis and subsequent development of cirrhosis is by targeting the liver with CCL_4 [57] or other chemotoxins, such as thioacetamide (TAA) [8,11,12]. For instance, biweekly administration of CCL_4 for six weeks led to increased circulating aminotransferase and alkaline phosphatase levels in Balb/C mice [97]. In addition, CCL_4 caused a dose-dependent progression of liver fibrosis [97]. However, the exact pathophysiological mechanism underlying hepatic fibrogenesis, in particular the role of hepatic stellate cells, requires further investigation.

More recently, co-administration of TAA and western-type diet for eight weeks in wild-type C57BL/6 mice was shown to induce hepatic inflammation, severe diffuse fibrosis, and collagen deposition [98]. Nevertheless, due to significant reductions in body weight, these models do not optimally resemble humanized NASH etiology.

One prominent model developed to better understand the progression from NAFLD to HCC is the STAM model, in which neonates received a low dose of streptozotocin, followed by a HFD starting from four weeks of age [99]. At ~6 weeks, ~8–12 weeks, and ~16–20 weeks of age, these mice developed inflammation and hepatocellular ballooning, progressive fibrosis, and HCC, respectively [99]. Concomitantly, these mice had reduced body weight and insulin levels compared to HFD-fed mice [99]. These data imply that NAFLD progression is likely an artificial process that does not accurately reflect human disease pathology, thereby limiting its preclinical potential.

Similar to the clinical situation, many preclinical NAFLD studies in dietary and genetic models demonstrated increased severity in males [100,101]. However, it should be noted that sex differences may vary between models and genotypes [25,102]. For instance, we previously showed that female $Ldlr^{-/-}$ and APOE2ki mice fed HFD displayed a very early hepatic inflammatory response [25]. Similarly, it was demonstrated that female C57BL/6 wild-type mice fed a high-fructose diet developed greater hepatic inflammation despite having similar liver steatosis as compared to male mice [103]. Other studies showed that female juvenile NAFLD/NASH models displayed hepatic oxidative stress, whereas male animals rather developed hepatic inflammation [104]. In line with these results, it was more recently shown that high fat intake (60% kcal and 34.9% g fat, 20% kcal and 26.2% g protein, and 20% kcal and 26.3% g carbohydrate) by juvenile female mice contributed to NAFLD development, whereas similar fat intake by maternal-offspring (i.e., high-fat intake two weeks before conception and during gestation and lactation) resulted in the successful establishment of NASH [105]. These data suggest that maternal exposure, as well as the HFD component, contribute to the degree of NAFLD disease severity in juvenile female offspring [105].

2.4. Other Murine Models

Besides a role for genetic and dietary factors in preclinical NAFLD development, recent focus has also discretely shifted towards the relevance of housing conditions, thereby introducing a novel concept of thermoneutral housing (30–32 °C) [106]. Compared to standard housing conditions, mice housed under thermoneutral conditions were not only shown to induce a pro-inflammatory immune response, but also to deteriorate HFD-induced NASH progression [106]. Additionally, mice displayed increased intestinal permeability and alterations in gut microbiome, features mimicking the human situation [106]. Although these hallmarks could also partially refute the sex bias that is often observed in murine models of NAFLD, there were no signs of hepatic fibrosis, neither in male nor in female C57BL/6 wild-type mice [106]. Altogether, these data propose that a dietary stimulus is prerequisite for liver fibrosis development.

It is well-known that the liver is a central metabolic organ, whose functions are capable of adapting to rhythmical changes of environment. Indeed, it has been previously shown that circadian rhythm is driving oscillations in hepatic triglyceride levels, inflammation, oxidative stress, mitochondrial dysfunction, and hepatic insulin resistance [107,108]. Moreover, it has been recently suggested that chronic disruption of circadian rhythm may spontaneously induce the progression from NAFLD to NASH, fibrosis, and HCC [20,109], similar to the human situation, pointing towards its translational value.

Last but not least, there has also been increased awareness on the validity and reproducibility of preclinical studies on NAFLD [110–112]. For instance, it has been shown that murine liver fibrosis is affected by sampling variation [8]. More recently, Jensen et al. [2] demonstrated that feeding wild-type C57BL/6 mice a high-fat/high-fructose/high-cholesterol diet (40%/20%/2%) for 16 weeks resulted in significant intraindividual differences in fibrosis score and several hepatic biomarkers. Nevertheless, differences in sample variation were absent in other routinely used NAFLD rodent models [2]. These data pointed towards the importance of standardizing sampling site location during preclinical liver biopsy procedures, thereby supporting the ability to compare experimental outcomes between individual murine NASH studies.

2.5. Rat NAFLD Models

In addition to the importance of murine models, preclinical studies on NAFLD pathogenesis are also frequently performed using rats. Rat models are thought to be more susceptible to HFD, and thus may display more severe and/or earlier histological features of NAFLD compared to mice [113]. A small selection of rat studies on NAFLD will be highlighted in this section.

Similar to mice, commonly used rat models refer to nutritional, genetic, and combined models (extensively reviewed elsewhere [114,115]), of which Sprague–Dawley [116,117], Wistar [118], and/or diabetic Zucker rats (fa/fa) [119] are well-known examples. For instance, Lieber et al. [120] and others [117] reported that Sprague–Dawley rats on a HFD (71% fat/11% carbohydrates/18% proteins) were able to develop insulin resistance, mild-to-marked steatosis, inflammation and/or fibrogenesis, thereby reproducing key features of human NASH. Yet, when fed a standard Lieber–DeCarli diet (35% fat, 47% carbohydrates, 18% proteins), rats displayed no signs of steatosis, inflammation, or fibrosis [120]. Diabetic Zucker rats, a well-characterized model of NAFLD, displayed similar features as its murine counterparts *ob/ob* and *db/db* mice, i.e., spontaneous development of severe obesity, steatosis, and insulin resistance [11]. Moreover, it was shown that Zucker rats are in need of an additional stimulus for onset of NASH [119]. Relevantly, when comparing 4 weeks of MCD diet between different rat models (i.e., Wistar, Long–Evans, and Sprague–Dawley rats), the Wistar strain was associated with the highest degree of hepatic fat accumulation [121], pointing either towards strain-dependency or the impact of dietary exposure time.

Altogether, rat models are useful tools for providing additional valuable insights into the complex pathogenesis of steatosis/NASH (but not HCC), even though dietary or chemical interventions in these animals do not fully resemble the human situation.

3. Therapeutic Approaches in Preclinical NAFLD Models

In addition to exploring NAFLD etiology, preclinical models are critically important for testing how potential therapeutic drugs can interfere with the progression of this chronic disease [115].

Previously, Zheng et al. [27] chronically exposed HFC-treated mice with Ezetimibe, which is known to reduce plasma LDL by selectively binding to the intestinal cholesterol transporter Niemann–Pick type C1-like 1. After four weeks of Ezetimibe, significant improvements in fatty liver were observed, which were associated with a decrease in hepatic triglycerides, cholesteryl esters, and free cholesterol [27]. Additionally, chronic treatment with Ezetimibe resulted in significant reductions in plasma ALT activity, pointing towards its ability to serve as a novel treatment for HFC-induced NAFLD [27].

Trevaskis et al. [51] treated HFD-induced wild-type C57BL/6 and *ob/ob* mice with GLP-1R agonist AC3174, an exenatide analog. AC3174 treatment significantly reduced intrahepatic lipid accumulation, plasma triglycerides, and ALT levels, likely due to its contribution in weight loss [51]. Additionally, data suggested that AC3174 modestly improved the histological severity of fibrosis, which was demonstrated by a decrease in liver collagen-1 protein. Altogether, these findings suggest that AC3174 may play a beneficial role in the treatment of key aspects of fibrotic NASH.

Domitrovic et al. [97] investigated the therapeutic effect of luteolin in the context of liver fibrosis. Luteolin is a member of the flavonoid family, which has shown to exhibit hepatoprotective activity in acute liver damage, amongst others [122]. Administration of luteolin to CCL$_4$-treated mice resulted in a dose-dependent reduction in hepatic fibrosis [97]. Although studies on the impact of luteolin in a more chronic model of liver fibrosis are desired, these data pointed towards therapeutic application of this drug in patients with hepatic fibrosis [97]. Similarly, in a study of Ganbold et al. [3], it was recently shown that administration of isorhamnetin, another natural flavonoid to human-like NASH mice, resulted in improved steatosis, liver injury, and fibrosis, pointing towards its therapeutic potential in NASH.

More recently, Khurana et al. [117] studied the role of inhibiting extracellular cathepsin D, a lysosomal enzyme that plays a role in lipid-related disorders, including NAFLD [123,124]. Using HFD-fed Sprague–Dawley rats, it was shown that inhibition of extracellular cathepsin D improved hepatic steatosis and reduced plasma levels of insulin and hepatic transaminases [117]. These data suggest that modulation of extracellular cathepsins may serve as a novel therapeutic modality for NAFLD [117].

Gehrke et al. [125] recently investigated eight to ten week-old wild-type C57BL/6 male mice that were fed an obesogenic diet (fructose/glucose supplementation in drinking water). In this study, mice were either challenged with voluntary wheel running or were kept on a sedentary lifestyle intervention [125]. Similar to well-known forced exercise models [126], voluntary wheel running protected these mice from HFD-induced pro-inflammatory and pro-fibrogenic states, as shown by decreased hepatic macrophage infiltration and improved fatty acid and glucose homeostasis. These data were in line with Kawanishi et al. [126], showing that exercise training reduced macrophage infiltration and adipose tissue inflammation by attenuating neutrophil infiltration in HFD-fed C57BL/6 mice. Thus, it is very likely that physical exercise exhibits beneficial effects and compensates for shortcomings of certain therapeutic approaches [125,126].

Table 1. Overview of commonly used dietary, genetic, chemically-induced, and other murine models of non-alcoholic steatohepatitis (NASH).

Type of Mouse Model	Treatment or Intervention	Phenotypical Outcome and Relevance to Human Disease	Author(s)
Dietary Models			
High-fat diet (HFD)	HFD containing 60% fat administered to C57BL6/J	After 10-12w, induction of obesity, insulin resistance and hyperlipidemia. After long-term exposure (36w), no or only minimal signs of inflammation and fibrosis. After chronic feeding (80w), hepatic steatosis, cell injury, portal & lobular inflammation and fibrosis.	Velázquez et al. [17], Ito et al. [19], Chen et al. [20], Vonghia et al. [21]
Atherogenic diet	Diet containing 1.25% cholesterol and 0.5% cholate	Increased plasma and liver lipid levels. From 6–24 weeks, induction NASH with hepatocellular ballooning in a time-dependent manner.	Matsuzawa et al. [24]
High-fat atherogenic diet	HFD containing 1.25% cholesterol and 0.5% cholate	Exacerbated NASH features including hepatic insulin resistance, oxidative stress, activation of hepatic stellate cells.	Matsuzawa et al. [24], Montandon et al. [41], Larter et al. [42]
High-fat/high-cholesterol diet (HFC)	HFC containing 21% milk butter, 0.2% cholesterol	After short-term HFC diet, only steatosis in C57BL/6 mice. Steatosis with severe inflammation in female Ldlr-/- and APOE2ki hyperlipidemic mice. After seven days, severe hepatic inflammation but no steatosis in male hyperlipidemic mice. After seven months, development of obesity, hepatomegaly, hepatic steatosis and varying degrees of steatohepatitis in C57BL/6 mice.	Wouters et al. [25,26] Zheng et al. [27]
High-fat/high-cholesterol/high-fructose diet (AMLN)	Diet containing 40% high-fat and 22% fructose, supplemented with ~18% trans-fat and 2% cholesterol	After 26–30w, marked steatosis, moderate lobular inflammation and hepatocellular ballooning in C57BL/6 and ob/ob mice.	Clapper et al. [28], Kristiansen et al. [29]

Table 1. *Cont.*

Type of Mouse Model	Treatment or Intervention	Phenotypical Outcome and Relevance to Human Disease	Author(s)
Gubra amylin diet (GAN)	High-fat (40 kcal-%, of which 0% trans-fat and 46% saturated fatty acids by weight), fructose (22%), sucrose (10%), cholesterol (2%)	After 8-16w, more pronounced weight gain and a highly similar phenotype of biopsy-confirmed fibrotic NASH in C57BL/6 and *ob/ob* mice.	Boland et al. [33]
High-fat/high-fructose/ high-cholesterol	Composed of 41% fat, 30% fructose, 2% cholesterol	Induction NASH in various models.	Abe et al. [34], Kennedy et al. [35], Suto et al. [36]
Soybean-oil-based Western-type diet	Western-type diet containing 25g/100 g n-6-PUFA-rich soybean oil +/- 0.75% cholesterol	After long-term exposure (20w), hepatic steatosis, inflammation and fibrosis, weight gain, insulin resistance, hepatic lipid peroxidation and oxidative stress in C57BL/6 mice.	Henkel et al. [37]
High-caloric cholesterol-free HFD	Composed of lard (21g/100g)/soy-bean oil (3g/100g)/5% fructose in drinking water	Only mild steatosis. No signs of hepatic inflammation and fibrosis.	Wouters et al. [25,26], Henkel et al. [37], Subramanian et al. [38], Mari et al. [39], Savard et al. [40]
Choline-deficient diet	C57BL/6 mice were fed HFD (45% of calories) for 8 weeks. During the final 4 weeks, diets were choline-deficient (or choline-supplemented)	Amplified liver fat accumulation, while improved glucose tolerance.	Raubenheimer et al. [48]
Methionine/choline-deficient diet (MCD)	Diet lacking methionine and choline, but containing high sucrose (40%) and moderate fat (10%)	After 2w, severe steatohepatitis with elevated serum AST and ALT levels. After 10w, additional Kupffer cell infiltration and irreversible fibrosis. After 1.5-4w, no signs of insulin resistance.	Santhekadur et al. [12], Montandon et al. [41], Itagaki et al. [47], Rinella et al. [52], Al Rajabi et al. [53]
Choline-deficient L-amino acid-defined diet (CDAA)	Choline-deficient L-amino acid-defined diet containing carbohydrates (68,5%), proteins (17,4%) and fats (14%)	Within a few weeks, fatty liver followed by mild features of NASH in C57BL/6J mice. After >20w, mild-to-moderate fibrosis and insulin resistance.	Van Herck et al. [11], Matsumoto et al. [54], Miura et al. [55]
Choline-deficient L-amino acid-defined diet on high-fat diet (CDAHFD)	Choline-deficient, L-amino acid-defined, HFD consisting of 60 kcal% fat and 0.1% methionine by weight	Excessive liver fat accumulation, increased circulating liver enzymes and progressive hepatic fibrosis.	Matsumoto et al. [54]
High-fat/high-fructose diet (ALIOS)	HFD with fructose-containing drinking water. Additional administration of a low weekly dose of intraperitoneal carbon tetrachloride (CCl$_4$)	After 16w, substantial steatosis with necro-inflammatory changes and increased ALT levels. No difference in steatosis degree or ALT levels if compared to without additional fructose. Development of progressive stages of human-like fatty liver disease.	Tetri et al. [56], Tsuchida et al. [57]
Diet-induced animal model of non-alcoholic fatty liver disease (DIAMOND)	High fat/carbohydrate diet (Western diet) with 42% kcal from fat, containing cholesterol (0.1%), with a high fructose/glucose solution (23.1 g/L d-fructose +18.9 g/L d-glucose)	After 16w, obesity, liver injury, dyslipidemia and insulin resistance, sustained up to 52w. Parent strains 129S1/SvImJ or C57BL/6 lacked insulin resistance and steatohepatitis or developed delayed insulin resistance.	Santhekadur et al. [12], Asgharpour et al. [58]

Table 1. *Cont.*

Type of Mouse Model	Treatment or Intervention	Phenotypical Outcome and Relevance to Human Disease	Author(s)
High-fat diet + glucose/ fructose-enriched drinking water	Obesogenic diet containing ((35.5% w/w) crude fat (58 kJ%), 22.8 MJ/kg = 5.45 kcal/g) and fructose (55% w/v) and glucose (45% w/v) enriched drinking water. After 8 weeks of dietary feeding, mice were randomly assigned to a voluntary wheel running group or a sedentary group.	Voluntary wheel running prevented HFD-induced pro-inflammatory / fibrogenic states in C57BL/6 mice. Hepatic steatosis was prevented by alterations in key liver metabolic processes.	Gehrke et al. [125]
Genetic Models			
Leptin deficiency (*ob/ob*)	Leptin-deficient (*ob/ob*) mice are predisposed to develop NASH and fibrosis, whereas not when maintained on regular chow diet. Treatment with high-fat/high-fructose/ high-cholesterol diet.	Lack the ability to spontaneously develop hepatic inflammation. After 12-26w, increased adiposity, total cholesterol and elevated plasma liver enzymes upon diet high in trans-fat (40%), fructose (22%) and cholesterol (2%). After treatment with high-fat/high-fructose/high-cholesterol diet, development of metabolic, histologic and transcriptomic features similar to human NASH.	Kristiansen et al. [29], Abe et al. [34], Trevaskis et al. [51]
Leptin resistance (*db/db*)	*db/db* mice are deficient in the leptin receptor, with dramatic elevations in circulating leptin concentrations. Dietary intervention with an MCD diet for 4 weeks.	Lack the ability to spontaneously develop hepatic inflammation and thus needs to be combined with a nutritional model for NASH. After 4w MCD diet, mice displayed marked hepatic inflammation and fibrosis.	Kennedy et al. [35], Sahai et al. [45], Hummel et al. [50]
MS-NASH (FATZO/Pco)	Mice spontaneous development of obesity	After 20w of fructose-supplemented diet, hepatic steatosis, lobular inflammation, ballooning and fibrosis.	Sun et al. [62]
Apolipoprotein E2 knock-in (APOE2)	Murine ApoE replaced by the human APOE2 gene	After 12w of HFC, steatosis in conjunction with early but not sustained hepatic inflammation.	Wouters et al. [25,26], Bieghs et al. [63]
ApoE deficiency (*ApoE$^{-/-}$*)	Complete deficiency in the murine ApoE gene	After 7w of Western diet, abnormal glucose tolerance, hepatomegaly, weight gain and full spectrum of NASH, while lacking humanized lipoprotein profiles.	Schierwagen et al. [64]
Low-density lipoprotein receptor deficiency (*Ldlr$^{-/-}$*)	Complete deficiency of the murine Ldl receptor, an important gene regulating the transport of non-modified lipids into macrophages	After 3-12w of HFC diet, resemblance to lifestyle-induced early-onset hepatic inflammation. High and low levels of circulating LDL and HDL, respectively, closely mimicked the human lipoprotein profile. Development of mild fibrosis.	Wouters et al. [25,26], Bieghs et al. [63]
Microsomal prostaglandin E synthase 1 (mPGES1) deficiency	Mice with global deletion of mPGES-133 were backcrossed on C57BL/6J	TNFα-dependent inflammatory response in murine liver. Increased severity of diet-induced murine NASH.	Henkel et al. [65]
Patatin-like phospholipase domain-containing 3 (PNPLA-3) knock-in	Mice carried I148M mutation in the Pnpla3 gene and were fed a high-sucrose or HFD diet for 4 weeks	Accumulation of PNPLA3 on lipid droplets. Development of hepatic steatosis.	Smagris et al. [72]
Transmembrane 6 superfamily member 2 knockdown (mTm6s2-shRNA8)	Adeno-associated virus-mediated short hairpin RNA knockdown of Tm6sf2 in liver of C57BL/6J mice	Increased hepatic fat content and decreased VLDL secretion, recapitulating the effects observed in humans carrying the TM6SF2-167Lys mutation	Kozlitina et al. [74]

Table 1. *Cont.*

Type of Mouse Model	Treatment or Intervention	Phenotypical Outcome and Relevance to Human Disease	Author(s)
Gankyrin liver-specific knockout (GLKO)	Cre-Alb mice were backcrossed with LoxP-Gank mice	Gankyrin generally drives liver proliferation. After 6-7 months of HFD, higher degree of hepatic steatosis but prevention of fibrosis development in GLKO mice compared to wild-type mice.	Cast et al. [75]
Truncated mutation in Alström (Alms1) gene (*foz/foz*)	11-base pair truncating mutation in the Alström gene ALMS1. Lack of knowledge regarding the exact role of Alms1	After 6 months of HFD, MetS features, including obesity, hyperglycemia / lipidemia and insulin resistance. Mice spontaneously develop steatosis, hepatic inflammation and fibrosis.	Santhekadur et al. [12], Jiang et al. [14], Arsov et al. [77]
Fatty liver Shionogi	Spontaneous development of hepatic inflammation with rather a mild degree of fibrosis. Uncontrollable heterogeneity in disease onset	Backcrossing with *ob/ob* mice resulted in severe liver steatosis, inflammation, advanced fibrosis and spontaneous HCC	He et al. [82]
Hepatocyte-specific phosphatase and tensin homolog deficiency (*Pten$^{-/-}$*)	PTEN deficiency specific in the liver	After 40w of age, steatosis, inflammation and fibrosis in the liver. After 74-78w of age, HCC was present in 83% of males and 50% of female mice.	Watanabe et al. [83], Takakura et al. [84]
Augmenter of liver regeneration knock-out (*Alr$^{-/-}$*)	Liver-specific deletion of augmenter of liver regeneration	4-8w after birth, steatohepatitis with hepatocellular necrosis, ductular proliferation and fibrosis. 1y after birth, HCC in nearly 60% of the mice	Van Herck et al. [11], Gandhi et al. [89]
Melanocortin 4 receptor knockout (*Mc4r$^{-/-}$*)	Mice with targeted disruption of melanocortin 4 receptor, which is a seven-transmembrane G protein–coupled receptor that is expressed in the hypothalamic nuclei	Development of simple steatosis. Upon feeding HFD, development of human-like NASH, including obesity, insulin resistance and dyslipidemia. After 20w HFD, obesity and NASH with clear signs of moderate fibrosis, functionally mimicking the human NASH disease state.	Itoh et al. [90], Yamada et al. [91]
Chemically-induced Models			
Carbon tetrachloride (CCL$_4$)	Biweekly injections of CCl$_4$	After 6w, increased circulating liver enzymes and dose-dependent progression of liver fibrosis in Balb/C mice	Domitrovic et al. [97]
Thioacetamide (TAA)	Three times/week IP injection thioacetamide (75mg/kg) in combination with western-type diet	After 8w, hepatic inflammation, severe diffuse fibrosis and collagen deposition in C57BL/6 mice	Hansen et al. [8] Van Herck et al. [11] Santhekadur et al. [12]
Streptozotocin + high-fat diet (STAM)	200 µg streptozotocin at 2 days after birth and feeding ad libitum with high-fat diet at 4 weeks of age	Between 6-20w of age, hepatic inflammation, hepatocellular ballooning, progressive fibrosis and HCC. Reduced body weight and insulin levels compared to HFD-fed mice	Fujii et al. [99]
Other models			
C57BL/6 background	Mice were housed in separate specific pathogen-free units maintained at either 22°C (standard) or 30-33°C (thermoneutral)	After 24w of thermoneutral housing, exacerbated HFD-driven NAFLD pathogenesis. Increased intestinal permeability and alterations in gut microbiome, mimicking the human situation.	Giles et al. [106]
C57BL/6 background	Juvenile NASH model: immediately after weaning, mice were fed HFC diet for a total of 16 weeks (4, 8, 12 and 16 weeks of diet)	Hepatic oxidative stress in female juvenile NAFLD/NASH models, whereas hepatic inflammation in males	Marin et al. [104]

Table 1. *Cont.*

Type of Mouse Model	Treatment or Intervention	Phenotypical Outcome and Relevance to Human Disease	Author(s)
C57BL/6 background	Juvenile NAFLD/NASH model: HFD were administered 2 weeks before conception and during gestation and lactation	Offspring HFC intake resulted in NAFLD, maternal-offspring fat intake contributed to NASH in juvenile female mice	Zhou et al. [105]
Models with circadian oscillations (e.g., *Per1/2$^{-/-}$* or liver-specific *Bmal1* knockout mice)	The effects of feeding time and circadian clocks on murine liver	Circadian rhythm drives oscillations in hepatic triglyceride levels, inflammation, oxidative stress, mitochondrial dysfunction and hepatic insulin resistance. Chronic disruption of circadian rhythm may spontaneously induce the progression from NAFLD to NASH, fibrosis and HCC	Adamovich et al. [107], Jacobi et al. [108], Kettner et al. [109]
C57BL/6 background	Mice (and other rodent models) were fed a high-fat/high-fructose/high-cholesterol for 16 weeks	Significant intraindividual differences in fibrosis score and hepatic biomarkers pointed towards the importance of standardizing sampling site location during preclinical liver biopsy procedures	Jensen et al. [2]

4. Clinical Relevance: Comparisons with Clinical Data

In general, NAFLD is considered the hepatic manifestation of MetS. Consequently, well-established therapeutic compounds against T2D and impaired lipid metabolism are thought to exert beneficial effects that mitigate the pathological features of NASH. One such example is the nuclear receptor peroxisome proliferator-activated receptor (PPAR) (extensively reviewed elsewhere [127]), due to its involvement in regulating lipid metabolism and inflammation. For instance, it was previously shown that hepatic *Ppara* inversely correlated with insulin resistance and NASH severity [128]. Remarkably, in this clinical study, histological improvements were positively associated with *Ppara* expression in patients with NASH [128], pointing towards the therapeutic potential of PPARα-agonists. Fibrates, which activate PPARα, are the most effective class of agents for lowering elevated triglyceride-rich lipoproteins [129]. While fenofibrate did not ameliorate liver histology in biopsy-proven NAFLD, a selective PPARα agonist, also known as Pemafibrate, did improve liver function in patients with dyslipidemia [130], which was previously established in diet-induced murine models of NAFLD [131].

Another isoform of PPAR, PPAR-δ, is involved in dyslipidemia and activation of PPAR-δ by means of a selective agonist, referred to as seladelpar (MBX-8025), beneficially affected plasma lipid levels and showed favorable trends in insulin resistance and waist circumference in patients with dyslipidemia [132]. More recently, these data were further supported using in-vivo studies, showing that seladelpar improved glucose metabolism, as well as plasma and hepatic lipid levels in obese *foz/foz* mice [133]. Collectively, these data pointed towards seladelpar as a potential novel therapy for NASH.

Another strategy is based on insulin-sensing drugs, known as Thiazolidinediones, which target the PPAR-γ isoform [134]. Examples of PPAR-γ agonists are lobeglitazone, pioglitazone, and rosiglitazone, of which the latter two are currently off-label and off-market, respectively [127]. When diabetic patients with NAFLD were treated with lobeglitazone, patients showed improvements in hepatic steatosis, glycemic, and lipid profiles, as well as liver enzyme levels [134]. In line, it was shown that HFD-induced obese mice treated with lobeglitazone improved glucose homeostasis as well as hepatic and plasma lipid levels [135]. Hence, these data pointed towards lobeglitazone as a potential treatment option for NAFLD.

Relevantly, the use of elafibranor (dual PPAR-α/δ agonist, clinical phase III trial) as a single drug regime is thought to be promising with regard to NASH, as shown by significant improvements of human NASH pathology without deteriorating hepatic fibrosis [136]. These data were further corroborated by findings in rodent studies of NAFLD [137]. Additionally, the development of anti-fibrotic therapies has recently received increasing attention [138]. Therefore, due to its multifactorial character, current treatment modalities should focus on both the reversal of NASH [139] and fibrosis [138].

Strategies, which currently hold clinical potential in late-stage drug development, include specific complementary agonists, i.e., for PPAR receptor subtypes and farnesoid X receptor (FXR) [139]. Using AMLN diet-induced obese mice with biopsy-confirmed NASH, Roth et al. [139] demonstrated that combined treatment with Elafibrinor and obeticholic acid (FXR agonist) significantly ameliorated histological features of steatosis, inflammation and fibrosis. Additionally, compared to single regimens, combined treatment targeted hepatic molecular mechanisms, thereby further improving NASH and fibrogenesis [139].

To conclude, in addition to the selective—but relevant—approaches described above, additional therapeutic options for NAFLD have been studied in preclinical and/or clinical settings [16], or are currently under investigation.

5. Conclusions

Although current preclinical NAFLD models can be considered indispensable tools for studying chronic liver disease pathology, it should be noted that the majority of existing rodent models mainly focus on certain stages of the disease rather than the total spectrum. Additionally, it is noteworthy that the NAFLD disease progression greatly varies across different strains [140]. Therefore, depending on its research question, careful model selection is highly recommended. Such selection should also properly consider sex, age, and hormonal status and must be based on prior knowledge, as it will have a large impact on data interpretation and its translational potential. Thus, our common goal is to establish an ideal preclinical model that—in addition to developing hepatic inflammation and fibrosis, along with obesity, high cholesterol, and insulin resistance—also responds to promising therapeutic interventions. This implies that future studies should continue focusing on recapitulating the multifactorial character of human NAFLD in preclinical models.

Author Contributions: Conceptualization, writing—original draft preparation and writing—review and editing, figure preparation, Y.O. and R.S.-S.; funding acquisition, R.S.-S. All authors have read and agreed to the published version of the manuscript.

Abbreviations

ALIOS	American Lifestyle Induced Obesity Syndrome
ALMS1	Alström
ALR	Augmenter of liver regeneration
APOE2ki	Apolipoprotein E2 knock-in
CCl_4	Carbon tetrachloride
CD	Diet deficient for/low in choline
CDAA	Choline-deficient L-amino acid-defined diet
DIAMOND	Diet-induced animal model of non-alcoholic fatty liver disease
FLS	Fatty liver Shionogi
FXR	Farnesoid X receptor
Gank	Gankyrin
GFER	Growth Factor ERV1 homolog of *Saccharomyces cerevisiae*
HCC	Hepatocellular carcinoma
HFC	High-fat/high-cholesterol diet
HFD	High-fat diet
Ldlr	Low-density lipoprotein receptor
MAT1a	methionine adenosyltransferase 1A

MC4R	Melanocortin 4 receptor
MetS	Metabolic Syndrome
MS-NASH	Mice formerly known as FATZO/Pco
NAFLD	Non-alcoholic fatty liver disease
NASH	Non-alcoholic steatohepatitis
NEMO	NF-κB essential modulator
PNPLA3	Patatin-like phospholipase domain-containing 3
PPAR	Peroxisome proliferator-activated receptor
PTEN	Phosphatase and tensin homolog
T2D	Type 2 Diabetes
TAA	Thioacetamide
TM6SF2	Transmembrane 6 superfamily member 2
TNFα	Tumor necrosis factor α
TSOD	Tsumura-Suzuki Obese Diabetes

References

1. Younossi, Z.M.; Golabi, P.; de Avila, L.; Paik, J.M.; Srishord, M.; Fukui, N.; Qiu, Y.; Burns, L.; Afendy, A.; Nader, F. The global epidemiology of NAFLD and NASH in patients with type 2 diabetes: A systematic review and meta-analysis. *J. Hepatol.* **2019**, *71*, 793–801. [CrossRef] [PubMed]

2. Jensen, V.S.; Tveden-Nyborg, P.; Zacho-Rasmussen, C.; Quaade, M.L.; Ipsen, D.H.; Hvid, H.; Fledelius, C.; Wulff, E.M.; Lykkesfeldt, J. Variation in diagnostic NAFLD/NASH read-outs in paired liver samples from rodent models. *J. Pharmacol. Toxicol. Methods* **2019**, *101*, 106651. [CrossRef] [PubMed]

3. Ganbold, M.; Owada, Y.; Ozawa, Y.; Shimamoto, Y.; Ferdousi, F.; Tominaga, K.; Zheng, Y.W.; Ohkohchi, N.; Isoda, H. Isorhamnetin Alleviates Steatosis and Fibrosis in Mice with Nonalcoholic Steatohepatitis. *Sci. Rep.* **2019**, *9*, 16210. [CrossRef] [PubMed]

4. Li, B.; Zhang, C.; Zhan, Y.T. Nonalcoholic Fatty Liver Disease Cirrhosis: A Review of Its Epidemiology, Risk Factors, Clinical Presentation, Diagnosis, Management, and Prognosis. *Can. J. Gastroenterol. Hepatol.* **2018**, *2018*, 2784537. [CrossRef] [PubMed]

5. Anstee, Q.M.; Reeves, H.L.; Kotsiliti, E.; Govaere, O.; Heikenwalder, M. From NASH to HCC: Current concepts and future challenges. *Nat. Rev. Gastroenterol. Hepatol.* **2019**, *16*, 411–428. [CrossRef] [PubMed]

6. Wong, R.J.; Cheung, R.; Ahmed, A. Nonalcoholic steatohepatitis is the most rapidly growing indication for liver transplantation in patients with hepatocellular carcinoma in the U.S. *Hepatology* **2014**, *59*, 2188–2195. [CrossRef]

7. Younossi, Z.M.; Loomba, R.; Anstee, Q.M.; Rinella, M.E.; Bugianesi, E.; Marchesini, G.; Neuschwander-Tetri, B.A.; Serfaty, L.; Negro, F.; Caldwell, S.H.; et al. Diagnostic modalities for nonalcoholic fatty liver disease, nonalcoholic steatohepatitis, and associated fibrosis. *Hepatology* **2018**, *68*, 349–360. [CrossRef]

8. Hansen, H.H.; Feigh, M.; Veidal, S.S.; Rigbolt, K.T.; Vrang, N.; Fosgerau, K. Mouse models of nonalcoholic steatohepatitis in preclinical drug development. *Drug Discov. Today* **2017**. [CrossRef]

9. Haczeyni, F.; Yeh, M.M.; Ioannou, G.N.; Leclercq, I.A.; Goldin, R.; Dan, Y.Y.; Yu, J.; Teoh, N.C.; Farrell, G.C. Mouse models of non-alcoholic steatohepatitis: A reflection on recent literature. *J. Gastroenterol. Hepatol.* **2018**, *33*, 1312–1320. [CrossRef]

10. Lau, J.K.; Zhang, X.; Yu, J. Animal models of non-alcoholic fatty liver disease: Current perspectives and recent advances. *J. Pathol.* **2017**, *241*, 36–44. [CrossRef]

11. Van Herck, M.A.; Vonghia, L.; Francque, S.M. Animal Models of Nonalcoholic Fatty Liver Disease-A Starter's Guide. *Nutrients* **2017**, *9*, 1072. [CrossRef] [PubMed]

12. Santhekadur, P.K.; Kumar, D.P.; Sanyal, A.J. Preclinical models of non-alcoholic fatty liver disease. *J. Hepatol.* **2018**, *68*, 230–237. [CrossRef] [PubMed]

13. Jahn, D.; Kircher, S.; Hermanns, H.M.; Geier, A. Animal models of NAFLD from a hepatologist's point of view. *Biochim. Biophys. Acta Mol. Basis Dis.* **2019**, *1865*, 943–953. [CrossRef] [PubMed]

14. Jiang, M.; Wu, N.; Chen, X.; Wang, W.; Chu, Y.; Liu, H.; Li, W.; Chen, D.; Li, X.; Xu, B. Pathogenesis of and major animal models used for nonalcoholic fatty liver disease. *J. Int. Med. Res.* **2019**, *47*, 1453–1466. [CrossRef] [PubMed]

15. Palladini, G.; Di Pasqua, L.G.; Berardo, C.; Siciliano, V.; Richelmi, P.; Perlini, S.; Ferrigno, A.; Vairetti, M. Animal Models of Steatosis (NAFLD) and Steatohepatitis (NASH) Exhibit Hepatic Lobe-Specific Gelatinases Activity and Oxidative Stress. *Can. J. Gastroenterol. Hepatol.* **2019**, *2019*, 5413461. [CrossRef]

16. Zhong, F.; Zhou, X.; Xu, J.; Gao, L. Rodent Models of Nonalcoholic Fatty Liver Disease. *Digestion* **2019**, 1–14. [CrossRef]

17. Velazquez, K.T.; Enos, R.T.; Bader, J.E.; Sougiannis, A.T.; Carson, M.S.; Chatzistamou, I.; Carson, J.A.; Nagarkatti, P.S.; Nagarkatti, M.; Murphy, E.A. Prolonged high-fat-diet feeding promotes non-alcoholic fatty liver disease and alters gut microbiota in mice. *World J. Hepatol.* **2019**, *11*, 619–637. [CrossRef]

18. Jacobs, A.; Warda, A.S.; Verbeek, J.; Cassiman, D.; Spincemaille, P. An Overview of Mouse Models of Nonalcoholic Steatohepatitis: From Past to Present. *Curr. Protoc. Mouse Biol.* **2016**, *6*, 185–200. [CrossRef]

19. Ito, M.; Suzuki, J.; Tsujioka, S.; Sasaki, M.; Gomori, A.; Shirakura, T.; Hirose, H.; Ito, M.; Ishihara, A.; Iwaasa, H.; et al. Longitudinal analysis of murine steatohepatitis model induced by chronic exposure to high-fat diet. *Hepatol. Res.* **2007**, *37*, 50–57. [CrossRef]

20. Chen, K.; Ma, J.; Jia, X.; Ai, W.; Ma, Z.; Pan, Q. Advancing the understanding of NAFLD to hepatocellular carcinoma development: From experimental models to humans. *Biochim. Biophys. Acta Rev. Cancer* **2019**, *1871*, 117–125. [CrossRef]

21. Vonghia, L.; Ruyssers, N.; Schrijvers, D.; Pelckmans, P.; Michielsen, P.; De Clerck, L.; Ramon, A.; Jirillo, E.; Ebo, D.; De Winter, B.; et al. CD4+ROR gamma t++ and Tregs in a Mouse Model of Diet-Induced Nonalcoholic Steatohepatitis. *Mediators Inflamm.* **2015**, *2015*, 239623. [CrossRef] [PubMed]

22. Chen, Y.H.; Chiu, C.C.; Hung, S.W.; Huang, W.C.; Lee, Y.P.; Liu, J.Y.; Huang, Y.T.; Chen, T.H.; Chuang, H.L. Gnotobiotic mice inoculated with Firmicutes, but not Bacteroidetes, deteriorate nonalcoholic fatty liver disease severity by modulating hepatic lipid metabolism. *Nutr. Res.* **2019**, *69*, 20–29. [CrossRef] [PubMed]

23. Raman, M.; Ahmed, I.; Gillevet, P.M.; Probert, C.S.; Ratcliffe, N.M.; Smith, S.; Greenwood, R.; Sikaroodi, M.; Lam, V.; Crotty, P.; et al. Fecal microbiome and volatile organic compound metabolome in obese humans with nonalcoholic fatty liver disease. *Clin. Gastroenterol. Hepatol.* **2013**, *11*, 868–875 e861-863. [CrossRef] [PubMed]

24. Matsuzawa, N.; Takamura, T.; Kurita, S.; Misu, H.; Ota, T.; Ando, H.; Yokoyama, M.; Honda, M.; Zen, Y.; Nakanuma, Y.; et al. Lipid-induced oxidative stress causes steatohepatitis in mice fed an atherogenic diet. *Hepatology* **2007**, *46*, 1392–1403. [CrossRef] [PubMed]

25. Wouters, K.; van Gorp, P.J.; Bieghs, V.; Gijbels, M.J.; Duimel, H.; Lutjohann, D.; Kerksiek, A.; van Kruchten, R.; Maeda, N.; Staels, B.; et al. Dietary cholesterol, rather than liver steatosis, leads to hepatic inflammation in hyperlipidemic mouse models of nonalcoholic steatohepatitis. *Hepatology* **2008**, *48*, 474–486. [CrossRef] [PubMed]

26. Wouters, K.; van Bilsen, M.; van Gorp, P.J.; Bieghs, V.; Lutjohann, D.; Kerksiek, A.; Staels, B.; Hofker, M.H.; Shiri-Sverdlov, R. Intrahepatic cholesterol influences progression, inhibition and reversal of non-alcoholic steatohepatitis in hyperlipidemic mice. *FEBS Lett.* **2010**, *584*, 1001–1005. [CrossRef]

27. Zheng, S.; Hoos, L.; Cook, J.; Tetzloff, G.; Davis, H., Jr.; van Heek, M.; Hwa, J.J. Ezetimibe improves high fat and cholesterol diet-induced non-alcoholic fatty liver disease in mice. *Eur. J. Pharmacol.* **2008**, *584*, 118–124. [CrossRef]

28. Clapper, J.R.; Hendricks, M.D.; Gu, G.; Wittmer, C.; Dolman, C.S.; Herich, J.; Athanacio, J.; Villescaz, C.; Ghosh, S.S.; Heilig, J.S.; et al. Diet-induced mouse model of fatty liver disease and nonalcoholic steatohepatitis reflecting clinical disease progression and methods of assessment. *Am. J. Physiol. Gastrointest Liver Physiol.* **2013**, *305*, G483–G495. [CrossRef]

29. Kristiansen, M.N.; Veidal, S.S.; Rigbolt, K.T.; Tolbol, K.S.; Roth, J.D.; Jelsing, J.; Vrang, N.; Feigh, M. Obese diet-induced mouse models of nonalcoholic steatohepatitis-tracking disease by liver biopsy. *World J. Hepatol.* **2016**, *8*, 673–684. [CrossRef]

30. Larter, C.Z.; Yeh, M.M. Animal models of NASH: Getting both pathology and metabolic context right. *J. Gastroenterol. Hepatol.* **2008**, *23*, 1635–1648. [CrossRef]

31. Leclercq, I.A.; Farrell, G.C.; Schriemer, R.; Robertson, G.R. Leptin is essential for the hepatic fibrogenic response to chronic liver injury. *J. Hepatol.* **2002**, *37*, 206–213. [CrossRef]

32. US. Food Drug Administration. Final Determination Regarding Partially Hydrogenated Oils (Removing Trans Fat). Available online: https://www.federalregister.gov/documents/2018/05/21/2018-10714/final-determination-regarding-partially-hydrogenated-oils (accessed on 21 May 2018).

33. Boland, M.L.; Oro, D.; Tolbol, K.S.; Thrane, S.T.; Nielsen, J.C.; Cohen, T.S.; Tabor, D.E.; Fernandes, F.; Tovchigrechko, A.; Veidal, S.S.; et al. Towards a standard diet-induced and biopsy-confirmed mouse model of non-alcoholic steatohepatitis: Impact of dietary fat source. *World J. Gastroenterol.* **2019**, *25*, 4904–4920. [CrossRef] [PubMed]

34. Abe, N.; Kato, S.; Tsuchida, T.; Sugimoto, K.; Saito, R.; Verschuren, L.; Kleemann, R.; Oka, K. Longitudinal characterization of diet-induced genetic murine models of non-alcoholic steatohepatitis with metabolic, histological, and transcriptomic hallmarks of human patients. *Biol. Open* **2019**, *8*. [CrossRef] [PubMed]

35. Kennedy, A.J.; Ellacott, K.L.; King, V.L.; Hasty, A.H. Mouse models of the metabolic syndrome. *Dis. Model. Mech.* **2010**, *3*, 156–166. [CrossRef]

36. Suto, J.; Matsuura, S.; Imamura, K.; Yamanaka, H.; Sekikawa, K. Genetic analysis of non-insulin-dependent diabetes mellitus in KK and KK-Ay mice. *Eur. J. Endocrinol.* **1998**, *139*, 654–661. [CrossRef] [PubMed]

37. Henkel, J.; Coleman, C.D.; Schraplau, A.; Jhrens, K.; Weber, D.; Castro, J.P.; Hugo, M.; Schulz, T.J.; Kramer, S.; Schurmann, A.; et al. Induction of steatohepatitis (NASH) with insulin resistance in wildtype B6 mice by a western-type diet containing soybean oil and cholesterol. *Mol. Med.* **2017**, *23*, 70–82. [CrossRef]

38. Subramanian, S.; Goodspeed, L.; Wang, S.; Kim, J.; Zeng, L.; Ioannou, G.N.; Haigh, W.G.; Yeh, M.M.; Kowdley, K.V.; O'Brien, K.D.; et al. Dietary cholesterol exacerbates hepatic steatosis and inflammation in obese LDL receptor-deficient mice. *J. Lipid Res.* **2011**, *52*, 1626–1635. [CrossRef]

39. Mari, M.; Caballero, F.; Colell, A.; Morales, A.; Caballeria, J.; Fernandez, A.; Enrich, C.; Fernandez-Checa, J.C.; Garcia-Ruiz, C. Mitochondrial free cholesterol loading sensitizes to TNF- and Fas-mediated steatohepatitis. *Cell Metab.* **2006**, *4*, 185–198. [CrossRef]

40. Savard, C.; Tartaglione, E.V.; Kuver, R.; Haigh, W.G.; Farrell, G.C.; Subramanian, S.; Chait, A.; Yeh, M.M.; Quinn, L.S.; Ioannou, G.N. Synergistic interaction of dietary cholesterol and dietary fat in inducing experimental steatohepatitis. *Hepatology* **2013**, *57*, 81–92. [CrossRef]

41. Montandon, S.A.; Somm, E.; Loizides-Mangold, U.; de Vito, C.; Dibner, C.; Jornayvaz, F.R. Multi-technique comparison of atherogenic and MCD NASH models highlights changes in sphingolipid metabolism. *Sci. Rep.* **2019**, *9*, 16810. [CrossRef]

42. Larter, C.Z.; Yeh, M.M.; Haigh, W.G.; Williams, J.; Brown, S.; Bell-Anderson, K.S.; Lee, S.P.; Farrell, G.C. Hepatic free fatty acids accumulate in experimental steatohepatitis: Role of adaptive pathways. *J. Hepatol.* **2008**, *48*, 638–647. [CrossRef] [PubMed]

43. Weltman, M.D.; Farrell, G.C.; Liddle, C. Increased hepatocyte CYP2E1 expression in a rat nutritional model of hepatic steatosis with inflammation. *Gastroenterology* **1996**, *111*, 1645–1653. [CrossRef]

44. Fan, Y.; Zhang, W.; Wei, H.; Sun, R.; Tian, Z.; Chen, Y. Hepatic NK cells attenuate fibrosis progression of non-alcoholic steatohepatitis in dependent of CXCL10-mediated recruitment. *Liver Int.* **2019**. [CrossRef] [PubMed]

45. Sahai, A.; Malladi, P.; Pan, X.; Paul, R.; Melin-Aldana, H.; Green, R.M.; Whitington, P.F. Obese and diabetic db/db mice develop marked liver fibrosis in a model of nonalcoholic steatohepatitis: Role of short-form leptin receptors and osteopontin. *Am. J. Physiol. Gastrointest Liver Physiol.* **2004**, *287*, G1035–G1043. [CrossRef]

46. Sahai, A.; Malladi, P.; Melin-Aldana, H.; Green, R.M.; Whitington, P.F. Upregulation of osteopontin expression is involved in the development of nonalcoholic steatohepatitis in a dietary murine model. *Am. J. Physiol. Gastrointest Liver Physiol.* **2004**, *287*, G264–G273. [CrossRef]

47. Itagaki, H.; Shimizu, K.; Morikawa, S.; Ogawa, K.; Ezaki, T. Morphological and functional characterization of non-alcoholic fatty liver disease induced by a methionine-choline-deficient diet in C57BL/6 mice. *Int. J. Clin. Exp. Pathol.* **2013**, *6*, 2683–2696.

48. Raubenheimer, P.J.; Nyirenda, M.J.; Walker, B.R. A choline-deficient diet exacerbates fatty liver but attenuates insulin resistance and glucose intolerance in mice fed a high-fat diet. *Diabetes* **2006**, *55*, 2015–2020. [CrossRef]

49. Ikejima, K.; Okumura, K.; Lang, T.; Honda, H.; Abe, W.; Yamashina, S.; Enomoto, N.; Takei, Y.; Sato, N. The role of leptin in progression of non-alcoholic fatty liver disease. *Hepatol. Res.* **2005**, *33*, 151–154. [CrossRef]

50. Hummel, K.P.; Dickie, M.M.; Coleman, D.L. Diabetes, a new mutation in the mouse. *Science* **1966**, *153*, 1127–1128. [CrossRef]

51. Trevaskis, J.L.; Griffin, P.S.; Wittmer, C.; Neuschwander-Tetri, B.A.; Brunt, E.M.; Dolman, C.S.; Erickson, M.R.; Napora, J.; Parkes, D.G.; Roth, J.D. Glucagon-like peptide-1 receptor agonism improves metabolic, biochemical, and histopathological indices of nonalcoholic steatohepatitis in mice. *Am. J. Physiol. Gastrointest Liver Physiol.* **2012**, *302*, G762–G772. [CrossRef]

52. Rinella, M.E.; Green, R.M. The methionine-choline deficient dietary model of steatohepatitis does not exhibit insulin resistance. *J. Hepatol.* **2004**, *40*, 47–51. [CrossRef] [PubMed]

53. Al Rajabi, A.; Castro, G.S.; da Silva, R.P.; Nelson, R.C.; Thiesen, A.; Vannucchi, H.; Vine, D.F.; Proctor, S.D.; Field, C.J.; Curtis, J.M.; et al. Choline supplementation protects against liver damage by normalizing cholesterol metabolism in Pemt/Ldlr knockout mice fed a high-fat diet. *J. Nutr.* **2014**, *144*, 252–257. [CrossRef] [PubMed]

54. Matsumoto, M.; Hada, N.; Sakamaki, Y.; Uno, A.; Shiga, T.; Tanaka, C.; Ito, T.; Katsume, A.; Sudoh, M. An improved mouse model that rapidly develops fibrosis in non-alcoholic steatohepatitis. *Int. J. Exp. Pathol.* **2013**, *94*, 93–103. [CrossRef] [PubMed]

55. Miura, K.; Kodama, Y.; Inokuchi, S.; Schnabl, B.; Aoyama, T.; Ohnishi, H.; Olefsky, J.M.; Brenner, D.A.; Seki, E. Toll-like receptor 9 promotes steatohepatitis by induction of interleukin-1beta in mice. *Gastroenterology* **2010**, *139*, 323–334.e327. [CrossRef] [PubMed]

56. Tetri, L.H.; Basaranoglu, M.; Brunt, E.M.; Yerian, L.M.; Neuschwander-Tetri, B.A. Severe NAFLD with hepatic necroinflammatory changes in mice fed trans fats and a high-fructose corn syrup equivalent. *Am. J. Physiol. Gastrointest Liver Physiol.* **2008**, *295*, G987–G995. [CrossRef] [PubMed]

57. Tsuchida, T.; Lee, Y.A.; Fujiwara, N.; Ybanez, M.; Allen, B.; Martins, S.; Fiel, M.I.; Goossens, N.; Chou, H.I.; Hoshida, Y.; et al. A simple diet- and chemical-induced murine NASH model with rapid progression of steatohepatitis, fibrosis and liver cancer. *J. Hepatol.* **2018**, *69*, 385–395. [CrossRef] [PubMed]

58. Asgharpour, A.; Cazanave, S.C.; Pacana, T.; Seneshaw, M.; Vincent, R.; Banini, B.A.; Kumar, D.P.; Daita, K.; Min, H.K.; Mirshahi, F.; et al. A diet-induced animal model of non-alcoholic fatty liver disease and hepatocellular cancer. *J. Hepatol.* **2016**, *65*, 579–588. [CrossRef]

59. Neff, E.P. Farewell, FATZO: A NASH mouse update. *Lab. Anim. (NY)* **2019**, *48*, 151. [CrossRef]

60. Alexander, J.; Chang, G.Q.; Dourmashkin, J.T.; Leibowitz, S.F. Distinct phenotypes of obesity-prone AKR/J, DBA2J and C57BL/6J mice compared to control strains. *Int. J. Obes. (Lond.)* **2006**, *30*, 50–59. [CrossRef]

61. Peterson, R.G.; Jackson, C.V.; Zimmerman, K.M.; Alsina-Fernandez, J.; Michael, M.D.; Emmerson, P.J.; Coskun, T. Glucose dysregulation and response to common anti-diabetic agents in the FATZO/Pco mouse. *PLoS ONE* **2017**, *12*, e0179856. [CrossRef]

62. Sun, G.; Jackson, C.V.; Zimmerman, K.; Zhang, L.K.; Finnearty, C.M.; Sandusky, G.E.; Zhang, G.; Peterson, R.G.; Wang, Y.J. The FATZO mouse, a next generation model of type 2 diabetes, develops NAFLD and NASH when fed a Western diet supplemented with fructose. *BMC Gastroenterol.* **2019**, *19*, 41. [CrossRef] [PubMed]

63. Bieghs, V.; Van Gorp, P.J.; Wouters, K.; Hendrikx, T.; Gijbels, M.J.; van Bilsen, M.; Bakker, J.; Binder, C.J.; Lutjohann, D.; Staels, B.; et al. LDL receptor knock-out mice are a physiological model particularly vulnerable to study the onset of inflammation in non-alcoholic fatty liver disease. *PLoS ONE* **2012**, *7*, e30668. [CrossRef] [PubMed]

64. Schierwagen, R.; Maybuchen, L.; Zimmer, S.; Hittatiya, K.; Back, C.; Klein, S.; Uschner, F.E.; Reul, W.; Boor, P.; Nickenig, G.; et al. Seven weeks of Western diet in apolipoprotein-E-deficient mice induce metabolic syndrome and non-alcoholic steatohepatitis with liver fibrosis. *Sci. Rep.* **2015**, *5*, 12931. [CrossRef] [PubMed]

65. Henkel, J.; Coleman, C.D.; Schraplau, A.; Johrens, K.; Weiss, T.S.; Jonas, W.; Schurmann, A.; Puschel, G.P. Augmented liver inflammation in a microsomal prostaglandin E synthase 1 (mPGES-1)-deficient diet-induced mouse NASH model. *Sci. Rep.* **2018**, *8*, 16127. [CrossRef]

66. Horrillo, R.; Planaguma, A.; Gonzalez-Periz, A.; Ferre, N.; Titos, E.; Miquel, R.; Lopez-Parra, M.; Masferrer, J.L.; Arroyo, V.; Claria, J. Comparative protection against liver inflammation and fibrosis by a selective cyclooxygenase-2 inhibitor and a nonredox-type 5-lipoxygenase inhibitor. *J. Pharmacol. Exp. Ther.* **2007**, *323*, 778–786. [CrossRef]

67. Karck, U.; Peters, T.; Decker, K. The release of tumor necrosis factor from endotoxin-stimulated rat Kupffer cells is regulated by prostaglandin E2 and dexamethasone. *J. Hepatol.* **1988**, *7*, 352–361. [CrossRef]

68. Park, J.Y.; Pillinger, M.H.; Abramson, S.B. Prostaglandin E2 synthesis and secretion: The role of PGE2 synthases. *Clin. Immunol.* **2006**, *119*, 229–240. [CrossRef]

69. Anstee, Q.M.; Day, C.P. The Genetics of Nonalcoholic Fatty Liver Disease: Spotlight on PNPLA3 and TM6SF2. *Semin. Liver Dis.* **2015**, *35*, 270–290. [CrossRef]

70. Romeo, S.; Kozlitina, J.; Xing, C.; Pertsemlidis, A.; Cox, D.; Pennacchio, L.A.; Boerwinkle, E.; Cohen, J.C.; Hobbs, H.H. Genetic variation in PNPLA3 confers susceptibility to nonalcoholic fatty liver disease. *Nat. Genet.* **2008**, *40*, 1461–1465. [CrossRef]

71. Pingitore, P.; Romeo, S. The role of PNPLA3 in health and disease. *Biochim. Biophys. Acta Mol. Cell Biol. Lipids* **2019**, *1864*, 900–906. [CrossRef]

72. Smagris, E.; BasuRay, S.; Li, J.; Huang, Y.; Lai, K.M.; Gromada, J.; Cohen, J.C.; Hobbs, H.H. Pnpla3I148M knockin mice accumulate PNPLA3 on lipid droplets and develop hepatic steatosis. *Hepatology* **2015**, *61*, 108–118. [CrossRef] [PubMed]

73. Chen, X.; Zhou, P.; De, L.; Li, B.; Su, S. The roles of transmembrane 6 superfamily member 2 rs58542926 polymorphism in chronic liver disease: A meta-analysis of 24,147 subjects. *Mol. Genet. Genomic Med.* **2019**, *7*, e824. [CrossRef] [PubMed]

74. Kozlitina, J.; Smagris, E.; Stender, S.; Nordestgaard, B.G.; Zhou, H.H.; Tybjaerg-Hansen, A.; Vogt, T.F.; Hobbs, H.H.; Cohen, J.C. Exome-wide association study identifies a TM6SF2 variant that confers susceptibility to nonalcoholic fatty liver disease. *Nat. Genet.* **2014**, *46*, 352–356. [CrossRef] [PubMed]

75. Cast, A.; Kumbaji, M.; D'Souza, A.; Rodriguez, K.; Gupta, A.; Karns, R.; Timchenko, L.; Timchenko, N. Liver Proliferation Is an Essential Driver of Fibrosis in Mouse Models of Nonalcoholic Fatty Liver Disease. *Hepatol. Commun.* **2019**, *3*, 1036–1049. [CrossRef]

76. Qian, Y.W.; Chen, Y.; Yang, W.; Fu, J.; Cao, J.; Ren, Y.B.; Zhu, J.J.; Su, B.; Luo, T.; Zhao, X.F.; et al. p28(GANK) prevents degradation of Oct4 and promotes expansion of tumor-initiating cells in hepatocarcinogenesis. *Gastroenterology* **2012**, *142*, 1547–1558.e1514. [CrossRef]

77. Arsov, T.; Silva, D.G.; O'Bryan, M.K.; Sainsbury, A.; Lee, N.J.; Kennedy, C.; Manji, S.S.; Nelms, K.; Liu, C.; Vinuesa, C.G.; et al. Fat aussie—A new Alstrom syndrome mouse showing a critical role for ALMS1 in obesity, diabetes, and spermatogenesis. *Mol. Endocrinol.* **2006**, *20*, 1610–1622. [CrossRef]

78. Collin, G.B.; Marshall, J.D.; Ikeda, A.; So, W.V.; Russell-Eggitt, I.; Maffei, P.; Beck, S.; Boerkoel, C.F.; Sicolo, N.; Martin, M.; et al. Mutations in ALMS1 cause obesity, type 2 diabetes and neurosensory degeneration in Alstrom syndrome. *Nat. Genet.* **2002**, *31*, 74–78. [CrossRef]

79. Soga, M.; Kishimoto, Y.; kawaguchi, J.; Nakai, Y.; Kawamura, Y.; Inagaki, S.; Katoh, K.; Oohara, T.; Makino, S.; Oshima, I. The FLS mouse: A new inbred strain with spontaneous fatty liver. *Lab. Anim. Sci.* **1999**, *49*, 269–275.

80. Semba, T.; Nishimura, M.; Nishimura, S.; Ohara, O.; Ishige, T.; Ohno, S.; Nonaka, K.; Sogawa, K.; Satoh, M.; Sawai, S.; et al. The FLS (fatty liver Shionogi) mouse reveals local expressions of lipocalin-2, CXCL1 and CXCL9 in the liver with non-alcoholic steatohepatitis. *BMC Gastroenterol.* **2013**, *13*, 120. [CrossRef]

81. Sugihara, T.; Koda, M.; Kishina, M.; Kato, J.; Tokunaga, S.; Matono, T.; Ueki, M.; Murawaki, Y. Fatty liver Shionogi-ob/ob mouse: A new candidate for a non-alcoholic steatohepatitis model. *Hepatol. Res.* **2013**, *43*, 547–556. [CrossRef]

82. He, L.; Tian, D.A.; Li, P.Y.; He, X.X. Mouse models of liver cancer: Progress and recommendations. *Oncotarget* **2015**, *6*, 23306–23322. [CrossRef] [PubMed]

83. Watanabe, S.; Horie, Y.; Kataoka, E.; Sato, W.; Dohmen, T.; Ohshima, S.; Goto, T.; Suzuki, A. Non-alcoholic steatohepatitis and hepatocellular carcinoma: Lessons from hepatocyte-specific phosphatase and tensin homolog (PTEN)-deficient mice. *J. Gastroenterol. Hepatol.* **2007**, *22* (Suppl. 1), S96–S100. [CrossRef]

84. Takakura, K.; Oikawa, T.; Tomita, Y.; Mizuno, Y.; Nakano, M.; Saeki, C.; Torisu, Y.; Saruta, M. Mouse models for investigating the underlying mechanisms of nonalcoholic steatohepatitis-derived hepatocellular carcinoma. *World J. Gastroenterol.* **2018**, *24*, 1989–1994. [CrossRef] [PubMed]

85. Chen, C.Y.; Chen, J.; He, L.; Stiles, B.L. PTEN: Tumor Suppressor and Metabolic Regulator. *Front. Endocrinol. (Lausanne)* **2018**, *9*, 338. [CrossRef] [PubMed]

86. Gandhi, C.R.; Chaillet, J.R.; Nalesnik, M.A.; Kumar, S.; Dangi, A.; Demetris, A.J.; Ferrell, R.; Wu, T.; Divanovic, S.; Stankeiwicz, T.; et al. Liver-specific deletion of augmenter of liver regeneration accelerates development of steatohepatitis and hepatocellular carcinoma in mice. *Gastroenterology* **2015**, *148*, 379–391.e374. [CrossRef] [PubMed]

87. Francavilla, A.; Vujanovic, N.L.; Polimeno, L.; Azzarone, A.; Iacobellis, A.; Deleo, A.; Hagiya, M.; Whiteside, T.L.; Starzl, T.E. The in vivo effect of hepatotrophic factors augmenter of liver regeneration, hepatocyte growth factor, and insulin-like growth factor-II on liver natural killer cell functions. *Hepatology* **1997**, *25*, 411–415. [CrossRef]

88. Ibrahim, S.; Weiss, T.S. Augmenter of liver regeneration: Essential for growth and beyond. *Cytokine Growth Factor Rev.* **2019**, *45*, 65–80. [CrossRef]

89. Gandhi, C.R.; Murase, N.; Starzl, T.E. Cholera toxin-sensitive GTP-binding protein-coupled activation of augmenter of liver regeneration (ALR) receptor and its function in rat kupffer cells. *J. Cell Physiol.* **2010**, *222*, 365–373. [CrossRef]

90. Itoh, M.; Suganami, T.; Nakagawa, N.; Tanaka, M.; Yamamoto, Y.; Kamei, Y.; Terai, S.; Sakaida, I.; Ogawa, Y. Melanocortin 4 receptor-deficient mice as a novel mouse model of nonalcoholic steatohepatitis. *Am. J. Pathol.* **2011**, *179*, 2454–2463. [CrossRef]

91. Yamada, T.; Kashiwagi, Y.; Rokugawa, T.; Kato, H.; Konishi, H.; Hamada, T.; Nagai, R.; Masago, Y.; Itoh, M.; Suganami, T.; et al. Evaluation of hepatic function using dynamic contrast-enhanced magnetic resonance imaging in melanocortin 4 receptor-deficient mice as a model of nonalcoholic steatohepatitis. *Magn. Reson. Imaging* **2019**, *57*, 210–217. [CrossRef]

92. Denk, H.; Abuja, P.M.; Zatloukal, K. Animal models of NAFLD from the pathologist's point of view. *Biochim. Biophys. Acta Mol. Basis Dis.* **2019**, *1865*, 929–942. [CrossRef]

93. Nishida, T.; Tsuneyama, K.; Fujimoto, M.; Nomoto, K.; Hayashi, S.; Miwa, S.; Nakajima, T.; Nakanishi, Y.; Sasaki, Y.; Suzuki, W.; et al. Spontaneous onset of nonalcoholic steatohepatitis and hepatocellular carcinoma in a mouse model of metabolic syndrome. *Lab. Invest.* **2013**, *93*, 230–241. [CrossRef] [PubMed]

94. Bettermann, K.; Mehta, A.K.; Hofer, E.M.; Wohlrab, C.; Golob-Schwarzl, N.; Svendova, V.; Schimek, M.G.; Stumptner, C.; Thuringer, A.; Speicher, M.R.; et al. Keratin 18-deficiency results in steatohepatitis and liver tumors in old mice: A model of steatohepatitis-associated liver carcinogenesis. *Oncotarget* **2016**, *7*, 73309–73322. [CrossRef] [PubMed]

95. Luedde, T.; Beraza, N.; Kotsikoris, V.; van Loo, G.; Nenci, A.; De Vos, R.; Roskams, T.; Trautwein, C.; Pasparakis, M. Deletion of NEMO/IKKgamma in liver parenchymal cells causes steatohepatitis and hepatocellular carcinoma. *Cancer Cell* **2007**, *11*, 119–132. [CrossRef] [PubMed]

96. Cano, A.; Buque, X.; Martinez-Una, M.; Aurrekoetxea, I.; Menor, A.; Garcia-Rodriguez, J.L.; Lu, S.C.; Martinez-Chantar, M.L.; Mato, J.M.; Ochoa, B.; et al. Methionine adenosyltransferase 1A gene deletion disrupts hepatic very low-density lipoprotein assembly in mice. *Hepatology* **2011**, *54*, 1975–1986. [CrossRef]

97. Domitrovic, R.; Jakovac, H.; Tomac, J.; Sain, I. Liver fibrosis in mice induced by carbon tetrachloride and its reversion by luteolin. *Toxicol. Appl. Pharmacol.* **2009**, *241*, 311–321. [CrossRef]

98. Sharma, L.; Gupta, D.; Abdullah, S.T. Thioacetamide potentiates high cholesterol and high fat diet induced steato-hepatitic changes in livers of C57BL/6J mice: A novel eight weeks model of fibrosing NASH. *Toxicol. Lett.* **2019**, *304*, 21–29. [CrossRef]

99. Fujii, M.; Shibazaki, Y.; Wakamatsu, K.; Honda, Y.; Kawauchi, Y.; Suzuki, K.; Arumugam, S.; Watanabe, K.; Ichida, T.; Asakura, H.; et al. A murine model for non-alcoholic steatohepatitis showing evidence of association between diabetes and hepatocellular carcinoma. *Med. Mol. Morphol* **2013**, *46*, 141–152. [CrossRef]

100. Jena, P.K.; Sheng, L.; Liu, H.X.; Kalanetra, K.M.; Mirsoian, A.; Murphy, W.J.; French, S.W.; Krishnan, V.V.; Mills, D.A.; Wan, Y.Y. Western Diet-Induced Dysbiosis in Farnesoid X Receptor Knockout Mice Causes Persistent Hepatic Inflammation after Antibiotic Treatment. *Am. J. Pathol.* **2017**, *187*, 1800–1813. [CrossRef]

101. Norheim, F.; Hui, S.T.; Kulahcioglu, E.; Mehrabian, M.; Cantor, R.M.; Pan, C.; Parks, B.W.; Lusis, A.J. Genetic and hormonal control of hepatic steatosis in female and male mice. *J. Lipid Res.* **2017**, *58*, 178–187. [CrossRef]

102. Lonardo, A.; Nascimbeni, F.; Ballestri, S.; Fairweather, D.; Win, S.; Than, T.A.; Abdelmalek, M.F.; Suzuki, A. Sex Differences in Nonalcoholic Fatty Liver Disease: State of the Art and Identification of Research Gaps. *Hepatology* **2019**, *70*, 1457–1469. [CrossRef] [PubMed]

103. Spruss, A.; Henkel, J.; Kanuri, G.; Blank, D.; Puschel, G.P.; Bischoff, S.C.; Bergheim, I. Female mice are more susceptible to nonalcoholic fatty liver disease: Sex-specific regulation of the hepatic AMP-activated protein kinase-plasminogen activator inhibitor 1 cascade, but not the hepatic endotoxin response. *Mol. Med.* **2012**, *18*, 1346–1355. [CrossRef] [PubMed]

104. Marin, V.; Rosso, N.; Dal Ben, M.; Raseni, A.; Boschelle, M.; Degrassi, C.; Nemeckova, I.; Nachtigal, P.; Avellini, C.; Tiribelli, C.; et al. An Animal Model for the Juvenile Non-Alcoholic Fatty Liver Disease and Non-Alcoholic Steatohepatitis. *PLoS ONE* **2016**, *11*, e0158817. [CrossRef] [PubMed]

105. Zhou, L.; Liu, D.; Wang, Z.; Dong, H.; Xu, X.; Zhou, S. Establishment and Comparison of Juvenile Female Mouse Models of Nonalcoholic Fatty Liver Disease and Nonalcoholic Steatohepatitis. *Gastroenterol. Res. Pract.* **2018**, *2018*, 8929620. [CrossRef] [PubMed]

106. Giles, D.A.; Moreno-Fernandez, M.E.; Stankiewicz, T.E.; Graspeuntner, S.; Cappelletti, M.; Wu, D.; Mukherjee, R.; Chan, C.C.; Lawson, M.J.; Klarquist, J.; et al. Thermoneutral housing exacerbates nonalcoholic

fatty liver disease in mice and allows for sex-independent disease modeling. *Nat. Med.* **2017**, *23*, 829–838. [CrossRef] [PubMed]

107. Adamovich, Y.; Rousso-Noori, L.; Zwighaft, Z.; Neufeld-Cohen, A.; Golik, M.; Kraut-Cohen, J.; Wang, M.; Han, X.; Asher, G. Circadian clocks and feeding time regulate the oscillations and levels of hepatic triglycerides. *Cell Metab.* **2014**, *19*, 319–330. [CrossRef]

108. Jacobi, D.; Liu, S.; Burkewitz, K.; Kory, N.; Knudsen, N.H.; Alexander, R.K.; Unluturk, U.; Li, X.; Kong, X.; Hyde, A.L.; et al. Hepatic Bmal1 Regulates Rhythmic Mitochondrial Dynamics and Promotes Metabolic Fitness. *Cell Metab.* **2015**, *22*, 709–720. [CrossRef]

109. Kettner, N.M.; Voicu, H.; Finegold, M.J.; Coarfa, C.; Sreekumar, A.; Putluri, N.; Katchy, C.A.; Lee, C.; Moore, D.D.; Fu, L. Circadian Homeostasis of Liver Metabolism Suppresses Hepatocarcinogenesis. *Cancer Cell* **2016**, *30*, 909–924. [CrossRef]

110. Baker, M. 1,500 scientists lift the lid on reproducibility. *Nature* **2016**, *533*, 452–454. [CrossRef]

111. Begley, C.G.; Ellis, L.M. Drug development: Raise standards for preclinical cancer research. *Nature* **2012**, *483*, 531–533. [CrossRef]

112. Goodman, S.N.; Fanelli, D.; Ioannidis, J.P. What does research reproducibility mean? *Sci. Transl. Med.* **2016**, *8*, 341ps312. [CrossRef] [PubMed]

113. Zou, Y.; Li, J.; Lu, C.; Wang, J.; Ge, J.; Huang, Y.; Zhang, L.; Wang, Y. High-fat emulsion-induced rat model of nonalcoholic steatohepatitis. *Life Sci.* **2006**, *79*, 1100–1107. [CrossRef] [PubMed]

114. Kucera, O.; Cervinkova, Z. Experimental models of non-alcoholic fatty liver disease in rats. *World J. Gastroenterol.* **2014**, *20*, 8364–8376. [CrossRef] [PubMed]

115. Rodrigues, A.A.; Andrade, R.S.B.; Vasconcelos, D.F.P. Relationship between Experimental Diet in Rats and Nonalcoholic Hepatic Disease: Review of Literature. *Int. J. Hepatol.* **2018**, *2018*, 9023027. [CrossRef]

116. Maciejewska, D.; Lukomska, A.; Dec, K.; Skonieczna-Zydecka, K.; Gutowska, I.; Skorka-Majewicz, M.; Styburski, D.; Misiakiewicz-Has, K.; Pilutin, A.; Palma, J.; et al. Diet-Induced Rat Model of Gradual Development of Non-Alcoholic Fatty Liver Disease (NAFLD) with Lipopolysaccharides (LPS) Secretion. *Diagnostics (Basel)* **2019**, *9*, 205. [CrossRef]

117. Khurana, P.; Yadati, T.; Goyal, S.; Dolas, A.; Houben, T.; Oligschlaeger, Y.; Agarwal, A.K.; Kulkarni, A.; Shiri-Sverdlov, R. Inhibiting Extracellular Cathepsin D Reduces Hepatic Steatosis in Sprague(-)Dawley Rats (dagger). *Biomolecules* **2019**, *9*, 171. [CrossRef]

118. Maeso-Diaz, R.; Boyer-Diaz, Z.; Lozano, J.J.; Ortega-Ribera, M.; Peralta, C.; Bosch, J.; Gracia-Sancho, J. New Rat Model of Advanced NASH Mimicking Pathophysiological Features and Transcriptomic Signature of The Human Disease. *Cells* **2019**, *8*, 1062. [CrossRef]

119. Carmiel-Haggai, M.; Cederbaum, A.I.; Nieto, N. A high-fat diet leads to the progression of non-alcoholic fatty liver disease in obese rats. *FASEB J.* **2005**, *19*, 136–138. [CrossRef]

120. Lieber, C.S.; Leo, M.A.; Mak, K.M.; Xu, Y.; Cao, Q.; Ren, C.; Ponomarenko, A.; DeCarli, L.M. Model of nonalcoholic steatohepatitis. *Am. J. Clin. Nutr.* **2004**, *79*, 502–509. [CrossRef]

121. Kirsch, R.; Clarkson, V.; Shephard, E.G.; Marais, D.A.; Jaffer, M.A.; Woodburne, V.E.; Kirsch, R.E.; Hall Pde, L. Rodent nutritional model of non-alcoholic steatohepatitis: Species, strain and sex difference studies. *J. Gastroenterol. Hepatol.* **2003**, *18*, 1272–1282. [CrossRef]

122. Domitrovic, R.; Jakovac, H.; Milin, C.; Radosevic-Stasic, B. Dose- and time-dependent effects of luteolin on carbon tetrachloride-induced hepatotoxicity in mice. *Exp. Toxicol. Pathol.* **2009**, *61*, 581–589. [CrossRef]

123. Walenbergh, S.M.; Houben, T.; Rensen, S.S.; Bieghs, V.; Hendrikx, T.; van Gorp, P.J.; Oligschlaeger, Y.; Jeurissen, M.L.; Gijbels, M.J.; Buurman, W.A.; et al. Plasma cathepsin D correlates with histological classifications of fatty liver disease in adults and responds to intervention. *Sci. Rep.* **2016**, *6*, 38278. [CrossRef]

124. Houben, T.; Oligschlaeger, Y.; Hendrikx, T.; Bitorina, A.V.; Walenbergh, S.M.A.; van Gorp, P.J.; Gijbels, M.J.J.; Friedrichs, S.; Plat, J.; Schaap, F.G.; et al. Cathepsin D regulates lipid metabolism in murine steatohepatitis. *Sci. Rep.* **2017**, *7*, 3494. [CrossRef]

125. Gehrke, N.; Biedenbach, J.; Huber, Y.; Straub, B.K.; Galle, P.R.; Simon, P.; Schattenberg, J.M. Voluntary exercise in mice fed an obesogenic diet alters the hepatic immune phenotype and improves metabolic parameters—An animal model of life style intervention in NAFLD. *Sci. Rep.* **2019**, *9*, 4007. [CrossRef] [PubMed]

126. Kawanishi, N.; Niihara, H.; Mizokami, T.; Yada, K.; Suzuki, K. Exercise training attenuates neutrophil infiltration and elastase expression in adipose tissue of high-fat-diet-induced obese mice. *Physiol. Rep.* **2015**, *3*. [CrossRef] [PubMed]

127. Boeckmans, J.; Natale, A.; Rombaut, M.; Buyl, K.; Rogiers, V.; De Kock, J.; Vanhaecke, T.; R, M.R. Anti-NASH Drug Development Hitches a Lift on PPAR Agonism. *Cells* **2019**, *9*, 37. [CrossRef] [PubMed]

128. Francque, S.; Verrijken, A.; Caron, S.; Prawitt, J.; Paumelle, R.; Derudas, B.; Lefebvre, P.; Taskinen, M.R.; Van Hul, W.; Mertens, I.; et al. PPARalpha gene expression correlates with severity and histological treatment response in patients with non-alcoholic steatohepatitis. *J. Hepatol.* **2015**, *63*, 164–173. [CrossRef] [PubMed]

129. Shipman, K.E.; Strange, R.C.; Ramachandran, S. Use of fibrates in the metabolic syndrome: A review. *World J. Diabetes* **2016**, *7*, 74–88. [CrossRef] [PubMed]

130. Ishibashi, S.; Arai, H.; Yokote, K.; Araki, E.; Suganami, H.; Yamashita, S.; Group, K.S. Efficacy and safety of pemafibrate (K-877), a selective peroxisome proliferator-activated receptor alpha modulator, in patients with dyslipidemia: Results from a 24-week, randomized, double blind, active-controlled, phase 3 trial. *J. Clin. Lipidol.* **2018**, *12*, 173–184. [CrossRef]

131. Honda, Y.; Kessoku, T.; Ogawa, Y.; Tomeno, W.; Imajo, K.; Fujita, K.; Yoneda, M.; Takizawa, T.; Saito, S.; Nagashima, Y.; et al. Pemafibrate, a novel selective peroxisome proliferator-activated receptor alpha modulator, improves the pathogenesis in a rodent model of nonalcoholic steatohepatitis. *Sci. Rep.* **2017**, *7*, 42477. [CrossRef]

132. Bays, H.E.; Schwartz, S.; Littlejohn, T., 3rd; Kerzner, B.; Krauss, R.M.; Karpf, D.B.; Choi, Y.J.; Wang, X.; Naim, S.; Roberts, B.K. MBX-8025, a novel peroxisome proliferator receptor-delta agonist: Lipid and other metabolic effects in dyslipidemic overweight patients treated with and without atorvastatin. *J. Clin. Endocrinol. Metab* **2011**, *96*, 2889–2897. [CrossRef] [PubMed]

133. Haczeyni, F.; Wang, H.; Barn, V.; Mridha, A.R.; Yeh, M.M.; Haigh, W.G.; Ioannou, G.N.; Choi, Y.J.; McWherter, C.A.; Teoh, N.C.; et al. The selective peroxisome proliferator-activated receptor-delta agonist seladelpar reverses nonalcoholic steatohepatitis pathology by abrogating lipotoxicity in diabetic obese mice. *Hepatol. Commun.* **2017**, *1*, 663–674. [CrossRef] [PubMed]

134. Lee, Y.H.; Kim, J.H.; Kim, S.R.; Jin, H.Y.; Rhee, E.J.; Cho, Y.M.; Lee, B.W. Lobeglitazone, a Novel Thiazolidinedione, Improves Non-Alcoholic Fatty Liver Disease in Type 2 Diabetes: Its Efficacy and Predictive Factors Related to Responsiveness. *J. Korean Med. Sci.* **2017**, *32*, 60–69. [CrossRef] [PubMed]

135. Choung, S.; Joung, K.H.; You, B.R.; Park, S.K.; Kim, H.J.; Ku, B.J. Treatment with Lobeglitazone Attenuates Hepatic Steatosis in Diet-Induced Obese Mice. *PPAR Res.* **2018**, *2018*, 4292509. [CrossRef] [PubMed]

136. Ratziu, V.; Harrison, S.A.; Francque, S.; Bedossa, P.; Lehert, P.; Serfaty, L.; Romero-Gomez, M.; Boursier, J.; Abdelmalek, M.; Caldwell, S.; et al. Elafibranor, an Agonist of the Peroxisome Proliferator-Activated Receptor-alpha and -delta, Induces Resolution of Nonalcoholic Steatohepatitis Without Fibrosis Worsening. *Gastroenterology* **2016**, *150*, 1147–1159.e1145. [CrossRef] [PubMed]

137. Tolbol, K.S.; Kristiansen, M.N.; Hansen, H.H.; Veidal, S.S.; Rigbolt, K.T.; Gillum, M.P.; Jelsing, J.; Vrang, N.; Feigh, M. Metabolic and hepatic effects of liraglutide, obeticholic acid and elafibranor in diet-induced obese mouse models of biopsy-confirmed nonalcoholic steatohepatitis. *World J. Gastroenterol.* **2018**, *24*, 179–194. [CrossRef]

138. Alukal, J.J.; Thuluvath, P.J. Reversal of NASH fibrosis with pharmacotherapy. *Hepatol. Int.* **2019**, *13*, 534–545. [CrossRef]

139. Roth, J.D.; Veidal, S.S.; Fensholdt, L.K.D.; Rigbolt, K.T.G.; Papazyan, R.; Nielsen, J.C.; Feigh, M.; Vrang, N.; Young, M.; Jelsing, J.; et al. Combined obeticholic acid and elafibranor treatment promotes additive liver histological improvements in a diet-induced ob/ob mouse model of biopsy-confirmed NASH. *Sci. Rep.* **2019**, *9*, 9046. [CrossRef]

140. Hui, S.T.; Kurt, Z.; Tuominen, I.; Norheim, F.; R, C.D.; Pan, C.; Dirks, D.L.; Magyar, C.E.; French, S.W.; Chella Krishnan, K.; et al. The Genetic Architecture of Diet-Induced Hepatic Fibrosis in Mice. *Hepatology* **2018**, *68*, 2182–2196. [CrossRef]

3

Depression and Cognitive Impairment—Extrahepatic Manifestations of NAFLD and NASH

Martina Colognesi †, Daniela Gabbia † and Sara De Martin *

Department of Pharmaceutical and Pharmacological Sciences, University of Padova, L.go Meneghetti 2, 35131 Padova, Italy; martina.colognesi@studenti.unipd.it (M.C.); daniela.gabbia@unipd.it (D.G.)
* Correspondence: sara.demartin@unipd.it
† M.C. and D.G. share first co-authorship.

Abstract: Non-alcoholic fatty liver disease (NAFLD) and its complication non-alcoholic steatohepatitis (NASH) are important causes of liver disease worldwide. Recently, a significant association between these hepatic diseases and different central nervous system (CNS) disorders has been observed in an increasing number of patients. NAFLD-related CNS dysfunctions include cognitive impairment, hippocampal-dependent memory impairment, and mood imbalances (in particular, depression and anxiety). This review aims at summarizing the main correlations observed between NAFLD development and these CNS dysfunctions, focusing on the studies investigating the mechanism(s) involved in this association. Growing evidences point at cerebrovascular alteration, neuroinflammation, and brain insulin resistance as NAFLD/NASH-related CNS manifestations. Since the pharmacological options available for the management of these conditions are still limited, further studies are needed to unravel the mechanism(s) of NAFLD/NASH and their central manifestations and identify effective pharmacological targets.

Keywords: non-alcoholic fatty liver disease; NAFLD; steatohepatitis; NASH; cognitive impairment; memory dysfunction; Alzheimer's disease; neurodegeneration

1. Introduction

Non-alcoholic fatty liver disease (NAFLD) is considered the hepatic manifestation of metabolic syndrome and is associated with progressive hepatocellular lipid accumulation, mostly of triglycerides, up to more than 10% of liver weight [1]. This disease comprises a wide range of liver disorders, from simple non-alcoholic fatty liver (NAFL) to non-alcoholic steatohepatitis (NASH) and, if not treated, can lead to threatening complications such as cirrhosis and hepatocellular carcinoma [2]. Generally, NAFLD is considered a benign and reversible condition, although one-third of NAFLD patients eventually progress to NASH, which is characterized by inflammation and hepatocellular injury [3]. While the causes involved in the establishment of NAFLD have been largely investigated, the main factors controlling the progression of NAFLD toward NASH remain pretty much unknown and are currently intensively studied. Many experimental evidences suggested that lipotoxicity, proinflammatory mediators, and oxidative stress may have a central role in this process [3], which can occur in the presence or absence of a high amount of dietary fat ingestion [1]. Moreover, the consumption of imbalanced diets (e.g., excessive fat and sugar intake), as well as the alteration of gut microbiome are involved in NAFLD development and progression [4–6]. In particular, high fat and high sugar diets, besides promoting the deposition of fat in the liver, could modify microbiome composition and affect gut barrier integrity, facilitating bacterial translocation and inflammation. Inflammation and oxidative stress have also shown to play a pivotal role in extrahepatic diseases, including many different central nervous system (CNS) diseases such as, for instance, Alzheimer's disease (AD). Accordingly, extensive evidences obtained in the last years have revealed that NAFLD may represent a risk factor for CNS impairment [7].

Several observations suggest that a correlation may exist between metabolic liver diseases, such as NAFLD and NASH, and CNS disorders, starting from the increased risk of developing AD, mild cognitive impairment (MCI), and dementia in patients with dyslipidemic disorders, and an association with neurodegeneration and cognitive deficits has been observed in patients with metabolic syndrome-related diseases such as type 2 diabetes mellitus (T2DM) and obesity [3].

In this review, we want to point the attention to depression and mild and severe cognitive impairment, which are becoming a serious health threat, and in recent years have been associated to NAFLD and NASH.

2. Cognitive Dysfunction and Brain Abnormalities

2.1. Depression

Depression is one of the most common CNS diseases involved in adult premature death and it is characterized by specific cognitive and somatic abnormalities over time. The common symptoms of patients with depressive disorders are mood imbalances or anhedonia [8], which are also associated with social dysfunction and cognitive and functional impairment [9].

Since depression is known to be associated with chronic liver disease (CLD) [10,11], and considering that nearly 30% of patients with NAFLD show major depressive disorder (MDD) with a prevalence higher than the general population [12], it is plausible to hypothesize that a correlation exists between NAFLD and depression. However, controversial results have been obtained by the different studies that tried to validate this hypothesis (Table 1). While dated population-based studies reported that NAFLD is absolutely not correlated to depressive disorders [10], other studies conducted in the same period or more recently reported the existence of a possible association between depression and NAFLD [12,13]. In particular, the study of Youssef and collaborators provided robust evidence of the correlation between depressive symptoms and hepatocyte ballooning, one of the main hallmarks of NAFLD progression, even after the adjustment for potential confounding factors such as age, sex, ethnicity, body mass index (BMI), diabetes mellitus, systemic hypertension, smoking, alcohol consumption, and anxiety symptoms. Indeed, a multivariate data analysis showed more severe hepatocyte ballooning in patients with mood disorders, validating the hypothesis of a NAFLD role in depressive symptoms [13]. Accordingly, Tomeno and collaborators suggested a correlation between the severity of steatosis and MDD comorbidity in NAFLD patients. These findings were confirmed by higher levels of serum markers of liver dysfunction such as aspartate aminotransferase (ALT), alanine aminotransferase (AST), γ-glutamyl transpeptidase (GGT), and high-sensitivity C-reactive protein (hs-CRP) in NAFLD patients affected by MDD [12]. Although the results of these pioneering studies need to be confirmed by other investigations, they pointed the attention on the relationship between NAFLD severity and MDD.

For a better understanding of the liver disease influence on depressive disorders, preclinical evaluations were performed in animal models of NASH to verify the presence of behavioral mood changes in these models. The forced swimming test was used in one of these studies to assess depressive-like behavior, like despair and anhedonia, in rats. Rats with NASH showed a lack of struggle to escape, in contrast with their normal attitude. This result demonstrated that NASH rats were affected by a sense of hopelessness, which is normally associated with depression [14].

Table 1. Principal clinical studies reporting an association between depressive disorders and NAFLD.

Study	Settings and Study Design	Subjects	Methods	Results and Conclusions
Lee et al. (2013) [10]	Cross-sectional national survey, population-based	10231 NHANES participants in the 18th year or older	PHQ-9 survey to screen depression associated with hematologic and biochemical tests and viral hepatitis	Depression and chronic hepatitis C are independently associated, but not metabolic syndrome
Tomeno et al. (2015) [12]	Population-based	258 participants	Blood test monitoring and lifestyle counseling for 48 weeks, with assessment of insulin resistance through HOMA-IR	32 NAFLD patients were comorbid with MDD and showed higher biochemical parameters (ALT, AST, GGT, ferritin, hs-CRP, and cholinesterase) than NAFLD patients without MDD. Only NAFLD patients without MDD improved their conditions with treatment.
Youssef et al. (2013) [13]	Cross-sectional analyses, population-based	567 participants aged 20 and older	HADS questionnaire to assess severity of depression and anxiety	Severe depressive symptoms were associated with increased hepatocyte ballooning
Elwing et al. (2006) [11]	Case-control comparison	36 patients undergoing cholecystectomy and 36 matched control subjects	Structured interview to assess psychiatric illnesses	Lifetime MDD has significantly increased rates in NASH subjects, in accordance with PHQ-9.
Filipović et al. (2018) [15]	Population-based	40 NAFLD positive participants aged from 34 to 57, and 36 controls aged from 39 to 53	3D T1-weighted MR images to measure gray and white matter volume and brain lateral ventricles, Serbian version of the MoCA test to assess cognitive functioning and Hamilton's depression rating scale to evaluate depression level	Cognitive status declined in NAFLD patients, according to the MoCA index. These patients had reduced gray and white matter volumes and higher risk of depression.

NHANES: National Health and Nutrition Examination Survey; PHQ-9: Patient Health Questionnaire; HOMA-IR: Homeostasis Model for the Assessment of Insulin Resistance; HADS: Hospital Anxiety & Depression Scale; MoCA: Montreal Cognitive Assessment.

Depression and anxiety have been associated not only with NAFLD, but they have also shown to be strictly involved in pathological features typical of NAFLD progression to NASH, such as insulin resistance and inflammation. The study of Elwing and collaborators tried to evaluate the correlation between these mood disorders and liver histological features. Their findings provide evidence that depression is directly associated with hepatic inflammatory markers, suggesting its active role in NASH progression [11]. One recent study investigated the possible changes of brain tissue volumes in NAFLD patients. They found a significant reduction of white and gray brain volumes and an increased volume of lateral ventricles, with respect to healthy patients. This ulterior remark suggests a higher risk of depression in NAFLD-diagnosed patients [15].

2.2. Cognitive Impairment

Mild cognitive impairment (MCI) is defined as an impairment in cognition more severe than that generally associated with normal memory and cognitive changes merely due to aging (clinically considered as "age-related cognitive decline"). However, this condition is less problematic than dementia or other cognitive deficits which significantly impair daily functions [16]. Among the different cognitive features which could be impaired, we will focus on memory, social functioning, visuospatial function, and executive functioning.

As far as metabolic syndrome and its components are concerned, including liver manifestations as NAFLD/NASH, many recent population-based studies have suggested their involvement in cognitive impairment, from mild ones up to dementia [17]. Although there are studies providing evidences that metabolic syndrome [18,19] and NASH [3,14] are associated with cognitive deficits, whether NAFLD may lead to cognitive impairment remains controversial (Table 2).

One of the first studies suggesting the presence of functional and cognitive impairment in NAFLD patients was a study by Elliott and collaborators [20]. The main conclusion they achieved was that NAFLD patients had a significantly worse cognitive function with respect to controls, supporting the idea that NAFLD may influence cognitive features.

A lead study in this field has been performed by Seo and collaborators and confirmed the hypothesis of the independent association between NAFLD and cognitive impairment after the analysis of the data obtained from the Third National Health and Nutrition Examination Survey (NHANES III). The authors considered patients with cognitive impairment, excluding possible confounding factors (e.g., BMI, waist circumference, diabetes mellitus, hypertension, hypercholesterolemia, history of acute myocardial infarction, heart failure, and stroke) and considering factors known to affect cognition, such as cardiovascular disease. They observed an increase of liver enzymes, surrogate marker of NAFLD presence and progression to NASH, even without histological signs of advanced liver dysfunction [21].

It is well known that screening tools like the Montreal Cognitive Assessment (MoCA) are quite useful and more sensitive than others for diagnosing forms of cognitive decline in old adults and patients with MCI [22]. Celikbilek and collaborators utilized for the first time the Turkish version of the MoCA test to investigate whether patients with NAFLD show more probability to manifest cognitive impairment than healthy subjects. The results showed a correlation between liver dysfunction and cognitive impairment, in particular, in the visuospatial and executive function domains, both associated with the prefrontal cortex (PFC) [23].

Recent studies tried to assess which brain region(s) may be affected by NAFLD and reported that these patients were characterized by lower levels of metabolic activity in some brain areas, e.g., PFC, hippocampus, and amygdala, due to low levels of dopamine in the PFC and cerebellum and of noradrenaline in the striatum [14]. Taken together, these observations validate the hypothesis of NAFLD implication in cognitive impairment.

Table 2. Principal clinical studies reported on cognitive impairment, MCI, and NAFLD patients.

Study	Settings and Study Design	Subjects	Methods	Results and Conclusions
Elliott et al. (2013) [20]	Cohort study	224 NAFLD participants and 100 controls	PHAQ and CFQ were used to evaluate functional and physical ability and cognitive abilities.	NAFLD patients showed significantly worse functional abilities, and they had more difficulties in specific daily activities than controls.
Seo et al. (2016) [21]	Cross-sectional population-based analysis	4472 participants aged from 20 to 59	Assessment of liver enzyme activity and cognitive evaluation using SRTT, SDLT, and SDST	NAFLD patients showed lower performance on the SDLT, and NAFLD resulted independently associated with lower cognitive performance.
Celikbilek et al. (2018) [23]	Prospective cross-sectional population-based analysis	70 participants and 73 age- and sex-matched controls aged from 18 to 70	Turkish version of the MoCA test to evaluate cognitive functions	Deficits were observed in each cognitive domain, mainly in the visuospatial and executive functioning. NAFLD patients reported significantly lower MoCA test scores.
An et al. (2019) [24]	Cross-sectional population-based analysis	23 NAFLD participants and 21 matched controls	BDI was used to assess depressive symptoms, and RBANS was used to characterize neurocognitive deficits.	BDI mean score indicated a moderate depression in NAFLD patients, and women reported significant association with visuospatial memory deficit.
Weinstein et al. (2019) [25]	Cross-sectional population-based analysis	1287 participants	Trail-making test to measure executive functioning. Similarity test was used to assess abstract reasoning skills, and the Hooper visual organization test was used to measure visual perception.	NAFLD and cognitive performances were not associated; however, poorer performances on the trail-making and similarities tests were linked to increased risk of advanced fibrosis in NAFLD participants.

PHAQ: Patient-Reported Outcomes Measurement Information System, Health Assessment Questionnaire; CFQ: Cognitive Failures Questionnaire; SRTT: Simple Reaction Time Test; SDLT: Serial Digit Learning Test; SDST: Symbol-Digit Substitution Test; BDI: Beck Depression Inventory; RBANS: Repeatable Battery for Assessment of Neuropsychological Status.

Another study investigated the possible correlation between cognitive status and NAFLD using the MoCA test, finding a lower MoCA score and a reduction in white and gray brain volumes in NAFLD patients [15]. In combination with the reduced gray and white volumes, these authors found an increase of lateral ventricles volumes, justifying the constant total brain volume in presence of different cognitive situations between the tested group. The main conclusion achieved by this study is that patients with NAFLD have a risk four times higher of manifesting lower cognitive abilities and depleted cognitive performance and deficit, and also confirmed the higher concentration of AST in NAFLD patients with cognitive deficit [15]. The correlation between higher levels of AST and ALT and poorer cognitive function, especially in visuospatial memory, was also supported by a recent population-based study conducted by An and collaborators [24].

Besides these results, there are also studies that found no correlation between NAFLD per se and cognitive impairment, as found in a cross-sectional study by Weinstein et al. [25], who associated poorer cognitive function (mainly in the executive areas) with an increased risk of advanced liver fibrosis but not NAFLD. These results suggest that the association between NAFLD and cognition may be influenced by the specific cognitive brain domains studied and also by the type of liver dysfunction.

Finally, to which extent sleep apnea and chronic intermittent hypoxia, which are known to result in cognitive impairment [26] and also to be associated with the metabolic syndrome and NAFLD/NASH [27], contributes to the cognitive impairment found in NAFLD still remains to be elucidated.

2.3. Neurodegenerative Diseases: Alzheimer's Disease

Alzheimer's disease is a neurodegenerative disorder which may derive from MCI progression [22] and it is characterized by the progressive atrophy of cortical and medial temporal structures, CNS areas involved in memory and learning deficits [28]. It belongs to a series of neurodegenerative disease provoking pathophysiological brain changes via accumulation of misfolded proteins, in particular, peptide variants of amyloid-β (Aβ). Progressive protein deposition causes amyloid and senile plaques formation with synaptic dysfunction, dendritic spines loss, and neuronal death [7].

The AD etiology remains unclear, but there are many possible mechanisms, other than aging, proposed to explain its development. Recently, a number of studies provided evidence of a strict correlation between metabolic syndrome-associated diseases, such as diabetes mellitus and NAFLD, and neurodegenerative disorders, like AD [29]. Indeed, de la Monte and collaborators introduced the concept that AD could be considered a neurodegenerative disorder mediated by insulin resistance, since similar abnormalities were found in both pathologies [28]. NAFLD is known to be associated with a dysregulated lipid metabolism and increased cellular oxidative stress, and these same characteristics are present in AD, underlining their possible interconnection. Furthermore, epidemiological data suggested that dyslipidemic and insulin-dependent diseases play a key role as cofactors of AD pathogenesis [3].

The hypothesis of a correlation between AD and NAFLD is very recent, and most studies are performed in animal models and not in human patients. One aspect implicated in the development of metabolic syndrome, NAFLD, and potentially AD is the consumption of a high fat diet (HFD). A number of experimental studies used this type of diet in animal models to verify whether an association exists between AD and metabolic syndrome related diseases [30]. One of the first studies conducted in mice chronically fed with HFD showed a time-dependent decline in brain weight with respect to controls. Subtle histopathological abnormalities like neuronal loss foci and cellular apoptosis were also found in brain tissue, pointing to a correlation between HFD-induced NAFLD and mild neuropathological brain lesions [31]. Kim and collaborators evaluated the possible impact of NAFLD in AD pathogenesis, using an AD transgenic mouse model. Their findings suggested an acceleration in neurodegeneration and in Aβ plaque formation after HFD-induced acute inflammation and NAFLD development [30]. The fact that HFD and fructose-rich diets may quicken AD cognitive decline has also been confirmed in recent experimental studies [32–34].

A population-based study was carried out to assess whether different biological markers, together with neuropsychological evaluations, could provide a robust method to measure MCI and early AD progression (Table 3). The authors of this study considered different covariates in their evaluations, such as age, sex, BMI, years of education, and APOE ε4 status, and the results they obtained suggested that ALT and AST to ALT ratio, whose levels increased in NAFLD patients, were directly associated with poor cognition and greater Aβ deposition in brain areas [35].

Currently, there is a great interest in confirming the existence of a correlation between NAFLD and AD, probably because these diseases are widespread worldwide, and an effective pharmacological treatment is still missing for both of them. New approaches are in the phase of optimization, as suggested by Karbalaei and collaborators, who used a systems biology method to investigate the genes involved in both NAFLD and AD pathophysiological pathways, providing another evidence of their reciprocal interconnection [36].

Table 3. Principal clinical study reported on the Alzheimer's disease and NAFLD connection.

Study	Settings and Study Design	Subjects	Methods	Results and Conclusions
Nho et al. (2019) [35]	Cohort study	1581 participants aged around 70	Evaluation of cerebrospinal fluid biomarkers and brain atrophy (magnetic resonance), and scores for executive functioning and memory	Increased ALT and AST to ALT ratio in AD patients were linked to poor cognition.

3. Molecular and Pathophysiological Pathways Connecting NAFLD/NASH to Cognitive Impairment

The pathogenesis of NAFLD and NASH is a quite complex process involving multiple pathways and risk factors, first of all being diet imbalances. The progressive lipid deposition in the liver leads to the alteration of lipid metabolism/lipid peroxidation, insulin resistance, oxidative stress, and inflammatory damage. This promotes a state of peripheral insulin resistance and low-grade systemic inflammation. For this reason, an increasing amount of evidence suggests that NAFLD and NASH not only affect liver function, but also induce multiple extrahepatic manifestations that also involve the central nervous system, e.g., depression, cognitive impairment, AD, and dementia. Moreover, emerging evidence has demonstrated the link between microbiome composition and gut impairment, and the development of both liver diseases and cognitive dysfunctions [37,38]. It could be hypothesized that the same detrimental stimuli that lead to NAFLD and NASH in the liver could induce cognitive impairment or AD-type neurodegeneration in the brain.

Many signaling pathways are demonstrated to be altered in both NAFLD/NASH and CNS dysfunction (depression, cognitive impairment, dementia, and AD), suggesting that these diseases share, at least in part, the same pathogenetic mechanisms. Some studies reported conflicting results and whether there is a causal relation between liver damage and the development of cognitive dysfunction or if steatosis triggers for other subsequent deleterious pathogenetic mechanisms remains to be fully understood [23,39].

The main pathways involved in the NALFD/NASH-related brain dysfunction are summarized in Figure 1. Three are the main pathological aspects accounted to link NAFLD/NASH to cognitive impairment, i.e., cerebrovascular alteration, neuroinflammation, and brain insulin resistance. Accordingly, the study of Karbalaei et al. suggested three putative groups of genes involved in both AD and NAFLD related to carbohydrate metabolism, long fatty acid metabolism, and interleukin signaling pathways [36].

One of the first brain area affected by early stage chronic liver diseases is the cerebellum; then, brain injury could progress to the hippocampus or prefrontal cortex (PFC), brain areas crucial for cognition, memory, learning, and mood regulation [40–43].

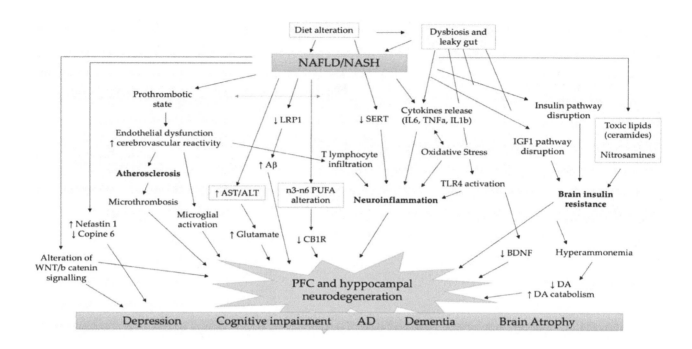

Figure 1. Main pathophysiological pathways involved in NAFLD/NASH and cognitive impairment.

The histological analysis of NASH patients' cerebella revealed the presence of parenchymal microthrombi, neurodegeneration in the Purkinje layer, and glial alteration in the molecular layer, in addition to the activation of microglia and astrocytes of white matter. Some of these features are also observed in some neurodegenerative and vascular diseases, e.g., AD, vascular dementia, and atherosclerosis [44].

Petta and collaborators observed in NAFLD patients the presence of cerebral lesions in PFC white matter, whose prevalence increases as liver function worsens, e.g., in NASH and advanced fibrosis, probably due to the proinflammatory and proatherogenic state typical of these advanced stages of liver diseases [45]. This is coherent with the fact that liver steatosis is characterized by a proinflammatory state that promotes atherosclerosis, endothelial dysfunction, platelet, and microglia activation in the brain. These alterations induce micro- and macrovascular damage, which is responsible for clinical and subclinical cerebrovascular dysfunctions [39]. The activation of inflammatory pathways characteristic of NAFLD and NASH induces the production and release of some inflammatory, prothrombotic, and oxidative stress mediators, e.g., the cytokines IL6, TNFα, and IL1β. Moreover, the increased production of reactive oxygen species could sustain the inflammatory cascade, further increasing IL6 release, neuroinflammation, and neurodegeneration [30]. It has been demonstrated that the peripheral inflammation observed in NASH patients may lead to endothelial damage and formation of microthrombi in the brain parenchyma, leading to neuroinflammation. It has been hypothesized that this phenomenon can be due to infiltrating CD4+ T lymphocytes that have been observed in the cerebellar meninges of these patients [44]. In addition, Ghareeb and collaborators observed an alteration in neurotransmitter activities induced by NAFLD, in addition to oxidative stress and metabolic dysfunction, and suggested that this may represent a risk factor for cognitive dysfunction and neurodegeneration [46]. In detail, they observed an increased activity of acetylcholine esterase (AChE) and monoamine oxidase (MAO) in NAFLD liver and brain tissues with respect to controls, accompanied to an increase of ATPase activity, and the inflammatory markers IL6 and TNF-α in the brain.

The Western diet (WD), a diet rich in fat and sugar, is considered one of the main risk factors for NAFLD/NASH, and its implication in the context of neuropsychiatric disorders and cognitive decline is a raising evidence. In the brain, it has been observed that WD is able to increase the activity of the endocannabinoid (eCB) system in the limbic areas controlling emotions, due to the increase of phospholipidic n-6/n-3 PUFA ratio in neuronal membranes and of n-6 PUFAs in the cytoplasm of hippocampal neurons. Cytoplasmatic n-6 PUFAs could be transformed into eCBs, lipid mediators binding to CB1 receptors (CB1R), reducing GABA release from interneurons located in CA1 area and altering theta oscillations. As a consequence of these alterations, WD could lead to an increase vulnerability to neuropsychiatric disorders and cognitive decline [47]. Moreover, an excessive consumption of fructose, a monosaccharide mainly used as sweetening agent in soft drinks, in addition to systemic metabolic alterations, was able to induce oxidative stress, thereby causing lipid peroxidation and protein nitrosylation in the hippocampus and reducing the expression of synaptic proteins, leading to impaired synaptic function, thus affecting learning and memory in a long-lived animal model [48]. Accordingly, many reports investigating the association between obesity and cognitive impairment have reported that the consumption of high-fat and high-sugar diet is able to increase oxidative stress, inflammation, and AChE activity, leading to cerebrovascular changes and neuronal loss in the hippocampus, disrupt myelination and axonal transmission, and decrease of dopamine (DA) and serotonin (5-HT) in the hippocampus, two of the key neurotransmitters involved in learning and memory processes [33,34,49,50].

Several pieces of evidence have demonstrated that unhealthy diets, e.g., the Western diet or high fructose intake, could greatly influence gut microbiome composition by decreasing anti-inflammatory autochthonous bacteria and increasing proinflammatory pathological ones. This affects intestinal permeability ("leaky gut") and leads to an increase of LPS/endotoxin entry into portal and systemic circulation [38]. This process could worsen liver steatosis and induce NASH progression by causing a widespread pro-inflammatory status. CNS function can also be impaired by these events through the gut–brain axis [51–53]. These studies further suggest the key role of the consumption of unbalanced diets and gut dysbiosis in the development of NAFLD/NASH, cognitive impairment, and AD.

An interesting review on the influence of liver dysfunction on AD progression suggested that chronic liver diseases may worsen amyloid burden due to an imbalance in peripheral amyloid-β (Aβ) clearance, leading to higher Aβ circulating levels. This can be due to a low hepatic expression of low-density lipoprotein receptor-related protein 1 (LRP-1), necessary for Aβ clearance, consequent to liver dysfunction and chronic inflammation. Furthermore, these features were proposed to negatively affect blood–brain barrier (BBB) integrity, thus contributing to a vicious cycle in Aβ clearance [7].

An impaired Wnt/β-catenin signaling pathway was reported to be involved in the pathogenesis of depression and AD [54,55]; thus, the dysregulated expression of proteins of this pathway observed in NAFLD rats could also be responsible for related cognitive impairment [56].

Another study demonstrated that the behavioral and cognitive impairments observed in rats with NAFLD could be linked to an imbalance of nesfatin-1 and copine 6 in the hippocampus and PFC [56]. Nesfatin-1 is able to regulate appetite, glucose, and energy metabolism, but also plays a role in mood and cognitive function [57,58]; thus, its increased plasma levels in NAFLD could be responsible for the observed cognitive dysfunction. Copine 6, a calcium sensor, plays an important role in brain-derived neurotrophic factor (BDNF)-dependent changes in dendritic spines, regulating neurotransmission, and promoting synaptic plasticity, learning and memory [59,60]. A decrease of copine 6 expression was related to depression-like behavior and immune activation and was also observed in NAFLD rats [56,61]. Another hypothesized mechanism leading to an increased risk of dementia and cognitive dysfunction in NAFLD/NASH subjects is related to chronic hyperglycemia and brain insulin resistance. It has been proposed that peripheral insulin resistance could trigger cognitive function through a liver–brain axis of neurodegeneration due to an excessive peripheral production of neurotoxic lipids, e.g., ceramides and nitrosamines, that pass across the blood–brain barrier (BBB) and affect neuronal activity, particularly in the hippocampus and PFC [3]. In the CNS, insulin orchestrates a network of pro-growth and pro-survival signals by activating intracellular pathways, e.g., insulin and insulin-like growth factor type 1 (IGF-1) signaling, thus promoting mitogenesis, cell survival, energy metabolism, and motility. Studies using different experimental models have demonstrated that NASH could increase the hepatic production of ceramides, nitrosamines, and related molecules, causing insulin resistance, oxidative stress, and brain injury. Liver-derived cytotoxic lipids enter the circulation, activate proinflammatory cytokine-mediated injury, and disrupt endothelial cell-to-cell junctions, thus increasing BBB permeability and penetrating in the CNS. Moreover, myelin degradation further increases endogenous ceramide production, exacerbating brain insulin resistance, neuroinflammation, oxidative stress, and neurotransmitter paucity, thus leading to neurocognitive deficits [3,31,62].

Recent evidences have demonstrated a close correlation between the alteration of gut microbiota (dysbiosis) and NASH development due to the increased intestinal permeability to lipopolysaccharide (LPS) that activates Toll-like receptor 4 (TLR4) of hepatic Kupffer cells (KCs) and hepatic stellate cells (HSCs), triggering the pro-inflammatory cytokine cascade that induces and maintains NASH. In the brain, the LPS-activated inflammatory cascade induces a decrease in BDNF expression, reduces the number of viable cells in the pyramidal layer, and promotes neurodegeneration and atrophy of hippocampal neurons, thus affecting CNS function and causing degenerative dementia and cognitive impairment [63].

A recent study of Higarza and collaborators demonstrated that a high-fat, high-cholesterol diet induces not only NASH but also dysbiosis, decreasing microbial short chain fatty acid (SCFA) production and increasing ammonia. Since hyperammonemia has been correlated to neuroinflammation and cognitive impairment, these authors suggested that diet-induced dysbiosis disrupts brain metabolism and function, factors contributing to the behavioral deficits observed in NASH. Additionally, they observed an increased DA catabolism in this NASH model, causing a drop of DA levels in the PFC and an increase of DOPA/DA ratio in the cerebellum. This suggests that insulin resistance could lead to dopaminergic dysfunction and a reduction of mitochondrial oxidative activity [14].

4. Pharmacological Strategies to Improve NAFLD/NASH-Related Cognitive Impairment

Although the increasing prevalence of NAFLD/NASH has made the need of effective treating options a priority, no therapy for NAFLD patients has been yet approved, and weight loss and increased physical activity remain the two gold standard interventions [64]. Several pharmacological agents have been studied and/or are in the pipeline for their effect on metabolic targets, the anti-inflammatory pathway, or fibrogenesis. Four agents (a PPARα/δ agonist, a FXR agonist, a CCR2/CCR5 antagonist, and an ASK1 inhibitor) are undergoing phase III clinical trials to be evaluated for their ability to reduce insulin resistance and the proinflammatory cascades responsible for NASH progression [65]. In this context, the development of a pharmacological option active also on the brain manifestations of NAFLD/NASH is a great challenge for scientists. Some interventions have been proposed in the last few years; nevertheless, their real usefulness as clinical pharmacological treatments needs to be further demonstrated.

Since insulin resistance is a distinctive feature of both steatohepatitis and AD, some studies have proposed the use of insulin-sensitizing agents, such as PPAR agonists, that are able to activate insulin-responsive genes and their signaling pathways to treat liver and brain insulin resistance-mediated diseases [66]. Early treatment with PPAR agonists has shown to effectively prevent brain atrophy, neurodegeneration, and its associated learning and memory impairment, preserving neurons expressing the insulin receptor and IGF receptor and maintaining cholinergic homeostasis and myelin expression [67,68]. Their antioxidant activity in the CNS was also reported to further sustain their therapeutic use in the content of oxidative stress-related diseases such as NAFLD, NASH, and AD.

Other studies demonstrated that in early stage AD patients, an improvement or stabilization of their cognitive impairment was obtained with intranasal insulin administration, leading to increased brain insulin levels [69–72].

Some studies have reported that chromium picolinate is able to improve insulin sensitivity by reducing glucose and insulin levels in overweight or obese subjects, and to increase HDL cholesterol and decrease LDL levels, thus controlling metabolic syndrome risk factors [73,74]. Moreover, this agent could improve cognitive function in elderly people, reducing semantic interference on learning, recall, and memory [75,76]. These positive effects on the insulin signaling pathway, both at the systemic and central level, suggest the use of chromium picolinate as a dietary supplement in NAFLD-related cognitive impairment and AD, even though clinical studies need to be performed to support this hypothesis.

The use of dietary supplements is widely exploited to support the dietary interventions in patients with metabolic syndrome, obesity, and NAFLD. A recent study on resveratrol, a polyphenol naturally present in grapes, blueberries, raspberries, and mulberries, has reported the improvement of both liver metabolic dysfunction and behavioral and cognitive impairments in a rat model of NAFLD [77]. Resveratrol administration to NAFLD rats is able to ameliorate the imbalanced expression of copine 6, p-catenin, and p-GSK3β in the hippocampus and PFC, restoring normal protein levels and improving the altered Wnt/β-catenin signaling pathway. This study further supports previous evidences on the effect of resveratrol in reducing Aβ plaque formation associated with AD [78].

Another study investigating the effect of *Curcuma* derivatives demonstrated their ability in improving high-fat and high-sugar diet-induced obesity, oxidative stress, memory impairment, and neurodegeneration. These effects have been attributed to the antioxidant properties and anticholinesterase activity of curcuminoids and terpenoids present in the tested extract. Furthermore, they increased serotonin and dopamine levels, exerting neuroprotection of hippocampal neurons [79].

Since several pieces of evidence suggested that liver steatosis may negatively affect cognitive performance in AD subjects, n3-PUFA supplementation can be considered as an option to improve NAFLD-related brain dysfunction, since these fatty acids are able to improve liver n3/n6 PUFA imbalance and modulate many neuronal functions, protecting them from oxidative stress and inhibiting signaling pathways responsible for tau phosphorylation in AD and dementia patients [80].

As stated before, the gut–brain axis and dysbiosis could play a role in the cognitive impairment of NAFLD and NASH patients. Starting from the observation that probiotics have demonstrated to improve NASH by decreasing LPS-induced pro-inflammatory cytokines, such as IL6 and TNF-α [81], a study of Mohammed et al. investigated the effect of *Lactobacillus plantarum* (*LP EMCC-1039*) administration on cognitive performance and liver function in dysbiosis-induced NASH in rats. *LP EMCC-1039* supplementation was correlated to an improvement of cognitive function in these animals due to the modulation of TLR4/BDNF signaling pathway, and an increase of viable cells and of the thickness of the pyramidal layer was observed [63].

5. Conclusions

In conclusion, increasing evidences suggest that a correlation exists between NAFLD/NASH and CNS diseases or dysfunctions such as depression, MCI, AD, and dementia. Growing evidences point at cerebrovascular alteration, neuroinflammation, and brain insulin resistance as NAFLD/NASH-related CNS manifestations. Unfortunately, the pharmacological options available for the management of these conditions are still limited, both in number and in efficacy. Further experimental and clinical studies are needed to gain new insights about the mechanism(s) of NAFLD/NASH and their central manifestations and identify effective pharmacological targets, after the comprehension of the complex mechanisms involved in the NAFLD/NASH, including the regulation of the gut–brain axis by diet and microbiome composition.

Author Contributions: Writing—original draft preparation, M.C., D.G.; writing—review and editing, S.D.M. All authors have read and agreed to the published version of the manuscript.

References

1.   Engin, A. Non-Alcoholic Fatty Liver Disease. In *Obesity and Lipotoxicity*; Engin, A.B., Engin, A., Eds.; Advances in Experimental Medicine and Biology; Springer International Publishing: Cham, Switzerland, 2017; Volume 960, pp. 443–467, ISBN 978-3-319-48380-1.

2.   Ekstedt, M.; Nasr, P.; Kechagias, S. Natural History of NAFLD/NASH. *Curr. Hepatol. Rep.* **2017**, *16*, 391–397. [CrossRef] [PubMed]

3.   De la Monte, S.M.; Longato, L.; Tong, M.; Wands, J.R. Insulin resistance and neurodegeneration: Roles of obesity, type 2 diabetes mellitus and non-alcoholic steatohepatitis. *Curr. Opin. Investig. Drugs* **2009**, *10*, 1049–1060. [PubMed]

4.   Elshaghabee, F.M.F.; Rokana, N.; Panwar, H.; Heller, K.J.; Schrezenmeir, J. Probiotics for dietary management of non-alcoholic fatty liver disease. *Environ. Chem. Lett.* **2019**, *17*, 1553–1563. [CrossRef]

5.   Gabbia, D.; Roverso, M.; Guido, M.; Sacchi, D.; Scaffidi, M.; Carrara, M.; Orso, G.; Russo, F.P.; Floreani, A.; Bogialli, S.; et al. Western Diet-Induced Metabolic Alterations Affect Circulating Markers of Liver Function before the Development of Steatosis. *Nutrients* **2019**, *11*, 1602. [CrossRef]

6.   Gabbia, D.; Saponaro, M.; Sarcognato, S.; Guido, M.; Ferri, N.; Carrara, M.; De Martin, S. Fucus vesiculosus and Ascophyllum nodosum Ameliorate Liver Function by Reducing Diet-Induced Steatosis in Rats. *Mar. Drugs* **2020**, *18*, 62. [CrossRef]

7.   Estrada, L.D.; Ahumada, P.; Cabrera, D.; Arab, J.P. Liver Dysfunction as a Novel Player in Alzheimer's Progression: Looking Outside the Brain. *Front. Aging Neurosci.* **2019**, *11*, 174. [CrossRef]

8.   Kaltenboeck, A.; Harmer, C. The neuroscience of depressive disorders: A brief review of the past and some considerations about the future. *Brain Neurosci. Adv.* **2018**, *2*. [CrossRef]

9.   Gonda, X.; Pompili, M.; Serafini, G.; Carvalho, A.F.; Rihmer, Z.; Dome, P. The role of cognitive dysfunction in the symptoms and remission from depression. *Ann. Gen. Psychiatry* **2015**, *14*, 27. [CrossRef]

10. Lee, K.; Otgonsuren, M.; Younoszai, Z.; Mir, H.M.; Younossi, Z.M. Association of Chronic Liver Disease with Depression: A Population-Based Study. *Psychosomatics* **2013**, *54*, 52–59. [CrossRef]

11. Elwing, J.E.; Lustman, P.J.; Wang, H.L.; Clouse, R.E. Depression, Anxiety, and Nonalcoholic Steatohepatitis. *Psychosom. Med.* **2006**, *68*, 563–569. [CrossRef]

12. Tomeno, W.; Kawashima, K.; Yoneda, M.; Saito, S.; Ogawa, Y.; Honda, Y.; Kessoku, T.; Imajo, K.; Mawatari, H.; Fujita, K.; et al. Non-alcoholic fatty liver disease comorbid with major depressive disorder: The pathological features and poor therapeutic efficacy: Fatty liver comorbid with depression. *J. Gastroenterol. Hepatol.* **2015**, *30*, 1009–1014. [CrossRef]

13. Youssef, N.A.; Abdelmalek, M.F.; Binks, M.; Guy, C.D.; Omenetti, A.; Smith, A.D.; Diehl, A.M.E.; Suzuki, A. Associations of depression, anxiety and antidepressants with histological severity of nonalcoholic fatty liver disease. *Liver Int.* **2013**, *33*, 1062–1070. [CrossRef]

14. Higarza, S.G.; Arboleya, S.; Gueimonde, M.; Gómez-Lázaro, E.; Arias, J.L.; Arias, N. Neurobehavioral dysfunction in non-alcoholic steatohepatitis is associated with hyperammonemia, gut dysbiosis, and metabolic and functional brain regional deficits. *PLoS ONE* **2019**, *14*, e0223019. [CrossRef]

15. Filipović, B.; Marković, O.; Đurić, V.; Filipović, B. Cognitive Changes and Brain Volume Reduction in Patients with Nonalcoholic Fatty Liver Disease. *Can. J. Gastroenterol. Hepatol.* **2018**, *2018*, 9638797. [CrossRef] [PubMed]

16. Sanford, A.M. Mild Cognitive Impairment. *Clin. Geriatr. Med.* **2017**, *33*, 325–337. [CrossRef]

17. Celikbilek, A.; Celikbilek, M. Cognitive impairment in patients with nonalcoholic fatty liver disease with liver fibrosis. *Liver Int.* **2020**, *40*, 1239. [CrossRef] [PubMed]

18. Panza, F.; Frisardi, V.; Seripa, D.; P Imbimbo, B.; Sancarlo, D.; D'Onofrio, G.; Addante, F.; Paris, F.; Pilotto, A.; Solfrizzi, V. Metabolic Syndrome, Mild Cognitive Impairment and Dementia. *CAR* **2011**, *8*, 492–509. [CrossRef]

19. Levin, B.E.; Llabre, M.M.; Dong, C.; Elkind, M.S.V.; Stern, Y.; Rundek, T.; Sacco, R.L.; Wright, C.B. Modeling Metabolic Syndrome and Its Association with Cognition: The Northern Manhattan Study. *J. Int. Neuropsychol. Soc.* **2014**, *20*, 951–960. [CrossRef]

20. Elliott, C.; Frith, J.; Day, C.P.; Jones, D.E.J.; Newton, J.L. Functional Impairment in Alcoholic Liver Disease and Non-alcoholic Fatty Liver Disease Is Significant and Persists over 3 Years of Follow-Up. *Dig. Dis. Sci.* **2013**, *58*, 2383–2391. [CrossRef] [PubMed]

21. Seo, S.W.; Gottesman, R.F.; Clark, J.M.; Hernaez, R.; Chang, Y.; Kim, C.; Ha, K.H.; Guallar, E.; Lazo, M. Nonalcoholic fatty liver disease is associated with cognitive function in adults. *Neurology* **2016**, *86*, 1136–1142. [CrossRef]

22. Jongsiriyanyong, S.; Limpawattana, P. Mild Cognitive Impairment in Clinical Practice: A Review Article. *Am. J. Alzheimers Dis. Other Demen.* **2018** *33*, 500–507. [CrossRef] [PubMed]

23. Celikbilek, A.; Celikbilek, M.; Bozkurt, G. Cognitive assessment of patients with nonalcoholic fatty liver disease. *Eur. J. Gastroenterol. Hepatol.* **2018**, *30*, 944–950. [CrossRef] [PubMed]

24. An, K.; Starkweather, A.; Sturgill, J.; Salyer, J.; Sterling, R.K. Association of CTRP13 With Liver Enzymes and Cognitive Symptoms in Nonalcoholic Fatty Liver Disease. *Nurs. Res.* **2019**, *68*, 29–38. [CrossRef] [PubMed]

25. Weinstein, G.; Davis-Plourde, K.; Himali, J.J.; Zelber-Sagi, S.; Beiser, A.S.; Seshadri, S. Non-alcoholic fatty liver disease, liver fibrosis score and cognitive function in middle-aged adults: The Framingham Study. *Liver Int.* **2019**, *39*, 1713–1721. [CrossRef] [PubMed]

26. Vanek, J.; Prasko, J.; Genzor, S.; Ociskova, M.; Kantor, K.; Holubova, M.; Slepecky, M.; Nesnidal, V.; Kolek, A.; Sova, M. Obstructive sleep apnea, depression and cognitive impairment. *Sleep Med.* **2020**, *72*, 50–58. [CrossRef]

27. Parikh, M.P.; Gupta, N.M.; McCullough, A.J. Obstructive Sleep Apnea and the Liver. *Clin. Liver Dis.* **2019**, *23*, 363–382. [CrossRef]

28. De la Monte, S.M. Insulin Resistance and Neurodegeneration: Progress Towards the Development of New Therapeutics for Alzheimer's Disease. *Drugs* **2017**, *77*, 47–65. [CrossRef]

29. De la Monte, S.M.; Tong, M. Brain metabolic dysfunction at the core of Alzheimer's disease. *Biochem. Pharm.* **2014**, *88*, 548–559. [CrossRef]

30. Kim, D.-G.; Krenz, A.; Toussaint, L.E.; Maurer, K.J.; Robinson, S.-A.; Yan, A.; Torres, L.; Bynoe, M.S. Non-alcoholic fatty liver disease induces signs of Alzheimer's disease (AD) in wild-type mice and accelerates pathological signs of AD in an AD model. *J. Neuroinflamm.* **2016**, *13*, 1. [CrossRef]

31. Lyn-Cook, L.E.; Lawton, M.; Tong, M.; Silbermann, E.; Longato, L.; Jiao, P.; Mark, P.; Wands, J.R.; Xu, H.; de la Monte, S.M. Hepatic ceramide may mediate brain insulin resistance and neurodegeneration in type 2 diabetes and non-alcoholic steatohepatitis. *J. Alzheimers Dis.* **2009**, *16*, 715–729. [CrossRef]

32. Pinçon, A.; De Montgolfier, O.; Akkoyunlu, N.; Daneault, C.; Pouliot, P.; Villeneuve, L.; Lesage, F.; Levy, B.I.; Thorin-Trescases, N.; Thorin, É.; et al. Non-Alcoholic Fatty Liver Disease, and the Underlying Altered Fatty Acid Metabolism, Reveals Brain Hypoperfusion and Contributes to the Cognitive Decline in APP/PS1 Mice. *Metabolites* **2019**, *9*, 104. [CrossRef] [PubMed]

33. Beilharz, J.E.; Maniam, J.; Morris, M.J. Diet-Induced Cognitive Deficits: The Role of Fat and Sugar, Potential Mechanisms and Nutritional Interventions. *Nutrients* **2015**, *7*, 6719–6738. [CrossRef]

34. Guimarães, C.A.; Biella, M.S.; Lopes, A.; Deroza, P.F.; Oliveira, M.B.; Macan, T.P.; Streck, E.L.; Ferreira, G.C.; Zugno, A.I.; Schuck, P.F. In vivo and in vitro effects of fructose on rat brain acetylcholinesterase activity: An ontogenetic study. *Acad. Bras. Cienc.* **2014**, *86*, 1919–1926. [CrossRef]

35. Nho, K.; Kueider-Paisley, A.; Ahmad, S.; MahmoudianDehkordi, S.; Arnold, M.; Risacher, S.L.; Louie, G.; Blach, C.; Baillie, R.; Han, X.; et al. Association of Altered Liver Enzymes With Alzheimer Disease Diagnosis, Cognition, Neuroimaging Measures, and Cerebrospinal Fluid Biomarkers. *JAMA Netw. Open* **2019**, *2*, e197978. [CrossRef]

36. Karbalaei, R.; Allahyari, M.; Rezaei-Tavirani, M.; Asadzadeh-Aghdaei, H.; Zali, M.R. Protein-protein interaction analysis of Alzheimer's disease and NAFLD based on systems biology methods unhide common ancestor pathways. *Gastroenterol. Hepatol. Bed. Bench.* **2018**, *11*, 27–33. [PubMed]

37. Hu, X.; Wang, T.; Jin, F. Alzheimer's disease and gut microbiota. *Sci. China Life Sci.* **2016**, *59*, 1006–1023. [CrossRef] [PubMed]

38. Fukui, H. Role of Gut Dysbiosis in Liver Diseases: What Have We Learned So Far? *Diseases* **2019**, *7*, 58. [CrossRef]

39. Lombardi, R.; Fargion, S.; Fracanzani, A.L. Brain involvement in non-alcoholic fatty liver disease (NAFLD): A systematic review. *Dig. Liver Dis.* **2019**, *51*, 1214–1222. [CrossRef]

40. Felipo, V.; Ordoño, J.F.; Urios, A.; El Mlili, N.; Giménez-Garzó, C.; Aguado, C.; González-Lopez, O.; Giner-Duran, R.; Serra, M.A.; Wassel, A.; et al. Patients with minimal hepatic encephalopathy show impaired mismatch negativity correlating with reduced performance in attention tests. *Hepatology* **2012**, *55*, 530–539. [CrossRef]

41. Felipo, V.; Urios, A.; Giménez-Garzó, C.; Cauli, O.; Andrés-Costa, M.-J.; González, O.; Serra, M.A.; Sánchez-González, J.; Aliaga, R.; Giner-Durán, R.; et al. Non invasive blood flow measurement in cerebellum detects minimal hepatic encephalopathy earlier than psychometric tests. *World J. Gastroenterol.* **2014**, *20*, 11815–11825. [CrossRef]

42. Butz, M.; Timmermann, L.; Braun, M.; Groiss, S.J.; Wojtecki, L.; Ostrowski, S.; Krause, H.; Pollok, B.; Gross, J.; Südmeyer, M.; et al. Motor impairment in liver cirrhosis without and with minimal hepatic encephalopathy. *Acta Neurol. Scand.* **2010**, *122*, 27–35. [CrossRef] [PubMed]

43. Giménez-Garzó, C.; Garcés, J.J.; Urios, A.; Mangas-Losada, A.; García-García, R.; González-López, O.; Giner-Durán, R.; Escudero-García, D.; Serra, M.A.; Soria, E.; et al. The PHES battery does not detect all cirrhotic patients with early neurological deficits, which are different in different patients. *PLoS ONE* **2017**, *12*, e0171211. [CrossRef] [PubMed]

44. Balzano, T.; Forteza, J.; Borreda, I.; Molina, P.; Giner, J.; Leone, P.; Urios, A.; Montoliu, C.; Felipo, V. Histological Features of Cerebellar Neuropathology in Patients With Alcoholic and Nonalcoholic Steatohepatitis. *J. Neuropathol. Exp. Neurol.* **2018**, *77*, 837–845. [CrossRef] [PubMed]

45. Petta, S.; Tuttolomondo, A.; Gagliardo, C.; Zafonte, R.; Brancatelli, G.; Cabibi, D.; Cammà, C.; Di Marco, V.; Galvano, L.; La Tona, G.; et al. The Presence of White Matter Lesions Is Associated With the Fibrosis Severity of Nonalcoholic Fatty Liver Disease. *Medicine (Baltimore)* **2016**, *95*, e3446. [CrossRef]

46. Ghareeb, D.A.; Hafez, H.S.; Hussien, H.M.; Kabapy, N.F. Non-alcoholic fatty liver induces insulin resistance and metabolic disorders with development of brain damage and dysfunction. *Metab. Brain Dis.* **2011**, *26*, 253. [CrossRef]

47. Dagnino-Subiabre, A. Stress and Western diets increase vulnerability to neuropsychiatric disorders: A common mechanism. *Nutr. Neurosci.* **2019**, 1–11. [CrossRef]

48. Rivera, D.S.; Lindsay, C.B.; Codocedo, J.F.; Carreño, L.E.; Cabrera, D.; Arrese, M.A.; Vio, C.P.; Bozinovic, F.; Inestrosa, N.C. Long-Term, Fructose-Induced Metabolic Syndrome-Like Condition Is Associated with Higher Metabolism, Reduced Synaptic Plasticity and Cognitive Impairment in Octodon degus. *Mol. Neurobiol.* **2018**, *55*, 9169–9187. [CrossRef]

49. Singh, D.P.; Kondepudi, K.K.; Bishnoi, M.; Chopra, K. Altered Monoamine Metabolism in High Fat Diet Induced Neuropsychiatric Changes in Rats. *J. Obes. Weight Loss Ther.* **2014**, *4*, 1–5. [CrossRef]

50. Castellani, G.; Contarini, G.; Mereu, M.; Albanesi, E.; Devroye, C.; D'Amore, C.; Ferretti, V.; De Martin, S.; Papaleo, F. Dopamine-mediated immunomodulation affects choroid plexus function. *Brain Behav. Immun.* **2019**, *81*, 138–150. [CrossRef]

51. Paik, Y.-H.; Schwabe, R.F.; Bataller, R.; Russo, M.P.; Jobin, C.; Brenner, D.A. Toll-Like receptor 4 mediates inflammatory signaling by bacterial lipopolysaccharide in human hepatic stellate cells. *Hepatology* **2003**, *37*, 1043–1055. [CrossRef]

52. Baothman, O.A.; Zamzami, M.A.; Taher, I.; Abubaker, J.; Abu-Farha, M. The role of Gut Microbiota in the development of obesity and Diabetes. *Lipids Health Dis.* **2016**, *15*, 108. [CrossRef] [PubMed]

53. Takeda, S.; Sato, N.; Morishita, R. Systemic inflammation, blood-brain barrier vulnerability and cognitive/non-cognitive symptoms in Alzheimer disease: Relevance to pathogenesis and therapy. *Front. Aging Neurosci.* **2014**, *6*, 171. [CrossRef] [PubMed]

54. Folke, J.; Pakkenberg, B.; Brudek, T. Impaired Wnt Signaling in the Prefrontal Cortex of Alzheimer's Disease. *Mol. Neurobiol.* **2019**, *56*, 873–891. [CrossRef] [PubMed]

55. Xu, L.-Z.; Xu, D.-F.; Han, Y.; Liu, L.-J.; Sun, C.-Y.; Deng, J.-H.; Zhang, R.-X.; Yuan, M.; Zhang, S.-Z.; Li, Z.-M.; et al. BDNF-GSK-3β-β-Catenin Pathway in the mPFC Is Involved in Antidepressant-Like Effects of Morinda officinalis Oligosaccharides in Rats. *Int. J. Neuropsychopharmacol.* **2017**, *20*, 83–93. [CrossRef]

56. Chen, Z.; Xu, Y.-Y.; Wu, R.; Han, Y.-X.; Yu, Y.; Ge, J.-F.; Chen, F.-H. Impaired learning and memory in rats induced by a high-fat diet: Involvement with the imbalance of nesfatin-1 abundance and copine 6 expression. *J. Neuroendocr.* **2017**, *29*. [CrossRef] [PubMed]

57. Ge, J.-F.; Xu, Y.-Y.; Qin, G.; Peng, Y.-N.; Zhang, C.-F.; Liu, X.-R.; Liang, L.-C.; Wang, Z.-Z.; Chen, F.-H. Depression-like Behavior Induced by Nesfatin-1 in Rats: Involvement of Increased Immune Activation and Imbalance of Synaptic Vesicle Proteins. *Front. Neurosci.* **2015**, *9*, 429. [CrossRef] [PubMed]

58. Ge, J.-F.; Xu, Y.-Y.; Qin, G.; Pan, X.-Y.; Cheng, J.-Q.; Chen, F.-H. Nesfatin-1, a potent anorexic agent, decreases exploration and induces anxiety-like behavior in rats without altering learning or memory. *Brain Res.* **2015**, *1629*, 171–181. [CrossRef]

59. Reinhard, J.R.; Kriz, A.; Galic, M.; Angliker, N.; Rajalu, M.; Vogt, K.E.; Ruegg, M.A. The calcium sensor Copine-6 regulates spine structural plasticity and learning and memory. *Nat. Commun.* **2016**, *7*, 11613. [CrossRef]

60. Burk, K.; Ramachandran, B.; Ahmed, S.; Hurtado-Zavala, J.I.; Awasthi, A.; Benito, E.; Faram, R.; Ahmad, H.; Swaminathan, A.; McIlhinney, J.; et al. Regulation of Dendritic Spine Morphology in Hippocampal Neurons by Copine-6. *Cereb. Cortex.* **2018**, *28*, 1087–1104. [CrossRef]

61. Han, Y.-X.; Tao, C.; Gao, X.-R.; Wang, L.; Jiang, F.-H.; Wang, C.; Fang, K.; Chen, X.-X.; Chen, Z.; Ge, J.-F. BDNF-Related Imbalance of Copine 6 and Synaptic Plasticity Markers Couples With Depression-Like Behavior and Immune Activation in CUMS Rats. *Front. Neurosci.* **2018**, *12*, 731. [CrossRef]

62. Tong, M.; Neusner, A.; Longato, L.; Lawton, M.; Wands, J.R. Nitrosamine Exposure Causes Insulin Resistance Diseases: Relevance to Type 2 Diabetes Mellitus, Non-Alcoholic Steatohepatitis, and Alzheimer's Disease. *J. Alzheimer's Dis.* **2010**, *37*, 827–844.

63. Mohammed, S.K.; Magdy, Y.M.; El-Waseef, D.A.; Nabih, E.S.; Hamouda, M.A.; El-Kharashi, O.A. Modulation of hippocampal TLR4/BDNF signal pathway using probiotics is a step closer towards treating cognitive impairment in NASH model. *Physiol. Behav.* **2020**, *214*, 112762. [CrossRef] [PubMed]

64. Younossi, Z.M. Non-alcoholic fatty liver disease—A global public health perspective. *J. Hepatol.* **2019**, *70*, 531–544. [CrossRef] [PubMed]

65. Alkhouri, N.; Scott, A. An update on the pharmacological treatment of nonalcoholic fatty liver disease: Beyond lifestyle modifications. *Clin. Liver Dis.* **2018**, *11*, 82–86. [CrossRef]

66. De la Monte, S.M. Brain Insulin Resistance and Deficiency as Therapeutic Targets in Alzheimer's Disease. *Curr. Alzheimer Res.* **2012**, *9*, 35–66. [CrossRef]

67. De la Monte, S.M.; Tong, M.; Lester-Coll, N.; Plater, J.; Wands, J.R. Therapeutic rescue of neurodegeneration in experimental type 3 diabetes: Relevance to Alzheimer's disease. *J. Alzheimer's Dis.* **2006**, *10*, 89–109. [CrossRef]

68. Landreth, G. Therapeutic use of agonists of the nuclear receptor PPARgamma in Alzheimer's disease. *Curr. Alzheimer Res.* **2007**, *4*, 159–164. [CrossRef]

69. Reger, M.A.; Watson, G.S.; Frey, W.H.; Baker, L.D.; Cholerton, B.; Keeling, M.L.; Belongia, D.A.; Fishel, M.A.; Plymate, S.R.; Schellenberg, G.D.; et al. Effects of intranasal insulin on cognition in memory-impaired older adults: Modulation by APOE genotype. *Neurobiol. Aging* **2006**, *27*, 451–458. [CrossRef]

70. Benedict, C.; Hallschmid, M.; Hatke, A.; Schultes, B.; Fehm, H.L.; Born, J.; Kern, W. Intranasal insulin improves memory in humans. *Psychoneuroendocrinology* **2004**, *29*, 1326–1334. [CrossRef]

71. Benedict, C.; Hallschmid, M.; Schmitz, K.; Schultes, B.; Ratter, F.; Fehm, H.L.; Born, J.; Kern, W. Intranasal insulin improves memory in humans: Superiority of insulin aspart. *Neuropsychopharmacology* **2007**, *32*, 239–243. [CrossRef]

72. Watson, G.S.; Cholerton, B.A.; Reger, M.A.; Baker, L.D.; Plymate, S.R.; Asthana, S.; Fishel, M.A.; Kulstad, J.J.; Green, P.S.; Cook, D.G.; et al. Preserved cognition in patients with early Alzheimer disease and amnestic mild cognitive impairment during treatment with rosiglitazone: A preliminary study. *Am. J. Geriatr. Psychiatry* **2005**, *13*, 950–958. [CrossRef] [PubMed]

73. De Martin, S.; Gabbia, D.; Carrara, M.; Ferri, N. The Brown Algae Fucus vesiculosus and Ascophyllum nodosum Reduce Metabolic Syndrome Risk Factors: A Clinical Study. *Nat. Prod. Commun.* **2018**, *13*, 1691–1694. [CrossRef]

74. Havel, P.J. A scientific review: The role of chromium in insulin resistance. *Diabetes Educ.* **2004**, *30* (Suppl. S3), 2–14.

75. Krikorian, R.; Eliassen, J.C.; Boespflug, E.L.; Nash, T.A.; Shidler, M.D. Improved cognitive-cerebral function in older adults with chromium supplementation. *Nutr. Neurosci.* **2010**, *13*, 116–122. [CrossRef]

76. Smorgon, C.; Mari, E.; Atti, A.R.; Dalla Nora, E.; Zamboni, P.F.; Calzoni, F.; Passaro, A.; Fellin, R. Trace elements and cognitive impairment: An elderly cohort study. *Arch. Gerontol. Geriatr.* **2004**, *38*, 393–402. [CrossRef]

77. Chen, X.-X.; Xu, Y.-Y.; Wu, R.; Chen, Z.; Fang, K.; Han, Y.-X.; Yu, Y.; Huang, L.-L.; Peng, L.; Ge, J.-F. Resveratrol Reduces Glucolipid Metabolic Dysfunction and Learning and Memory Impairment in a NAFLD Rat Model: Involvement in Regulating the Imbalance of Nesfatin-1 Abundance and Copine 6 Expression. *Front. Endocrinol.* **2019**, *10*, 434. [CrossRef]

78. Karuppagounder, S.S.; Pinto, J.T.; Xu, H.; Chen, H.-L.; Beal, M.F.; Gibson, G.E. Dietary supplementation with resveratrol reduces plaque pathology in a transgenic model of Alzheimer's disease. *Neurochem. Int.* **2009**, *54*, 111–118. [CrossRef]

79.   Rao, L.S.N.; Kilari, E.K.; Kola, P.K. Protective effect of Curcuma amada acetone extract against high-fat and high-sugar diet-induced obesity and memory impairment. *Nutr. Neurosci.* **2019**, 1–14. [CrossRef]
80.   Cole, G.M.; Ma, Q.-L.; Frautschy, S.A. Omega-3 fatty acids and dementia. *Prostaglandins Leukot. Essent. Fat. Acids* **2009**, *81*, 213–221. [CrossRef]
81.   Medina, J.; Fernández-Salazar, L.I.; García-Buey, L.; Moreno-Otero, R. Approach to the pathogenesis and treatment of nonalcoholic steatohepatitis. *Diabetes Care* **2004**, *27*, 2057–2066. [CrossRef]

4

Role of Serum Uric Acid and Ferritin in the Development and Progression of NAFLD

Rosa Lombardi, Giuseppina Pisano and Silvia Fargion *

Department of Pathophysiology and Transplantation, IRCCS "Ca' Granda" IRCCS Foundation, Poiliclinico Hospital, University of Milan, Centro delle Malattie Metaboliche del Fegato, Milan 20122, Italy; rosalombardi@hotmail.it (R.L.); pinaz81@hotmail.com (G.P.)
* Correspondence: silvia.fargion@unimi.it

Academic Editors: Amedeo Lonardo and Giovanni Targher

Abstract: Nonalcoholic fatty liver disease (NAFLD), tightly linked to the metabolic syndrome (MS), has emerged as a leading cause of chronic liver disease worldwide. Since it is potentially progressive towards non-alcoholic steatohepatitis (NASH) and hepatic fibrosis, up to cirrhosis and its associated complications, the need for predictive factors of NAFLD and of its advanced forms is mandatory. Despite the current "gold standard" for the assessment of liver damage in NAFLD being liver biopsy, in recent years, several non-invasive tools have been designed as alternatives to histology, of which fibroscan seems the most promising. Among the different serum markers considered, serum uric acid (SUA) and ferritin have emerged as possible predictors of severity of liver damage in NAFLD. In fact, as widely described in this review, they share common pathogenetic pathways and are both associated with hepatic steatosis and MS, thus suggesting a likely synergistic action. Nevertheless, the power of these serum markers seems to be too low if considered alone, suggesting that they should be included in a wider perspective together with other metabolic and biochemical parameters in order to predict liver damage.

Keywords: SUA; liver damage; fibrosis; NASH; serum markers; oxidative stress; insulin resistance; metabolic syndrome

1. Introduction

Nonalcoholic fatty liver disease (NAFLD), tightly linked to metabolic syndrome (MS), has emerged as a leading cause of chronic liver disease worldwide with a rapidly growing prevalence in the general population, ranging between 20% and 30%, and paralleling the epidemics of obesity and type 2 diabetes mellitus (T2DM) all over the world [1,2]. NAFLD encompasses a clinical-pathologic spectrum of liver diseases ranging from simple steatosis to nonalcoholic steatohepatitis (NASH), the more aggressive form of NAFLD, which can progress to cirrhosis and its associated complications [3,4].

Unfortunately, the only validated method to diagnose NASH, the potentially evolving form of NAFLD, is liver biopsy. Nonetheless, this procedure is limited by intra and inter-observer variability, sampling errors and invasiveness, thus letting impossible its feasibility in such a large number of patients with NAFLD. Several scores have been designed in the attempt to diagnose NASH and fibrosis stage without histological data, but the debate on their real utility is still ongoing [5]. Fibroscan is emerging as a reliable tool to identify fibrosis in a non-invasive way, but still the large "grey area" of its results does not allow one to discriminate the entity of fibrosis in a large portion of patients with NAFLD [6].

During the last few years, among the several parameters evaluated as possible predictors of NAFLD, serum uric acid (SUA) and ferritin have emerged. In fact, increasing evidence has shown that SUA levels as well as high ferritin are associated with the metabolic insulin resistance syndrome, higher body fat content and more severe liver damage.

2. Uric Acid

Serum uric acid (SUA) is a product of purine metabolism in humans and originates from hypoxanthine after a double enzyme catalysis by xanthine oxidase (XO) in the liver. Its production is regulated by the endogenous (nucleoproteins originating from cellular metabolism) and exogenous (dietary) precursor proteins delivered to the liver, whereas its excretion is controlled by the kidneys through renal plasma flow, glomerular filtration and proximal tubular exchange. Therefore, an impairment in this balance, caused by either an over generation of uric acid, like in MS and diets rich in fructose and purines or by a reduction in its excretion, as in acute renal failure or consequent to some drugs (ciclosporin, ethambutol, pyrazinamide, and cytotoxic chemotherapy), can lead to high SUA levels [7,8].

3. Serum Uric Acid and Metabolic Syndrome Clinical Manifestations

SUA is the most common and well-studied risk factor for developing gout. In addition, beyond contributing to the pathogenesis of gout, arthritis, and chronic nephropathy, hyperuricemia is associated with the so-called "cardio-metabolic diseases" including cardiovascular disease and all the metabolic diseases associated with MS [9]. Several studies reported a significantly higher prevalence of MS (up to 60%) and its components such as hypertension, hyperinsulinemia, hypertriglyceridemia and diabetes in the hyperuricemic population, suggesting that hyperuricemia might be an indicator for early diagnosis of MS and of its different clinical manifestations [10–12]. Moreover, a meta-analysis of prospective cohort studies provided strong evidence that a high level of SUA is a risk factor for developing T2DM in middle-aged and older people, independently of other established metabolic risk features [13].

4. Serum Uric Acid and Nonalcoholic Fatty Liver Disease (NAFLD)

Lonardo *et al.* [14] firstly described an association between NAFLD and serum uric acid levels in a small case-control study of Italian patients with ultrasound-diagnosed NAFLD.

The relationship between SUA and NAFLD was then confirmed in cross-sectional and prospective studies in which SUA resulted to be an independent risk factor for NAFLD [15,16]. More recently in two different meta-analyses of prospective studies including very large numbers of participants, it was shown a significant higher risk of NAFLD in subjects with higher SUA compared to those with lower levels. A linear dose-response effect between SUA and NAFLD was reported with each 1 mg increase of SUA leading to 21% rise in NAFLD risk [17,18]. Moreover, in patients with established coronary artery disease, hyperuricemia was reported to be a potent predictor of mortality in overweight or obese patients in whom liver steatosis was highly prevalent [19].

The mutual relationship between NAFLD and SUA was shown in another study aimed at exploring the causal relationship and underlying mechanisms linking NAFLD and hyperuricemia. By analyzing prospectively a cohort of 5541 patients, NAFLD resulted strongly associated with the risk of developing hyperuricemia over a period of seven years. In a second part of the same study, xantine oxidase was demonstrated to be the mediator of this relationship through the activation of the ucleotide-binding oligomerization domain-like (NOD-like) receptor family pyrin domain containing 3 (NLRP3) inflammasome [20] in both in HepG2 cells and mice, as explained in the next pharagraph. However, a major limitation of these study designs is their inability to show the biological mechanisms underpinning the association between SUA and NAFLD. Furthermore, experimental animal models supporting this association do not always mirror human biology.

Interestingly, Sirota *et al.* [21] examined the association between SUA levels and NAFLD in a large population-based study from the United States including 10,732 non-diabetic adults who participated in the National Health and Nutrition Examination Survey 1988–1994. The Authors found that the odds ratio for NAFLD was significantly higher in patients with the highest SUA values (3rd and 4th quartiles) compared to subjects in the lowest quartiles. In addition, after adjusting for the known risk factors, uric acid (4th quartile) remained significantly associated with NAFLD. Thus, they concluded that elevated SUA level is independently associated with ultrasound-diagnosed NAFLD and with increasing severity of NAFLD as evaluated by ultrasonography. These data were in line with previous results by Petta *et al.* [22] obtained in a group of patients with histologically proven NAFLD. They had demonstrated that hyperuricemia was associated with histological features of liver disease, representing an independent risk factor for higher grade of steatosis, lobular inflammation and higher NAFLD Activity Score (NAS), the histological score routinely used for the diagnosis and grading of NASH. Thus, these data confirm and extend the results obtained in Asiatic subjects also to Caucasian patients, consolidating the relationship between NAFLD and SUA.

Finally, Afzali *et al.* [23], on the basis of the observation that elevated SUA levels strongly reflect and may even cause oxidative stress, insulin resistance (IR), and MS, and that experimental, and in *in vitro* models indicate that uric acid is able to induce inflammatory responses, all known risk factors involved in the pathogenesis and in the progression of liver disease of different etiology, addressed the question whether the baseline SUA level was associated with the incidence of hospitalization or death due to cirrhosis. These authors analyzed 5518 participants from the first National Health and Nutrition Examination Survey during a mean follow-up of 12.9 years (range 5.4–21 years) and demonstrated that subjects with the higher uric acid values had a higher risk of cirrhosis related hospitalization or death even after adjustment for important causes and risk factors of chronic liver disease. In addition, patients with higher SUA levels had a greater probability of elevated serum ALT and GGT. They suggested that the negative effect of SUA was mediated by the induction by uric acid of endothelial dysfunction, IR, oxidative stress and systemic inflammation, which are known risk factors for the development and progression of liver disease of different etiology. However, despite this fascinating hypothesis, a major limitation of these results obtained in clinical studies is that the direct demonstration in patients with NAFLD of the mechanisms underpinning the negative effect of SUA is still missing.

5. Relationship between Uric Acid and NAFLD/Metabolic Syndrome: Possible Mechanisms

Accumulating clinical evidence suggests that hyperuricemia is strongly associated with MS/NAFLD, and abnormal glucose metabolism and IR, as well as oxidative stress and NLRP3 inflammasome involvement, have been pointed out as possible linking conditions [11,24]. The possible interactions of the different mechanisms involved are schematically depicted in Figure 1.

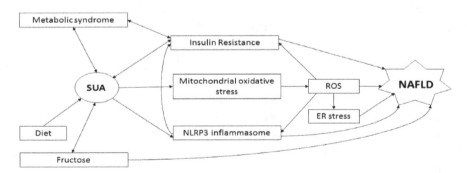

Figure 1. Pathogenetic pathways of the association between serum uric acid and NAFLD. Abbreviations: SUA, serum uric acid; ROS, reactive oxygen species; ER, endoplasmic reticulum; NAFLD, non-alcoholic fatty liver disease.

Furthermore, a very recent study by a Chinese group, has focused on the progression of NAFLD in hyperuricemic subjects, showing a key role of perturbations of phospholipases, purine nucleotide degradation and Liver X receptor/retinoid X receptor. In particular, they demonstrated an increase in oxidative stress and IR driven by an upregulation of phospatidic acid and cholesterol ester metabolism and a downregulation of the acid uric precursor, namely inosin [25].

5.1. Interaction between Uric Acid and Insulin

Insulin acts on the proximal renal tubule fostering acid uric reabsorption and increasing renal cellular metabolism, thus leading to hyperuricemia. Indeed, elevated SUA levels may prompt the development of IR by reducing endothelial nitric oxide (NO) bioavailability and supply to cells [26].

In addition, in an experimental model, mice fed with hyperuricemia-inducing diet (HUA) presented significantly lower insulin sensitivity and impaired glucose metabolism compared to those with a standard diet, as well as higher levels of both serum and intrahepatic triglycerides. In particular, hyperuricemia inhibited a protein kinase B (AKT) response to insulin by decreasing its phosphorylation and conversely increasing the phosphorylation of the insulin receptor substrate-1 (IRS1) in liver, muscle and fat tissue, thus fostering the onset of IR. This effect seems to be secondary to uric acid induced radical oxygen species (ROS) and activation of the NLRP3 inflammasome [27,28]. These data were confirmed also in HepG2 cell cultures exposed to different concentrations of uric acid. Not surprisingly, administration of probenecid, a uric acid transport inhibitor into cells, or the antioxidant *N*-acetylcisteine, diminished intracellular triglycerides accumulation and improved insulin-signaling.

5.2. Uric Acid and Lipid Metabolism

Beyond hyperinsulinemia, uric acid is responsible of mitochondrial oxidative stress [29], sterol regulatory element-binding protein 1 (SREBP-1) activation induced by endoplasmic reticulum (ER) stress [30] and NLRP3 inflammasome involvement [31], all causative factors of lipid metabolism impairment.

Moreover, evidence suggests that uric acid could originate from fructose metabolism, which is well known for inducing hepatic steatosis being directly metabolized to triglycerides in the liver [32], and be responsible for mitochondrial oxidative stress. In turn, SUA amplifies the lipogenic effect of fructose by upregulating its metabolic enzymatic reactions [33]. In cultured HepG2 cellular lines exposed to fructose, increased intracellular levels of uric acid and triglycerides were registered. Interestingly, allopurinol effectively prevented the formation of uric acid after exposure to fructose [29].

5.3. Mitochondrial and Endoplasmic Reticulum (ER) Oxidative Stress

Oxidative stress plays a key-role in steatosis induced by uric acid. In the study by Lanaspa *et al.* [29], cellular exposure to high SUA levels determined mitochondrial oxidative stress with generation of ROS by nicotinamide adenine dinucleotide phosphate (NADPH) oxidase. As a result, the activity of aconitase, an enzyme involved in the acid citric circle, was markedly reduced leading to accumulation of citrate, a substrate for hepatic *de novo* lipogenesis and subsequent intracellular fat generation.

Furthermore, ROS production promotes ER stress, which is determinant of fat accumulation in steatosis. In fact, alterations in its homeostasis have been demonstrated in human HepG2 cells and mice models of fatty liver [34,35]. ER is a site of protein folding and production of lipids and sterols. If a perturbation in this compartment occurs, misfolded and unfolded proteins accumulate and activate the unfolded protein response (UPR) signaling pathways, which regulate hepatic lipid metabolism and promote fat accumulation in the liver because of the expression of genes encoding for lipogenic enzymes driven by the transcriptional factor SREBP-1c. Uric acid has been shown to induce the expression of unfolded response protein (URP)-inducible and to increase the cleavage of SREBP-1c into the mature form and its nuclear translocation, thus enhancing the *de novo* lipogenesis. This data has been shown in both HepG2 cells and primary mice hepatocytes [30].

Despite these data, acute elevations seem to provide antioxidant protection, and uric acid contributes >50% of the antioxidant capacity of our organism. In fact, it has a direct effect on the inhibition of free radicals, protecting the cell membrane and DNA. The antioxidant activity of SUA also occurs in the brain, being a protector for several disease such as multiple sclerosis and neurodegenerative disease, as well as cardiac and renal toxicity [36]. Thus, an eventually beneficial action could be speculated also on the liver.

In addition, there is still no consensus if uric acid is a protective or a risk factor; however, it seems that the quantity and the duration of the concentration of the uric acid in the blood is essential for this answer, possibly being the acute increase in its protective levels whereas chronic elevated levels are dangerous.

5.4. The Ucleotide-Binding Oligomerization Domain-Like (NOD-Like) Receptor Family Pyrin Domain Containing 3 (NLRP3) Inflammasome

Another factor which has been reported to be strongly involved in the pathogenesis of uric acid toxicity is NLRP3 inflammasome, an intracellular multiprotein complex that is assembled and activated by pathogen-associated and damage-associated molecular patterns with subsequent production of pro-inflammatory and pro-fibrotic cytokines (IL-1β and IL-18). It plays a central role in obesity and IR and has been involved in dyslipidemia and lipid accumulation in hepatocytes [28,31]. The NLRP3 inflammasome is activated by uric acid, both directly and indirectly through ROS production [37] and recent evidence has demonstrated that it contributes to hepatic steatosis and insulin resistance in a murine model [28]. This suggestion was confirmed in cultured HepG2 and L02 cellular lines, where the NLRP3 inflammasome knock-down cells decreased the uric acid-induced hepatic free fatty acids (FFAs) accumulation [31].

In conclusion, SUA is able to regulate lipid production and to foster the onset of metabolic disorders and NAFLD through multifaceted pathways. Thereby, evidence is accumulating on the benefit of lowering SUA levels in NAFLD by using drugs commonly employed in the treatment of hyperuricemia, like allopurinol or probenecid.

6. Ferritin

Hyperferritinemia is a frequent finding in the general population, is detected in 30%–40% of the patients with MS/NAFLD, and has been suggested as a marker of severity of the disease.

The difficulty in the interpretation of increased ferritin is related to the multiple causes that can lead to its increase, initially identified as marker of iron overload, following the increase of transferrin saturation, and also in the presence of severe hepatic necrosis. Furthermore, other more frequent causes need to be considered, namely the presence of inflammation, since ferritin behaves as a protein of acute phase and it can also be induced in the setting of systemic inflammation, like in rheumatologi, infectious or neoplastic diseases, and alcohol abuse, where ferritin levels rapidly decrease with alcohol abstinence. However, enlarging the most common cause of hyperferritinemia identified in the last years is the presence of the MS, to which NAFLD is frequently associated.

7. Ferritin and Metabolic Syndrome Clinical Manifestations

Hyperferritinemia is detected in about one-third of patients with NAFLD and the MS and its levels seem to be directly correlated with the severity of IR [38,39].

The first reports on the relationship between ferritin, IR/T2DM and the MS study in Europe were published in the 1990s. In 1998, Ford et al. [40] reported the results of a case-control study in Europe, demonstrating that subjects with hyperferritinemia had a 2.4-fold higher risk of developing T2DM. In addition, Salonen [41] showed in a prospective study that increased ferritin levels precede the development of diabetes and Kim obtained the same results in a very large cohort of Korean subjects [42]. In addition, cross-sectional studies found that elevated ferritin levels were associated with central obesity [43], hypertension [44], and dyslipidemia [45], all manifestations of the MS. Moreover, Iwasaki highlighted an association between serum ferritin, visceral fat and subcutaneous adiposity and suggested that serum ferritin concentration may be a useful indicator of systemic fat content and degree of IR [46]. In addition, Alam *et al.* [47] demonstrated that obesity led to hyperferritinemia irrespective of actual body iron story, advocating a state of subclinical inflammation responsible for high levels of ferritin.

Others demonstrated in population-based studies that moderate to markedly increased ferritin concentrations represent a biological biomarker predictive of early death in a dose-dependent manner [48]. Thus, even if in this study, information on the presence of liver steatosis was lacking, it is very likely that ferritin may be a predictor of early death also in the setting of NAFLD.

8. Ferritin and NAFLD

The tight link between ferritin and insulin dysregulation was shown by Fernandez-Real [49], who proposed ferritin as a marker of IR. Zelber-Sagi *et al.* [50]demonstrated that among different metabolic features, insulin was the strongest predictor of increased serum ferritin levels and that the association between serum ferritin and MS was mediated by NAFLD.

A French group coined the term of *"dysmetabolic iron overload syndrome"* (DIOS), to indicate subjects with increased ferritin levels, with normal or only mildly increased transferrin saturation, in the presence of liver steatosis, IR and two or more components of the MS, along with moderate hepatic iron accumulation with the typical pattern of mixed parenchymal and mesenchymal iron deposition [51]. However, it was also observed that several patients with NAFLD, IR and manifestations of MS may have increased ferritin even in the absence of increased iron stores.

In addition, Kim *et al.* [42] reported that serum ferritin levels predict incident non-alcoholic fatty liver disease in healthy Korean men.

9. Relationship between Ferritin and NAFLD/Metabolic Syndrome: Possible Mechanisms

Numerous data demonstrate that hepatic iron accumulation could elicit the onset of metabolic imbalance and liver damage and figure out the DIOS or more recently called "insulin-resistance associated with iron overload syndrome".

The liver has a central role in iron metabolism as it is the principle source of hepcidin, the regulatory peptide hormone of iron homeostasis. In fact, in response to several stimuli, like excessive iron deposits, inflammatory signals (IL-6) or ER-stress, hepcidin is overexpressed and determines a reduction in iron intestinal absorption and an increase in iron retention from macrophage and hepatocytes [52,53]. In addition, hepatocyte necrosis, with subsequent erythrophagocytosis by macrophages, and the systemic inflammatory state induced by obesity and NAFLD itself, may predispose individuals to increased hepcidin levels.

Many mechanisms linking iron and liver damage have been described. Firstly, iron, once accumulated in the liver, causes oxidative stress through the Fenton and Haber–Weiss chemistry with production of ROS and damage to membranes, proteins and DNA. Secondly, ferritin itself, which is the expression of iron storage in the liver, behaves as a real pro-inflammatory cytokine directly activating the hepatic stellate cells via Nuclear Factor κB (NFκB) cascade and inducing fibrogenesis [54]. Nevertheless, the role of hepatic iron and progression of liver disease is still to be fully elucidated.

In addition, very recent data suggest a possible role of splenic iron accumulation in promoting liver damage. However, these results need further confirmations [55].

9.1. Pathogenesis of DIOS (Dysmetabolic Iron Overload Syndrome)

Several explanations for the correlation between high ferritin levels and NAFLD have been proposed, namely IR, erythrophagocytosis by hepatic macrophages and dysregulation of proteins and pathways involved in iron homeostasis. Among the latter, hepcidin seems to have a key role in iron accumulation in NAFLD [56,57], as increased levels of this peptide have been detected in these patients [58,59], as well in the paediatric NAFLD population [60]. Furthermore, an influence of genetic factors has been considered, in particular the heterozygosis state of β-thalassemia and mutations in the HFE gene responsible for hereditary hemochromatosis (HH) [38,61,62] (Figure 2).

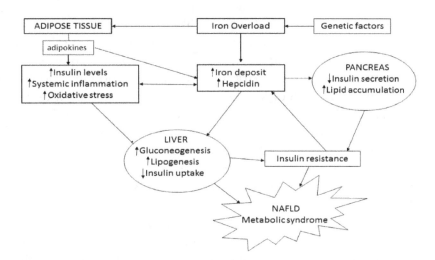

Figure 2. Pathogenetic pathways of the association between ferritin and NAFLD. Up arrow in the boxes: increase; down arrow in the boxes: decrease.

9.2. Hyperferritinemia and Insulin-Resistance

The relationship between hyperferritinemia and IR seems to be mutual. In fact, early *in vitro* studies have suggested that insulin might determine a rapid and marked stimulation of iron uptake by fat cells, by a redistribution of transferrin receptors from an intracellular membrane compartment to the cell surface [49]. On the other hand, systemic iron overload may prompt the onset of diabetes mellitus (DM) consequent to an impairment in pancreatic β-cells function due to intra-parenchymal iron deposition. In fact, because of oxidative stress, β-cells are less sensitive to glucose stimulation and die by to apoptosis with consequent reduction in insulin production [63].

The effect of iron overload on glucose metabolism has been investigated in animal models. In a study by Choi *et al.* [64], mice fed with a standard diet enriched in iron, presented higher levels of ferritin, hepcidin and inflammatory cytokines, as well as a higher degree of IR and metabolic dysregulations, mainly driven by an overexpression of genes involved in either gluconeogenesis or lipogenesis. These features were exasperated in mice fed with high fat diet (HFD) enriched with iron, suggesting a synergistic effect of fat and iron. The authors have speculated that insulin stimulates ferritin synthesis via inflammatory pathways and enhances hepcidin expression. On the other hand, iron interferes with insulin inhibition of glucose production by the liver and decreases the hepatic extraction and metabolism of insulin, leading to peripheral hyperinsulinemia. These data were confirmed by Dongiovanni *et al.* [65], who showed that an iron-enriched diet in mice led to the development of IR, probably due to the secretion of adipokines by the visceral adipose tissue consequent to iron accumulation.

Recent data by Vecchi *et al.* [66] further explored the relationship between glucose and iron metabolism and showed a new regulatory pathway in iron homeostasis driven by gluconeogenic stimuli and with the major actors being hepcdin and PPARGC1A, a transcriptional coactivator of genes involved in gluconeogenesis. Therefore, in conditions like NAFLD, obesity and T2DM, persistently activated gluceoneogenesis may result in overstimulation of hepcidin and iron accumulation.

The interplay between iron and insulin has been also confirmed by experimental data that showed how iron depletion could elicit an over expression and higher affinity of insulin receptors, as well as an increase in the expression of molecules involved in the intracellular signal cascade activated by insulin receptors and of genes involved in glucose uptake [57].

9.3. Hyperferritinemia and Adipose Tissue

The adipose tissue behaves as an endocrine organ, which under a condition of chronic inflammation, as in NAFLD, releases adipokines in the bloodstream, thus altering glucose and iron homeostasis and may determine a condition of subclinical inflammation itself [47,67]. Many adipokines play a central role in this scenario, namely adiponectin, leptin and resistin [57]. Adiponectin, which is an anti-steatotic and anti-inflammatory adipokine, is reduced in dysmetabolic conditions like NAFLD, IR and T2DM, and seems to predict the severity of liver inflammation and fibrosis. In fact, it has the capability of inducing the transcription of key genes in iron metabolism, like the hemeoxygenase-1 (HO-1), determining lower iron levels in hepatocytes, thus preventing apoptosis. Conversely, leptin, an adipokine involved in the control of food intake and energy consumption, seems to upregulate hepcidin synthesis, thus contributing to DIOS pathogenesis.

Finally, resistin is able to either impair glucose tolerance or reduce glucose uptake from muscular tissue or induce an inhibitor of insulin signaling namely SOCS3 (Suppressor of cytokine signaling 3), thus eliciting a condition of IR.

In line with this are the results by Beckry *et al.* [68] who have shown the ectopic expression of hepcidin in white adipose tissue of obese individuals and that of leptin, usually increased in obese subjects, was able to enhance hepcidin mRNA *in vitro*. In addition, Green *et al.* [69] have demonstrated how isolated primary rat adipocytes exposed to iron become insulin-resistant decreasing insulin mediated glucose transport and fostering lipolisis. On the other hand, a "portal vein theory" has been proposed and comprises the concept that visceral adipose tissue and/or the gut release into the portal vein increasing amounts of FFAs and pro-inflammatory factors, which, in turn, reach the liver and contribute to the onset of hepatic IR and steatosis. However, further studies are needed for a better comprehension of this casual link [70].

10. Hyperferritinemia and Severity of Liver Damage in NAFLD

Iron and ferritin have been hypothesized to foster the progression of organ damage, including hepatic and cardiovascular diseases.

In 2001, our group showed that hyperferritinemia with normal transferrin saturation was a hallmark of a glucose/lipid metabolism disorder and, when associated with multiple metabolic abnormalities and iron overload, identified patients at risk for NASH. Interestingly, we observed that patients in whom ferritin remained elevated despite lifestyle modifications (diet, weight loss, physical activity) differed from those whose ferritin normalized, presenting the former a more severe liver disease. We hypothesized that the increase of ferritin possibly reflected a synergistic induction of its synthesis because of increased iron stores, hepatic steatosis and subclinical inflammation. In contrast, when the increase in serum ferritin was a consequence only of altered lipid metabolism, it was reversible with diet and unrelated to iron stores [71].

Since then, several other studies analyzed the relationship between ferritin, iron overload and severity of liver damage in patients with NAFLD. Bugianesi *et al.* [38] demonstrated that increased ferritin levels are markers of severe histologic damage, but not of iron overload and that iron burden and HFE mutations do not contribute significantly to hepatic fibrosis in the majority of patients with NAFLD. Manousou *et al.* [72] evaluated in 111 NAFLD patients the relationship between serum ferritin and features of MS with respect to histological inflammation and/or fibrosis. Interestingly, ferritin resulted a good predictor of advanced liver disease, with respect to both NASH and fibrosis. In addition, Kowdley *et al.* [73] demonstrated that elevated serum ferritin is an independent predictor of histologic severity and advanced fibrosis among patients with NAFLD. He found in a cohort of 628 biopsy-proven NAFLD with hyperferritinemia that ferritin, besides being significantly associated with markers of liver damage (elevated serum ALT, AST and decreased platelets) and of iron overload (iron, transferrin-iron saturation and iron stain grade), was associated with more severe histologic features of NAFLD, including steatosis, hepatocellular ballooning, increased NAFLD Activity Score (NAS) and diagnosis of NASH. In addition, ferritin was also independently associated with advanced hepatic fibrosis and with higher NAS, the latter even among patients without hepatic iron deposition. The authors concluded that serum ferritin was useful to identify NAFLD patients at risk for NASH and advanced fibrosis.

These data were confirmed in a cohort of 108 Korean biopsy proven NAFLD patients in whom a positive correlation between ferritin level, metabolic alterations, liver fibrosis and NASH was found. Nevertheless, the association between ferritin and histology resulted weaker compared to another serum marker resulting from hepatocytes apoptosis, namely fragmented cytokeratin-18 (CK-18) [74].

Conversely, Angulo *et al.* [75] retrospectively analyzed in 1404 NAFLD patients the accuracy of serum ferritin in determining the presence and severity of liver fibrosis, and whether combining non-invasive fibrosis scoring systems with serum ferritin analysis could increase the accuracy of those tests. Although serum levels of ferritin correlated with more-severe liver fibrosis; however, either the performance of ferritin resulted unsatisfactorily for any grade of fibrosis or the accuracy of the non-invasive scores did not change with inclusion of serum ferritin. On the basis of adjusted multiple logistic regression analysis, they concluded that serum ferritin levels alone had a low level of diagnostic accuracy for the presence or severity of liver fibrosis in patients with NAFLD.

Similar results were reported by Yoneda *et al.* [76], who analyzed 1201 biopsy-proven NAFLD patients previously enrolled into the Japan Study Group of NAFLD and belonging to a large Japanese cohort database of NAFLD patients. By comparing serum ferritin levels and hepatic histology, the authors showed that ferritin increased with increasing histological grade of steatosis, lobular inflammation and ballooning and that at multivariate analyses it was independently associated with steatosis grade and fibrotic stage. However, ferritin showed a suboptimal performance as predictive test of any degree of liver fibrosis, possibly because several other factors including sex and metabolic features could have interfered. The conclusion of the study was that serum ferritin had a low diagnostic accuracy for detecting fibrosis in NAFLD patients when considered alone.

Nevertheless, ferritin has also been included in serum panels in order to detect liver damage non-invasively. One of these is the NAFIC score, which relies on ferritin, insulin and type IV collagen serum levels and which has been tested in a cohort of 147 biopsy-proven NAFLD and validated in another cohort of 355 patients from nine hepatologic centers in Japan. A cut-off of two has been identified to diagnose the presence of NASH in NAFLD patients, with a sensitivity and a specificity of 63% and 83%, respectively. Later, a new modified NAFIC score was created including higher insulin values that presented a better diagnostic performance (sensitivity 74%, specificity 75% and Area under Receiving Operating Characteristic—AUROC 0.801) [77].

Another score which includes ferritin as a variable is the FibroMeter NAFLD score. It consists of a panel of serum markers and has been shown to have a high diagnostic accuracy for staging liver fibrosis. In particular, in a study of 235 NAFLD patients, it showed an AUROC of 0.94 for significant fibrosis ($\geq$F2), 0.93 for severe fibrosis (F3), and 0.9 for cirrhosis [5,78].

In conclusion, increasing data aimed at pointing ferritin as possible predictive factor of liver damage are accumulating. Despite conflicting and still not conclusive results, it could be speculated that ferritin might be used as a surrogate marker, especially if combined with other metabolic and biochemical variables, to identify a more severe liver disease, even if with an intermediate sensitivity and specificity.

11. Does Hyperferritinemia Reflect Iron Overload?

In an attempt to clarify whether the increase in ferritin observed in patients with NAFLD reflects iron overload, studies were performed to define a possible association between ferritin and both liver siderosis and mutations in genes involved in iron metabolism. Interestingly, HFE mutations responsible for hereditary hemochromatosis resulted non significantly associated either to liver siderosis or hyperferritinemia and also liver damage did not result as being influenced by the presence of these mutations [62]. *Vice versa*, liver damage defined either by more severe fibrosis or presence of NASH, resulted as significantly associated with the presence of liver siderosis and β thalassemia traits [79]. However, the large majority of studies concluded that the increased ferritin values observed in patients with NAFLD reflect increased iron stores and acquired and genetic factors predisposing individuals to lipid and iron metabolism alterations in the presence of subclinical inflammation.

12. Iron Depletion in Patients with Hyperferritinemia, Metabolic Alterations and NAFLD

Iron is known for causing oxidative stress through the Fenton and Haber–Weiss chemistry with production of ROS and damage to membranes, proteins and DNA, thus being capable of inducing liver damage and fibrosis. Ferritin is the primary iron-storage protein and serum ferritin concentration has historically been used to predict severe fibrosis in chronic liver diseases.

Several studies showed that iron depletion therapy was followed by a reduction in plasma glucose and by an improvement of insulin sensitivity. Facchini *et al.* in 2002 [80] demonstrated in a small series of NAFLD patients, with and without increased ferritin levels, that iron removal in carbohydrate intolerant patients with clinical evidence of nonalcoholic fatty liver disease was able to improve insulin sensitivity in the short term (without changes in body weight). Fernandez-Real showed in a randomized trial that blood letting in high-ferritin T2DM improved insulin sensitivity and secretion [81]. In addition, Valenti *et al.* [82] demonstrated that iron depletion by venesection, in patients with moderate iron overload associated with NAFLD, determined a decrease of both IR and transaminases, as well as of ferritin levels.

Despite these encouraging data, confirmed also in following studies, the role of iron depletion in the improvement in liver histology and the natural history of liver disease is still under definition because of the lack of studies including a large number of patients.

13. Conclusions

NAFLD is recognized as the leading cause of chronic liver disease worldwide, and, in a percentage of cases, it is potentially progressive towards advanced fibrosis and severe complications. As a consequence, the need for predictive factors of NAFLD and especially of its progressive forms is mandatory. In recent years, SUA and ferritin have emerged as possible predictors of hepatic steatosis and liver damage. Interestingly, some studies have reported high SUA levels in patients with hyperferritinemia and *vice versa*, thus suggesting a mutual relationship and a synergistic action [83–85].

In fact, as extensively depicted in this review, SUA and ferritin share common pathogenic mechanisms, in particular oxidative stress and IR, and are associated with metabolic features, among the latter obesity and T2DM are the most important. Therefore, it could be speculated that both SUA and ferritin are the main actors in the multifaceted and complicated scenario of NAFLD and its dysmetabolic features.

However, given that the majority of studies are based on observational data, well-designed prospective studies including a large series of patients of different ethnicities are warranted before a definite role of SUA and ferritin in the pathogenesis of NAFLD can be established. In addition, it could be of interest to evaluate whether treating hyperuricemia and hyperferritinemia may lead to NAFLD improvement, and, in turn, whether regression of NAFLD is accompanied by a normalization of SUA and ferritin levels.

Author Contributions: Rosa Lombardi wrote the first version of the manuscript, Giuseppina Pisano made the extensive revision of literature and Silvia Fargion revised the final version of the manuscript.

References

1. Williams, C.D.; Stengel, J.; Asike, M.I.; Torres, D.M.; Shaw, J.; Contreras, M.; Landt, C.L.; Harrison, S.A. Prevalence of nonalcoholic fatty liver disease and nonalcoholic steatohepatitis among a largely middle-aged population utilizing ultrasound and liver biopsy: A prospective study. *Gastroenterology* **2011**, *140*, 124–131. [CrossRef] [PubMed]

2. Lonardo, A.; Ballestri, S.; Marchesini, G.; Angulo, P.; Loria, P. Nonalcoholic fatty liver disease: A precursor of the metabolic syndrome. *Dig. Liver Dis.* **2015**, *47*, 181–190. [CrossRef] [PubMed]

3. Anstee, Q.M.; Targher, G.; Day, C.P. Progression of NAFLD to diabetes mellitus, cardiovascular disease or cirrhosis. *Nat. Rev. Gastroenterol. Hepatol.* **2013**, *10*, 330–344. [CrossRef] [PubMed]

4.	Serfaty, L.; Lemoine, M. Definition and natural history of metabolic steatosis: Clinical aspects of NAFLD, NASH and cirrhosis. *Diabetes Metab.* **2008**, *34*, 634–637. [CrossRef]
5.	Buzzetti, E.; Lombardi, R.; de Luca, L.; Tsochatzis, E.A. Noninvasive assessment of fibrosis in patients with nonalcoholic fatty liver disease. *Int. J. Endocrinol.* **2015**, *2015*, 343828. [CrossRef] [PubMed]
6.	Tsochatzis, E.A.; Gurusamy, K.S.; Ntaoula, S.; Cholongitas, E.; Davidson, B.R.; Burroughs, A.K. Elastography for the diagnosis of severity of fibrosis in chronic liver disease: A meta-analysis of diagnostic accuracy. *J. Hepatol.* **2011**, *54*, 650–659. [CrossRef] [PubMed]
7.	Mount, D.B.; Kwon, C.Y.; Zandi-Nejad, K. Renal urate transport. *Rheum. Dis. Clin. N. Am.* **2006**, *32*, 313–331. [CrossRef] [PubMed]
8.	Richette, P.; Bardin, T. Gout. *Lancet* **2010**, *375*, 318–328. [CrossRef]
9.	Zhang, M.L.; Gao, Y.X.; Wang, X.; Chang, H.; Huang, G.W. Serum uric acid and appropriate cutoff value for prediction of metabolic syndrome among Chinese adults. *J. Clin. Biochem. Nutr.* **2013**, *52*, 38–42. [CrossRef] [PubMed]
10.	Choi, H.K.; Ford, E.S. Prevalence of the metabolic syndrome in individuals with hyperuricemia. *Am. J. Med.* **2007**, *120*, 442–447. [CrossRef] [PubMed]
11.	Kodama, S.; Saito, K.; Yachi, Y.; Asumi, M.; Sugawara, A.; Totsuka, K.; Saito, A.; Sone, H. Association between serum uric acid and development of type 2 diabetes. *Diabetes Care* **2009**, *32*, 1737–1742. [CrossRef] [PubMed]
12.	Lin, S.D.; Tsai, D.H.; Hsu, S.R. Association between serum uric acid level and components of the metabolic syndrome. *J. Chin. Med. Assoc.* **2006**, *69*, 512–516. [CrossRef]
13.	Lv, Q.; Meng, X.F.; He, F.F.; Chen, S.; Su, H.; Xiong, J.; Gao, P.; Tian, X.J.; Liu, J.S.; Zhu, Z.H.; et al. High serum uric acid and increased risk of type 2 diabetes: A systemic review and meta-analysis of prospective cohort studies. *PLoS ONE* **2013**, *8*, e56864.
14.	Lonardo, A.; Loria, P.; Leonardi, F.; Borsatti, A.; Neri, P.; Pulvirenti, M.; Verrone, A.M.; Bagni, A.; Bertolotti, M.; Ganazzi, D.; et al. Fasting insulin and uric acid levels but not indices of iron metabolism are independent predictors of non-alcoholic fatty liver disease. A case-control study. *Dig. Liver Dis.* **2002**, *34*, 204–211. [CrossRef]
15.	Li, Y.; Xu, C.; Yu, C.; Xu, L.; Miao, M. Association of serum uric acid level with non-alcoholic fatty liver disease: A cross-sectional study. *J. Hepatol.* **2009**, *50*, 1029–1034. [PubMed]
16.	Ryu, S.; Chang, Y.; Kim, S.G.; Cho, J.; Guallar, E. Serum uric acid levels predict incident nonalcoholic fatty liver disease in healthy Korean men. *Metabolism* **2011**, *60*, 860–866. [CrossRef] [PubMed]
17.	Liu, Z.; Que, S.; Zhou, L.; Zheng, S. Dose-response relationship of serum uric acid with metabolic syndrome and non-alcoholic fatty liver disease incidence: A meta-analysis of prospective studies. *Sci. Rep.* **2015**, *5*, 14325. [CrossRef] [PubMed]
18.	Yuan, H.; Yu, C.; Li, X.; Sun, L.; Zhu, X.; Zhao, C.; Zhang, Z.; Yang, Z. Serum uric acid levels and risk of metabolic syndrome: A dose-response meta-analysis of prospective studies. *J. Clin. Endocrinol. Metab.* **2015**, *100*, 4198–4207. [CrossRef] [PubMed]
19.	Chen, J.H.; Chuang, S.Y.; Chen, H.J.; Yeh, W.T.; Pan, W.H. Serum uric acid level as an independent risk factor for all-cause, cardiovascular, and ischemic stroke mortality: A Chinese cohort study. *Arthritis Rheum.* **2009**, *61*, 225–232. [CrossRef] [PubMed]
20.	Xu, C.; Wan, X.; Xu, L.; Weng, H.; Yan, M.; Miao, M.; Sun, Y.; Xu, G.; Dooley, S.; Li, Y.; et al. Xanthine oxidase in non-alcoholic fatty liver disease and hyperuricemia: One stone hits two birds. *J. Hepatol.* **2015**, *62*, 1412–1419. [CrossRef] [PubMed]
21.	Sirota, J.C.; McFann, K.; Targher, G.; Johnson, R.J.; Chonchol, M.; Jalal, D.I. Elevated serum uric acid levels are associated with non-alcoholic fatty liver disease independently of metabolic syndrome features in the United States: Liver ultrasound data from the National Health and Nutrition Examination Survey. *Metabolism* **2013**, *62*, 392–399. [CrossRef] [PubMed]
22.	Petta, S.; Camma, C.; Cabibi, D.; Di Marco, V.; Craxi, A. Hyperuricemia is associated with histological liver damage in patients with non-alcoholic fatty liver disease. *Aliment. Pharmacol. Ther.* **2011**, *34*, 757–766. [PubMed]
23.	Afzali, A.; Weiss, N.S.; Boyko, E.J.; Ioannou, G.N. Association between serum uric acid level and chronic liver disease in the United States. *Hepatology* **2010**, *52*, 578–589. [CrossRef] [PubMed]
24.	Abreu, E.; Fonseca, M.J.; Santos, A.C. Association between hyperuricemia and insulin resistance. *Acta Med. Port.* **2011**, *24*, 565–574. [PubMed]

25. Tan, Y.; Liu, X.; Zhou, K.; He, X.; Lu, C.; He, B.; Niu, X.; Xiao, C.; Xu, G.; Bian, Z.; *et al.* The potential biomarkers to identify the development of steatosis in hyperuricemia. *PLoS ONE* **2016**, *11*, e0149043. [CrossRef] [PubMed]

26. Li, C.; Hsieh, M.C.; Chang, S.J. Metabolic syndrome, diabetes, and hyperuricemia. *Curr. Opin. Rheumatol.* **2013**, *25*, 210–216. [CrossRef] [PubMed]

27. Zhu, Y.; Hu, Y.; Huang, T.; Zhang, Y.; Li, Z.; Luo, C.; Luo, Y.; Yuan, H.; Hisatome, I.; Yamamoto, T.; *et al.* High uric acid directly inhibits insulin signalling and induces insulin resistance. *Biochem. Biophys. Res. Commun.* **2014**, *447*, 707–714. [CrossRef] [PubMed]

28. Vandanmagsar, B.; Youm, Y.H.; Ravussin, A.; Galgani, J.E.; Stadler, K.; Mynatt, R.L.; Ravussin, E.; Stephens, J.M.; Dixit, V.D. The NLRP3 inflammasome instigates obesity-induced inflammation and insulin resistance. *Nat. Med.* **2011**, *17*, 179–188. [CrossRef] [PubMed]

29. Lanaspa, M.A.; Sanchez-Lozada, L.G.; Choi, Y.J.; Cicerchi, C.; Kanbay, M.; Roncal-Jimenez, C.A.; Ishimoto, T.; Li, N.; Marek, G.; Duranay, M.; *et al.* Uric acid induces hepatic steatosis by generation of mitochondrial oxidative stress: potential role in fructose-dependent and -independent fatty liver. *J. Biol. Chem.* **2012**, *287*, 40732–40744. [CrossRef] [PubMed]

30. Choi, Y.J.; Shin, H.S.; Choi, H.S.; Park, J.W.; Jo, I.; Oh, E.S.; Lee, K.Y.; Lee, B.H.; Johnson, R.J.; Kang, D.H. Uric acid induces fat accumulation via generation of endoplasmic reticulum stress and SREBP-1c activation in hepatocytes. *Lab. Investig.* **2014**, *94*, 1114–1125. [CrossRef] [PubMed]

31. Wan, X.; Xu, C.; Lin, Y.; Lu, C.; Li, D.; Sang, J.; He, H.; Liu, X.; Li, Y.; Yu, C. Uric acid regulates hepatic steatosis and insulin resistance through the NLRP3 inflammasome-dependent mechanism. *J. Hepatol.* **2015**. [CrossRef]

32. Ackerman, Z.; Oron-Herman, M.; Grozovski, M.; Rosenthal, T.; Pappo, O.; Link, G.; Sela, B.A. Fructose-induced fatty liver disease: hepatic effects of blood pressure and plasma triglyceride reduction. *Hypertension* **2005**, *45*, 1012–1018. [CrossRef] [PubMed]

33. Lanaspa, M.A.; Sanchez-Lozada, L.G.; Cicerchi, C.; Li, N.; Roncal-Jimenez, C.A.; Ishimoto, T.; Le, M.; Garcia, G.E.; Thomas, J.B.; Rivard, C.J.; *et al.* Uric acid stimulates fructokinase and accelerates fructose metabolism in the development of fatty liver. *PLoS ONE* **2012**, *7*, e47948. [CrossRef] [PubMed]

34. Pagliassotti, M.J. Endoplasmic reticulum stress in nonalcoholic fatty liver disease. *Annu. Rev. Nutr.* **2012**, *32*, 17–33. [CrossRef] [PubMed]

35. Zhang, C.; Chen, X.; Zhu, R.M.; Zhang, Y.; Yu, T.; Wang, H.; Zhao, H.; Zhao, M.; Ji, Y.L.; Chen, Y.H.; *et al.* Endoplasmic reticulum stress is involved in hepatic SREBP-1c activation and lipid accumulation in fructose-fed mice. *Toxicol. Lett.* **2012**, *212*, 229–240. [CrossRef] [PubMed]

36. De Oliveira, E.P.; Burini, R.C. High plasma uric acid concentration: causes and consequences. *Diabetol. Metab. Syndr.* **2012**, *4*, 12. [CrossRef] [PubMed]

37. Martinon, F.; Petrilli, V.; Mayor, A.; Tardivel, A.; Tschopp, J. Gout-associated uric acid crystals activate the NALP3 inflammasome. *Nature* **2006**, *440*, 237–241. [CrossRef] [PubMed]

38. Bugianesi, E.; Manzini, P.; D'Antico, S.; Vanni, E.; Longo, F.; Leone, N.; Massarenti, P.; Piga, A.; Marchesini, G.; Rizzetto, M. Relative contribution of iron burden, HFE mutations, and insulin resistance to fibrosis in nonalcoholic fatty liver. *Hepatology* **2004**, *39*, 179–187. [CrossRef] [PubMed]

39. Fernandez-Real, J.M.; Ricart-Engel, W.; Arroyo, E.; Balanca, R.; Casamitjana-Abella, R.; Cabrero, D.; Fernandez-Castaner, M.; Soler, J. Serum ferritin as a component of the insulin resistance syndrome. *Diabetes Care* **1998**, *21*, 62–68. [CrossRef] [PubMed]

40. Ford, E.S.; Cogswell, M.E. Diabetes and serum ferritin concentration among U.S. adults. *Diabetes Care* **1999**, *22*, 1978–1983. [CrossRef] [PubMed]

41. Salonen, J.T.; Tuomainen, T.P.; Nyyssonen, K.; Lakka, H.M.; Punnonen, K. Relation between iron stores and non-insulin dependent diabetes in men: Case-control study. *BMJ* **1998**, *317*, 727. [CrossRef] [PubMed]

42. Kim, C.W.; Chang, Y.; Sung, E.; Shin, H.; Ryu, S. Serum ferritin levels predict incident non-alcoholic fatty liver disease in healthy Korean men. *Metabolism* **2012**, *61*, 1182–1188. [CrossRef] [PubMed]

43. Gillum, R.F. Association of serum ferritin and indices of body fat distribution and obesity in Mexican American men—The third national health and nutrition examination survey. *Int. J. Obes. Relat. Metab. Disord.* **2001**, *25*, 639–645. [CrossRef] [PubMed]

44. Piperno, A.; Trombini, P.; Gelosa, M.; Mauri, V.; Pecci, V.; Vergani, A.; Salvioni, A.; Mariani, R.; Mancia, G. Increased serum ferritin is common in men with essential hypertension. *J. Hypertens.* **2002**, *20*, 1513–1518. [CrossRef] [PubMed]

45. Williams, M.J.; Poulton, R.; Williams, S. Relationship of serum ferritin with cardiovascular risk factors and inflammation in young men and women. *Atherosclerosis* **2002**, *165*, 179–184. [CrossRef]

46. Iwasaki, T.; Nakajima, A.; Yoneda, M.; Yamada, Y.; Mukasa, K.; Fujita, K.; Fujisawa, N.; Wada, K.; Terauchi, Y. Serum ferritin is associated with visceral fat area and subcutaneous fat area. *Diabetes Care* **2005**, *28*, 2486–2491. [CrossRef] [PubMed]

47. Alam, F.; Memon, A.S.; Fatima, S.S. Increased Body Mass Index may lead to Hyperferritinemia Irrespective of Body Iron Stores. *Pak. J. Med. Sci.* **2015**, *31*, 1521–1526. [PubMed]

48. Ellervik, C.; Marott, J.L.; Tybjaerg-Hansen, A.; Schnohr, P.; Nordestgaard, B.G. Total and cause-specific mortality by moderately and markedly increased ferritin concentrations: General population study and metaanalysis. *Clin. Chem.* **2014**, *60*, 1419–1428. [CrossRef] [PubMed]

49. Fernandez-Real, J.M.; Lopez-Bermejo, A.; Ricart, W. Cross-talk between iron metabolism and diabetes. *Diabetes* **2002**, *51*, 2348–2354. [CrossRef] [PubMed]

50. Zelber-Sagi, S.; Nitzan-Kaluski, D.; Halpern, Z.; Oren, R. NAFLD and hyperinsulinemia are major deter4.minants of serum ferritin levels. *J. Hepatol.* **2007**, *46*, 700–707. [CrossRef] [PubMed]

51. Moirand, R.; Mortaji, A.M.; Loreal, O.; Paillard, F.; Brissot, P.; Deugnier, Y. A new syndrome of liver iron overload with normal transferrin saturation. *Lancet* **1997**, *349*, 95–97. [CrossRef]

52. Corradini, E.; Meynard, D.; Wu, Q.; Chen, S.; Ventura, P.; Pietrangelo, A.; Babitt, J.L. Serum and liver iron differently regulate the bone morphogenetic protein 6 (BMP6)-SMAD signaling pathway in mice. *Hepatology* **2011**, *54*, 273–284. [CrossRef] [PubMed]

53. Vecchi, C.; Montosi, G.; Zhang, K.; Lamberti, I.; Duncan, S.A.; Kaufman, R.J.; Pietrangelo, A. ER stress controls iron metabolism through induction of hepcidin. *Science* **2009**, *325*, 877–880. [CrossRef] [PubMed]

54. Fargion, S.; Valenti, L.; Fracanzani, A.L. Beyond hereditary hemochromatosis: New insights into the relationship between iron overload and chronic liver diseases. *Dig. Liver Dis.* **2011**, *43*, 89–95. [CrossRef] [PubMed]

55. Murotomi, K.; Arai, S.; Uchida, S.; Endo, S.; Mitsuzumi, H.; Tabei, Y.; Yoshida, Y.; Nakajima, Y. Involvement of splenic iron accumulation in the development of nonalcoholic steatohepatitis in Tsumura Suzuki Obese Diabetes mice. *Sci. Rep.* **2016**, *6*, 22476. [CrossRef] [PubMed]

56. Corradini, E.; Pietrangelo, A. Iron and steatohepatitis. *J. Gastroenterol. Hepatol.* **2012**, *27*, 42–46. [CrossRef] [PubMed]

57. Dongiovanni, P.; Fracanzani, A.L.; Fargion, S.; Valenti, L. Iron in fatty liver and in the metabolic syndrome: a promising therapeutic target. *J. Hepatol.* **2011**, *55*, 920–932. [CrossRef] [PubMed]

58. Boga, S.; Alkim, H.; Alkim, C.; Koksal, A.R.; Bayram, M.; Yilmaz Ozguven, M.B.; Tekin Neijmann, S. The relationship of serum hemojuvelin and hepcidin levels with iron overload in nonalcoholic fatty liver disease. *J. Gastrointest. Liver Dis.* **2015**, *24*, 293–300.

59. Senates, E.; Yilmaz, Y.; Colak, Y.; Ozturk, O.; Altunoz, M.E.; Kurt, R.; Ozkara, S.; Aksaray, S.; Tuncer, I.; Ovunc, A.O. Serum levels of hepcidin in patients with biopsy-proven nonalcoholic fatty liver disease. *Metab. Syndr. Relat. Disord.* **2011**, *9*, 287–290. [CrossRef] [PubMed]

60. Demircioglu, F.; Gorunmez, G.; Dagistan, E.; Goksugur, S.B.; Bekdas, M.; Tosun, M.; Kizildag, B.; Kismet, E. Serum hepcidin levels and iron metabolism in obese children with and without fatty liver: Case-control study. *Eur. J. Pediatr.* **2014**, *173*, 947–951. [CrossRef] [PubMed]

61. Neri, S.; Pulvirenti, D.; Signorelli, S.; Ignaccolo, L.; Tsami, A.; Mauceri, B.; Misseri, M.; Interlandi, D.; Cutuli, N.; Castellino, P. The HFE gene heterozygosis H63D: A cofactor for liver damage in patients with steatohepatitis? Epidemiological and clinical considerations. *Intern. Med. J.* **2008**, *38*, 254–258. [CrossRef] [PubMed]

62. Valenti, L.; Dongiovanni, P.; Fracanzani, A.L.; Fargion, S. HFE mutations in nonalcoholic fatty liver disease. *Hepatology* **2008**, *47*, 1794–1795. [CrossRef] [PubMed]

63. McClain, D.A.; Abraham, D.; Rogers, J.; Brady, R.; Gault, P.; Ajioka, R.; Kushner, J.P. High prevalence of abnormal glucose homeostasis secondary to decreased insulin secretion in individuals with hereditary haemochromatosis. *Diabetologia* **2006**, *49*, 1661–1669. [CrossRef] [PubMed]

64. Choi, J.S.; Koh, I.U.; Lee, H.J.; Kim, W.H.; Song, J. Effects of excess dietary iron and fat on glucose and lipid metabolism. *J. Nutr. Biochem.* **2013**, *24*, 1634–1644. [CrossRef] [PubMed]

65. Dongiovanni, P.; Ruscica, M.; Rametta, R.; Recalcati, S.; Steffani, L.; Gatti, S.; Girelli, D.; Cairo, G.; Magni, P.; Fargion, S.; *et al.* Dietary iron overload induces visceral adipose tissue insulin resistance. *Am. J. Pathol.* **2013**, *182*, 2254–2263. [CrossRef] [PubMed]

66. Vecchi, C.; Montosi, G.; Garuti, C.; Corradini, E.; Sabelli, M.; Canali, S.; Pietrangelo, A. Gluconeogenic signals regulate iron homeostasis via hepcidin in mice. *Gastroenterology* **2014**, *146*, 1060–1069. [CrossRef] [PubMed]

67. Marra, F.; Bertolani, C. Adipokines in liver diseases. *Hepatology* **2009**, *50*, 957–969. [CrossRef] [PubMed]

68. Bekri, S.; Gual, P.; Anty, R.; Luciani, N.; Dahman, M.; Ramesh, B.; Iannelli, A.; Staccini-Myx, A.; Casanova, D.; Ben Amor, I.; *et al.* Increased adipose tissue expression of hepcidin in severe obesity is independent from diabetes and NASH. *Gastroenterology* **2006**, *131*, 788–796. [CrossRef] [PubMed]

69. Green, A.; Basile, R.; Rumberger, J.M. Transferrin and iron induce insulin resistance of glucose transport in adipocytes. *Metabolism* **2006**, *55*, 1042–1045. [CrossRef] [PubMed]

70. Item, F.; Konrad, D. Visceral fat and metabolic inflammation: the portal theory revisited. *Obes. Rev.* **2012**, *13*, 30–39. [CrossRef] [PubMed]

71. Fargion, S.; Mattioli, M.; Fracanzani, A.L.; Sampietro, M.; Tavazzi, D.; Fociani, P.; Taioli, E.; Valenti, L.; Fiorelli, G. Hyperferritinemia, iron overload, and multiple metabolic alterations identify patients at risk for nonalcoholic steatohepatitis. *Am. J. Gastroenterol.* **2001**, *96*, 2448–2455. [CrossRef] [PubMed]

72. Manousou, P.; Kalambokis, G.; Grillo, F.; Watkins, J.; Xirouchakis, E.; Pleguezuelo, M.; Leandro, G.; Arvaniti, V.; Germani, G.; Patch, D.; *et al.* Serum ferritin is a discriminant marker for both fibrosis and inflammation in histologically proven non-alcoholic fatty liver disease patients. *Liver Int.* **2011**, *31*, 730–739. [CrossRef] [PubMed]

73. Kowdley, K.V.; Belt, P.; Wilson, L.A.; Yeh, M.M.; Neuschwander-Tetri, B.A.; Chalasani, N.; Sanyal, A.J.; Nelson, J.E.; Network, N.C.R. Serum ferritin is an independent predictor of histologic severity and advanced fibrosis in patients with nonalcoholic fatty liver disease. *Hepatology* **2012**, *55*, 77–85. [CrossRef] [PubMed]

74. Kim, Y.S.; Jung, E.S.; Hur, W.; Bae, S.H.; Choi, J.Y.; Song, M.J.; Kim, C.W.; Jo, S.H.; Lee, C.D.; Lee, Y.S.; *et al.* Noninvasive predictors of nonalcoholic steatohepatitis in Korean patients with histologically proven nonalcoholic fatty liver disease. *Clin. Mol. Hepatol.* **2013**, *19*, 120–130. [CrossRef] [PubMed]

75. Angulo, P.; George, J.; Day, C.P.; Vanni, E.; Russell, L.; de la Cruz, A.C.; Liaquat, H.; Mezzabotta, L.; Lee, E.; Bugianesi, E. Serum ferritin levels lack diagnostic accuracy for liver fibrosis in patients with nonalcoholic fatty liver disease. *Clin. Gastroenterol. Hepatol.* **2014**, *12*, 1163–1169. [CrossRef] [PubMed]

76. Yoneda, M.; Thomas, E.; Sumida, Y.; Imajo, K.; Eguchi, Y.; Hyogo, H.; Fujii, H.; Ono, M.; Kawaguchi, T.; Schiff, E.R. Clinical usage of serum ferritin to assess liver fibrosis in patients with non-alcoholic fatty liver disease: Proceed with caution. *Hepatol. Res.* **2014**, *44*, E499–E502. [CrossRef] [PubMed]

77. Nakamura, A.; Yoneda, M.; Sumida, Y.; Eguchi, Y.; Fujii, H.; Hyogo, H.; Ono, M.; Suzuki, Y.; Kawaguchi, T.; Aoki, N.; *et al.* Modification of a simple clinical scoring system as a diagnostic screening tool for non-alcoholic steatohepatitis in Japanese patients with non-alcoholic fatty liver disease. *J. Diabetes Investig.* **2013**, *4*, 651–658. [CrossRef] [PubMed]

78. Cales, P.; Boursier, J.; Oberti, F.; Hubert, I.; Gallois, Y.; Rousselet, M.C.; Dib, N.; Moal, V.; Macchi, L.; Chevailler, A.; *et al.* FibroMeters: A family of blood tests for liver fibrosis. *Gastroenterol. Clin. Biol.* **2008**, *32*, 40–51. [CrossRef]

79. Valenti, L.; Canavesi, E.; Galmozzi, E.; Dongiovanni, P.; Rametta, R.; Maggioni, P.; Maggioni, M.; Fracanzani, A.L.; Fargion, S. β-Globin mutations are associated with parenchymal siderosis and fibrosis in patients with non-alcoholic fatty liver disease. *J. Hepatol.* **2010**, *53*, 927–933. [CrossRef] [PubMed]

80. Facchini, F.S.; Hua, N.W.; Stoohs, R.A. Effect of iron depletion in carbohydrate-intolerant patients with clinical evidence of nonalcoholic fatty liver disease. *Gastroenterology* **2002**, *122*, 931–939. [CrossRef] [PubMed]

81. Fernandez-Real, J.M.; Penarroja, G.; Castro, A.; Garcia-Bragado, F.; Hernandez-Aguado, I.; Ricart, W. Blood letting in high-ferritin type 2 diabetes: effects on insulin sensitivity and β-cell function. *Diabetes* **2002**, *51*, 1000–1004. [CrossRef] [PubMed]

82. Valenti, L.; Fracanzani, A.L.; Dongiovanni, P.; Bugianesi, E.; Marchesini, G.; Manzini, P.; Vanni, E.; Fargion, S. Iron depletion by phlebotomy improves insulin resistance in patients with nonalcoholic fatty liver disease and hyperferritinemia: evidence from a case-control study. *Am. J. Gastroenterol.* **2007**, *102*, 1251–1258. [CrossRef] [PubMed]

83. Chen, S.C.; Huang, Y.F.; Wang, J.D. Hyperferritinemia and hyperuricemia may be associated with liver function abnormality in obese adolescents. *PLoS ONE* **2012**, *7*, e48645. [CrossRef] [PubMed]
84. Ghio, A.J.; Ford, E.S.; Kennedy, T.P.; Hoidal, J.R. The association between serum ferritin and uric acid in humans. *Free Radic. Res.* **2005**, *39*, 337–342. [CrossRef] [PubMed]
85. Mainous, A.G., 3rd; Knoll, M.E.; Everett, C.J.; Matheson, E.M.; Hulihan, M.M.; Grant, A.M. Uric acid as a potential cue to screen for iron overload. *J. Am. Board Fam. Med.* **2011**, *24*, 415–421. [CrossRef] [PubMed]

5

Does Lysosomial Acid Lipase Reduction Play a Role in Adult Non-Alcoholic Fatty Liver Disease?

Francesco Baratta [1,†], Daniele Pastori [1,†], Licia Polimeni [1], Giulia Tozzi [2], Francesco Violi [3], Francesco Angelico [4,*,‡] and Maria Del Ben [3,‡]

[1]   Department of Internal Medicine and Medical Specialities and Department of Anatomical, Histological, Forensic Medicine and Orthopedics Sciences-Sapienza University, Rome 00185, Italy; francesco.baratta@uniroma1.it (F.B.); daniele.pastori@uniroma1.it (D.P.); licia.polimeni@uniroma1.it (L.P.)

[2]   Unit for Neuromuscular and Neurodegenerative Diseases, Children's Hospital and Research Institute "Bambino Gesù", Rome 00165, Italy; giulia.tozzi@opbg.net

[3]   Department of Internal Medicine and Medical Specialities, Sapienza University, Rome 00185, Italy; francesco.violi@uniroma1.it (F.V.); maria.delben@uniroma1.it (M.D.B.)

[4]   Department of Public Health and Infectious Diseases, Sapienza University, Policlinico Umberto I, I Clinica Medica, Viale del Policlinico 155, Rome 00161, Italy

*   Correspondence: francesco.angelico@uniroma1.it

†   These authors contributed equally to this work.

‡   Joint senior authors.

Academic Editor: Amedeo Lonardo

Abstract: Lysosomal Acid Lipase (LAL) is a key enzyme involved in lipid metabolism, responsible for hydrolysing the cholesteryl esters and triglycerides. Wolman Disease represents the early onset phenotype of LAL deficiency rapidly leading to death. Cholesterol Ester Storage Disease is a late onset phenotype that occurs with fatty liver, elevated aminotransferase levels, hepatomegaly and dyslipidaemia, the latter characterized by elevated LDL-C and low HDL-C. The natural history and the clinical manifestations of the LAL deficiency in adults are not well defined, and the diagnosis is often incidental. LAL deficiency has been suggested as an under-recognized cause of dyslipidaemia and fatty liver. Therefore, LAL activity may be reduced also in non-obese patients presenting non-alcoholic fatty liver disease (NAFLD), unexplained persistently elevated liver transaminases or with elevation in LDL cholesterol. In these patients, it could be indicated to test LAL activity. So far, very few studies have been performed to assess LAL activity in representative samples of normal subjects or patients with NAFLD. Moreover, no large study has been carried out in adult subjects with NAFLD or cryptogenic cirrhosis.

Keywords: lysosomial acid lipase; non-alcoholic fatty liver disease; Wolman Disease; cholesterol ester storage disease; hypercholesterolemia

1. Introduction

Non-alcoholic fatty liver disease (NAFLD) is a spectrum of disorders characterized by excessive hepatic fat accumulation that occurs in individuals in the absence of significant alcohol consumption or chronic viral infection. NAFLD is the most common hepatic disease involving a growing number of people worldwide. In the general population, the prevalence of NAFLD is about 20%–30%, and reaches 70%–90% in obese or diabetic patients [1]. The early stage of NAFLD is represented by simple steatosis, where the main histologic finding is the presence of fatty liver; in some cases simple steatosis my evolve in non-alcoholic steatohepatitis (NASH), where steatosis is associated with hepatocellular injury and inflammation with or without fibrosis.

Traditionally, NAFLD has been interpreted as a benign condition; however, more recent evidence suggests that NAFLD may progress to advanced liver disease such as cirrhosis, hepatocellular carcinoma, and end stage hepatic failure [2].

NAFLD is the result of many different pathogenic mechanisms which cause lipid accumulation into hepatocytes [3], increased oxidative stress, pro-inflammatory changes [4], and eventually fibrosis in a subset of individuals.

The mechanisms underlying the evolution of simple steatosis to NASH and/or liver cirrhosis are not yet clarified, and the progression of NAFLD is not predictable.

Nowadays, NAFLD is a major cause of cryptogenic cirrhosis, whose prevalence has increased over the last years especially in patients with a history of obesity and type 2 diabetes. NAFLD is the third most common indication for liver transplantation in the United States and is projected to eventually overtake the hepatitis C virus and alcoholic liver disease and to become the main cause of liver transplants [5].

2. Non-Alcoholic Fatty Liver Disease and Cardiovascular Disease

Prospective studies suggested that, in patients with NAFLD, cardiovascular disease (CVD) is the first cause of death [6]. Thus, atherosclerosis is the primary cause of morbidity for these subjects, and many of them will be suffering from CVD before the development of liver-related complications [7].

The association between NAFLD and CV risk has been largely investigated [8], but a definite explanation has not been provided. Among the proposed mechanisms, it has been suggested that NAFLD, especially in its more advanced forms, might act itself as a stimulus for the release of pro-atherogenic factors contributing actively to the onset of CVD [9].

The association of steatosis with different pro-atherogenic conditions is another plausible reason accounting for an increased CV risk [10]. Thus, patients with NAFLD disclosed systemic signs of atherosclerosis, such as increased carotid intima-media thickness and endothelial dysfunction [11].

Common metabolic disorders, such as dyslipidaemia, type 2 diabetes [12] and central obesity, have been associated with both simple liver steatosis and progressive NASH.

Besides, it has been also suggested that fatty liver can be considered an hepatic consequence of the insulin resistance related to the metabolic syndrome (MetS) [13,14], which is a highly pro-atherogenic condition that involves approximately 20% of the non-diabetic population in the western countries meeting the ATPIII diagnostic criteria [15].

Insulin resistance is a paramount pathophysiological moment in the MetS, and according to the "two hit" hypothesis, is also considered to play a central role in the first stage of fatty liver infiltration [16]. However, whether MetS with insulin resistance promotes fatty liver or whether NAFLD itself induces chronic hyperinsulinemia by impaired insulin degradation, is still under debate. The current opinion is that there is a strong bidirectional association between NAFLD and MetS [9].

However, not all NAFLD cases could be explained by insulin resistance; in fact, not all subjects with MetS will develop NAFLD and not all subjects with NAFLD have MetS or will develop it.

PNPLA3 and Non-Metabolic NAFLD

Patatin-like phospholipase domain-containing protein 3 (PNPLA3) is a gene encoding a lipase enzyme expressed in adipocytes. The mutation of PNPLA3, such as the PNPLA3 MM genotype, showed to be strongly associated with the presence of NAFLD and NASH [17]. Patients with PNPLA3 MM genotype do not show classical metabolic features commonly described in NAFLD patients with wild type genotype. In fact, normal peripheral and hepatic insulin sensitivity has been described in NAFLD patients with PNLPA3 mutation [18,19].

In addition, NAFLD patients with PNPLA3 mutation showed a lower CV risk compared to "metabolic" NAFLD patients, questioning as to whether NAFLD represents an independent CV risk factor.

3. Clinical Presentations of Genetic LAL Deficiency

Lysosomal Acid Lipase (LAL) deficiency is a rare autosomal recessive genetic disease characterized by the accumulation of cholesteryl esters (CE) and triglycerides in many tissues, caused by mutations of the gene encoding LAL, namely *LIPA* gene [20]. The most common *LIPA* gene mutation is the E8SJM variant, and its frequency is 0.0025 in the general population; this translates into a carrier frequency of about one in 200 in Western countries [21].

LAL deficiency is a heterogeneous disease and two main different phenotypes may be present; the Wolman Disease represents the early onset of LAL deficiency and manifests itself during the first six months of life, and it is rapidly fatal for the patient. Babies with LAL deficiency show growth retardation associated with malabsorption, hepatosplenomegaly, severe liver dysfunction, rapidly progressive anaemia and multi-organ failure. Adrenal calcification is the pathognomonic sign of Wolman Disease. The survival beyond one year of age is very rare.

Cholesterol Ester Storage Disease (CESD) is a late onset phenotype that occurs with fatty liver, elevated aminotransferase levels, hepatomegaly and dyslipidaemia characterized by elevated low-density lipoprotein cholesterol (LDL-C) and low high-density lipoprotein cholesterol (HDL-C) with or without triglyceride elevation. CESD may manifest in infancy, childhood or adulthood, and it remains often unrecognized since symptoms can overlap with other conditions. Patients have a more variable age of clinical presentation, ranging from five years to 44 years or over, and milder clinical courses [22].

The natural history and the clinical manifestations of the disease in children and adults are less well defined and the diagnosis is often incidental. Lipid abnormalities are common, and patients may present early signs of systemic atherosclerosis. Moreover, hepatomegaly and microvescicular steatosis with liver cell damage and splenomegaly are common features of the disease [23].

Clinical phenotype and the severity of LAL deficiency depend on the magnitude of the residual enzymatic activity. Therefore, finding steatosis and NASH in non-obese patients with lipid abnormalities may help in differentiating LAL deficiency from other metabolic causes of NAFLD such as MetS, type 2 diabetes, hypertriglyceridemia and central obesity [24].

4. Liver Histology in LAL Deficiency

The relationship between LAL deficiency and histological liver alterations was investigated only in subjects with CESD or Wolman Disease.

Based on available data, all patients with *LIPA* gene disorders have liver steatosis. Often, the differential diagnosis with other causes of fatty liver can be difficult and a definitive diagnosis can be done only by histological analysis of liver biopsy specimens.

In paraffin fixed specimen, the main feature is represented by a pervasive and homogeneous microvescicolar steatosis, although this aspect is not specific for CESD [23]. Conversely, in unfixed frozen samples, the finding of cholesterol ester crystals, using polarized light, is a distinctive feature of CESD [25].

Recently, Hůlková H. *et al.* [25] provided a new immunohistochemistry method to better identify CESD, in both paraffin-fixed and frozen biopsy specimen. The presence of luminal cathepsin D and membrane lysosomal markers namely lysosomal-associated membrane protein 1 and 2, and lysosomal integral membrane protein 2 around the lipid vacuoles, confirms the intra-lysosomal lipid accumulation. Moreover, the presence of macrophage with intracellular ceroid accumulation is another common histological finding in patients with CESD. The presence of this specific feature, namely ceroid induction, localized in lysosomes from macrophage, but not in those from hepatocytes, supports the diagnosis of CESD.

5. The Role of LAL in Lipid Metabolism

LAL is a key enzyme involved in intracellular lipid metabolism and trafficking; it is responsible for the intra-lysosomal hydrolysis of LDL CE and triglycerides into free cholesterol and free fatty acids [26]. Therefore, the reduction of LAL activity determines intra-lysosomal lipid accumulation and a consecutive reduction of free cholesterol in cytosol [27]. This can promote an increase of the activity of the sterol regulatory element-binding proteins (SREBPs), leading to increased lipogenesis, cholesterol biosynthesis and VLDL production. At the same time, there is also a reduction of the expression of liver X receptors (LXRs) leading to reduced efflux of cholesterol and HDL production. Therefore, abnormalities in serum lipids are induced.

The main evidence of lipid serum alterations, in LAL activity deficiency, derives from studies performed in patients with homozygous genetic disorders for *LIPA* gene.

The most common lipoprotein alterations in patients with homozygous LAL deficiency are type IIa (high LDL-C with normal triglycerides) and type IIb dyslipidaemias (high LDL-C and triglycerides), combined with low HDL-C. In these patients, dyslipidaemia has been associated with accelerated atherosclerosis. Therefore, in the presence of a type IIa dyslipidaemia, the differential diagnosis with heterozygous familial hypercholesterolemia (HeFH) is very important but not always easy to perform. The presence of family history for premature CVD and/or for hypercholesterolemia may contribute to make FH diagnosis. By contrast, in the absence of diagnostic criteria for HeFH, diagnosis of LAL deficiency should be suspected.

Further studies were carried out in heterozygous patients for *LIPA* gene mutation. A recent review on patients with different LIPA mutations [23], reported an increase of total and LDL-C, and most patients had a severe LDL-C elevation (>200 mg/dL). In 65 patients, HDL cholesterol was determined, and, in 57 of those, it was found to be reduced. Premature atherosclerosis was also documented in some patients. Based on the above study, it appears that the occurrence of lipid alterations and of accelerated atherosclerosis is similar in patients with LAL deficiency due to homozygous and heterozygous mutation of *LIPA* gene. LAL deficiency should more often be considered in dyslipidemic patients with combined hyperlipidemia and low HDL-C.

Only one study explored lipid data in patients with non-genetic LAL activity reduction. Authors reported a moderate elevation of total and LDL-C in NAFLD patients with lower LAL activity. No differences were reported in HDL-C and triglycerides.

All the above data suggest a negative correlation between LAL activity and total and LDL-C elevation.

6. The Role of LAL in Atherosclerosis

It has been recently hypothesized that changes in LAL activity could contribute to the atherosclerotic process. The formation and accumulation of foam cells within wall arteries is a key pathophysiological moment in the formation of atherosclerotic plaque [28].

Foam cells derived from oxidation of lipid products, mostly in the form of CE, that cannot be metabolized upon LDL receptor pathway and are recognized and removed by scavenger receptors expressed on macrophages and smooth muscular cells, leading to accumulation of cholesterol in these cells [27]. Thus, CE are physiologically hydrolysed in the lysosomes by LAL to generate free cholesterol, which, after being re-esterified in the endoplasmic reticulum, can form cytosolic lipid droplets. The accumulation of free cholesterol in lysosomes during the atherosclerotic process could inhibit LAL activity, causing accumulation of CE in cells. LAL is also present within the extracellular space of atherosclerotic intima [29].

Physiopathology findings have been confirmed by interventional studies on mice with recombinant human LAL, in which a reversal of atherosclerotic lesions have been observed [27].

7. Who Should Be Tested for LAL Activity?

LAL activity reduction should always be suspected in non-obese patients presenting with NAFLD and/or cryptogenic cirrhosis, unexplained persistently elevated liver transaminases or with elevation in LDL-C and decreased HDL-C (Table 1). An accurate anamnesis is necessary to exclude potential causes contributing to fatty liver, such as viral causes, alcohol abuse or the presence of familial hypercholesterolemia [24].

In these patients, it could be indicated to test LAL activity, using the dried blood spot (DBS) test. The DBS is a simple test used to determine LAL activity by comparing total lipase activity to lipase activity in the presence of a highly specific inhibitor (Lalistat 2) of LAL. It allows the differentiation of healthy subjects from affected individuals. All patients with LAL reduction ($\leq$0.40 nmol/spot/h) detected by DBS should perform genetic tests to detect LAL gene mutations [30].

Table 1. Clinical suspicion of lysosomal acid lipase (LAL) reduction.

Who Should Be Tested for LAL Activity?
Patients with unexplained:
•Liver Dysfunction ($\geq$1 of the following)
Persistent elevation of ALT
Presence of hepatomegaly
Hepatic steatosis
AND/OR
•Dislipidemia ($\geq$1 of the following)
High LDL-C ($\geq$160 mg/dL–4.1 mmol/L)
Low HDL-C ($\leq$40 mg/dL–1.0 mmol/L in males; $\leq$50 mg/dL–1.3 mmol/L in females)

8. Current Research Status on LAL Activity and NAFLD

Very few studies have been performed so far to assess LAL activity in representative samples of normal adult subjects or patients with NAFLD. Moreover, no large study has been carried out in adult subjects with NAFLD, and prevalence of *LIPA* gene mutation in this setting is unknown. Only one study investigated the clinical phenotype of patients with heterozygous mutations for *LIPA* genes. However, this study was focused only on lipid panel results and did not show data about hepatic condition or about other biochemical values [21].

In vitro, it has been demonstrated that several factors may modulate LAL activity [31]. In particular, enhanced LAL activity was associated with eicosanoids, gonadotropins and glucagon, and reduced activity was correlated with Lp(a), LDL remnants and oxidized LDL concentrations.

We recently reported, for the first time, reduced blood LAL activity in adult patients with NAFLD [32]. LAL activity was significantly reduced in 240 patients with NAFLD, as compared to 100 adult subjects [0.78 (0.61–1.01) *vs.* 1.15 (0.94–1.72) nmol/spot/h, $p < 0.001$]. NAFLD patients with LAL activity below median had higher values of serum total cholesterol ($p < 0.05$) and LDL-C ($p < 0.05$), and increased serum liver enzymes (ALT, $p < 0.001$; AST, $p < 0.01$; GGT, $p < 0.01$). We also observed a progressive decrease of LAL activity from patients with simple steatosis [0.84 (0.62–1.08) nmol/spot/h, $p < 0.001$ *vs.* HS] to those with biopsy-proven NASH [0.67 (0.51–0.77) nmol/spot/h, $p < 0.001$ *vs.* HS; $p < 0.001$, among groups].

However, at present, there are no data on certain epigenetic modulation of LAL activity *in vivo* models. Thus, studies are needed to better clarify mechanisms of epigenetic modulation of LAL activity and their potential role as therapeutic targets. For example, we do not know if an intervention on modifiable cardio-metabolic risk factors typically associated with NAFLD, such as metabolic syndrome, overweight, increased oxidative stress, may have a role in modulating LAL activity.

In addition, it is not known if the improvement in LAL activity may translate into a reduction of fatty liver content in adult NAFLD patients.

9. Future Directions

Altogether these data indicated that modifications in LAL activity are associated with dyslipidaemia and liver dysfunction [21]. In fact, both serum lipoprotein alterations and NAFLD are common and share many possible pathophysiological mechanisms. Moreover, it is not surprising that LAL activity reduction could be also an unrecognized contributing factor in the development and progression of NAFLD to cryptogenic cirrhosis.

Therefore, the identification of clinical and metabolic risk factors, especially those modifiable, which are able to modulate LAL activity, may have important clinical implications for the management of patients with NAFLD. Moreover, future research should also address epigenetic modulation of LAL activity and also take into consideration the effect of drug treatments. This would be particularly important to better understand the contribution of LAL in the complex scenario of NAFLD.

Recently, Burton BK *et al.* reported an impressive reduction of hepatic fat content as assessed by means of magnetic resonance imaging in patients with severe LAL deficiency treated for 20 weeks with enzyme replacement therapy with Sebelipase alfa [33]. These findings were paralleled by improvement in serum liver enzymes and lipid levels. The study was carried out in subjects with confirmed enzyme activity-based diagnosis performed by dried blood spots using the inhibitor Lalistat 2. Almost 50% of patients had bridging fibrosis at liver biopsy and 31% had cirrhosis.

These findings, together with those showing low LAL activity in patients with NAFLD and NASH [32], suggest a strong association between impaired LAL activity and fatty liver pathogenesis and progression. Thus, LAL activity seems to be linked to NAFLD through several mechanisms including lipid metabolism alterations, intra-hepatic fat accumulation and pro-atherosclerotic functions (Figure 1).

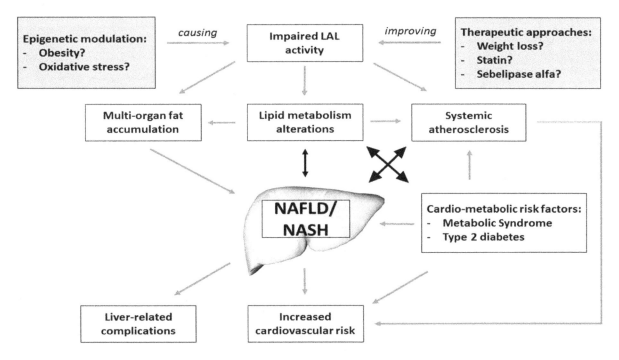

Figure 1. Putative mechanisms linking impaired LAL activity and NAFLD/NASH.

Finally, we speculate that LAL activity reduction may become a possible new target for the treatment of NAFLD. In fact, enzyme-replacement therapy may soon be available. This treatment will be indicated for patients with more severe, genetic LAL deficiency, where treatment will be lifesaving. However, in a recent clinical trial lead on CESD patients, treatment with sebelipase was associated with a significant reduction in fatty liver content in almost all treated patients [33]. Based on this evidence, we may speculate that, in the future, enzyme-replacement therapy could be also indicated for less severe LAL deficiency, especially in patients with more advanced forms of NAFLD, such as those with NASH or cryptogenic cirrhosis. Therefore, we believe that it is important to test NAFLD patients for LAL activity to identify a subgroup of patients at higher risk for liver disease progression.

Author Contributions: Francesco Baratta, Licia Polimeni, Giulia Tozzi and Daniele Pastori drafted the article or revised it critically. Maria Del Ben, Francesco Violi and Francesco Angelico gave final approval of the version to be published.

References

1.   Vernon, G.; Baranova, A.; Younossi, Z.M. Systematic review: The epidemiology and natural history of non-alcoholic fatty liver disease and non-alcoholic steatohepatitis in adults. *Aliment. Pharmacol. Ther.* **2011**, *34*, 274–285. [CrossRef] [PubMed]

2.   Kawano, Y.; Cohen, D.E. Mechanisms of hepatic triglyceride accumulation in non-alcoholic fatty liver disease. *J. Gastroenterol.* **2013**, *48*, 434–441. [CrossRef] [PubMed]

3.   Takaki, A.; Kawai, D.; Yamamoto, K. Multiple hits, including oxidative stress, as pathogenesis and treatment target in non-alcoholic steatohepatitis (NASH). *Int. J. Mol. Sci.* **2013**, *14*, 20704–20728. [CrossRef] [PubMed]

4.   Pastori, D.; Baratta, F.; Carnevale, R.; Cangemi, R.; del Ben, M.; Bucci, T.; Polimeni, L.; Labbadia, G.; Nocella, C.; Scardella, L.; *et al.* Similar reduction of cholesterol-adjusted vitamin e serum levels in simple steatosis and non-alcoholic steatohepatitis. *Clin. Transl. Gastroenterol.* **2015**, *6*, e113. [CrossRef] [PubMed]

5.   Kemmer, N.; Neff, G.W.; Franco, E.; Osman-Mohammed, H.; Leone, J.; Parkinson, E.; Cece, E.; Alsina, A. Nonalcoholic fatty liver disease epidemic and its implications for liver transplantation. *Transplantation* **2013**, *96*, 860–862. [CrossRef] [PubMed]

6.   Soderberg, C.; Stal, P.; Askling, J.; Glaumann, H.; Lindberg, G.; Marmur, J.; Hultcrantz, R. Decreased survival of subjects with elevated liver function tests during a 28-year follow-up. *Hepatology* **2010**, *51*, 595–602. [CrossRef] [PubMed]

7.   Ballestri, S.; Lonardo, A.; Bonapace, S.; Byrne, C.D.; Loria, P.; Targher, G. Risk of cardiovascular, cardiac and arrhythmic complications in patients with non-alcoholic fatty liver disease. *World J. Gastroenterol.* **2014**, *20*, 1724–1745. [CrossRef] [PubMed]

8.   Bhatia, L.S.; Curzen, N.P.; Calder, P.C.; Byrne, C.D. Non-alcoholic fatty liver disease: A new and important cardiovascular risk factor? *Eur. Heart J.* **2012**, *33*, 1190–1200. [CrossRef] [PubMed]

9.   Del Ben, M.; Baratta, F.; Polimeni, L.; Angelico, F. Non-alcoholic fatty liver disease and cardiovascular disease: Epidemiological, clinical and pathophysiological evidences. *Internal Emerg. Med.* **2012**, *7*, S291–S296. [CrossRef] [PubMed]

10.   Sookoian, S.; Castano, G.O.; Burgueno, A.L.; Rosselli, M.S.; Gianotti, T.F.; Mallardi, P.; Martino, J.S.; Pirola, C.J. Circulating levels and hepatic expression of molecular mediators of atherosclerosis in nonalcoholic fatty liver disease. *Atherosclerosis* **2010**, *209*, 585–591. [CrossRef] [PubMed]

11.   Pastori, D.; Loffredo, L.; Perri, L.; Baratta, F.; Scardella, L.; Polimeni, L.; Pani, A.; Brancorsini, M.; Albanese, F.; Catasca, E.; *et al.* Relation of nonalcoholic fatty liver disease and framingham risk score to flow-mediated dilation in patients with cardiometabolic risk factors. *Am. J. Cardiol.* **2015**, *115*, 1402–1406. [CrossRef] [PubMed]

12.   Targher, G.; Bertolini, L.; Padovani, R.; Rodella, S.; Tessari, R.; Zenari, L.; Day, C.; Arcaro, G. Prevalence of nonalcoholic fatty liver disease and its association with cardiovascular disease among type 2 diabetic patients. *Diabetes Care* **2007**, *30*, 1212–1218. [CrossRef] [PubMed]

13.   Targher, G.; Marra, F.; Marchesini, G. Increased risk of cardiovascular disease in non-alcoholic fatty liver disease: Causal effect or epiphenomenon? *Diabetologia* **2008**, *51*, 1947–1953. [CrossRef] [PubMed]

14.   Marchesini, G.; Bugianesi, E.; Forlani, G.; Cerrelli, F.; Lenzi, M.; Manini, R.; Natale, S.; Vanni, E.; Villanova, N.; Melchionda, N.; *et al.* Nonalcoholic fatty liver, steatohepatitis, and the metabolic syndrome. *Hepatology* **2003**, *37*, 917–923. [CrossRef] [PubMed]

15.   Del Ben, M.; Polimeni, L.; Baratta, F.; Pastori, D.; Loffredo, L.; Angelico, F. Modern approach to the clinical management of non-alcoholic fatty liver disease. *World J. Gastroenterol.* **2014**, *20*, 8341–8350. [PubMed]

16.   Day, C.P.; James, O.F. Steatohepatitis: A tale of two "hits"? *Gastroenterology* **1998**, *114*, 842–845. [CrossRef]

17. Wood, K.L.; Miller, M.H.; Dillon, J.F. Systematic review of genetic association studies involving histologically confirmed non-alcoholic fatty liver disease. *BMJ Open Gastroenterol.* **2015**, *2*, e000019. [CrossRef] [PubMed]

18. Del Ben, M.; Polimeni, L.; Brancorsini, M.; di Costanzo, A.; D'Erasmo, L.; Baratta, F.; Loffredo, L.; Pastori, D.; Pignatelli, P.; Violi, F.; *et al.* Non-alcoholic fatty liver disease, metabolic syndrome and patatin-like phospholipase domain-containing protein3 gene variants. *Eur. J. Intern. Med.* **2014**, *25*, 566–570. [CrossRef] [PubMed]

19. Della Corte, C.; Fintini, D.; Giordano, U.; Cappa, M.; Brufani, C.; Majo, F.; Mennini, C.; Nobili, V. Fatty liver and insulin resistance in children with hypobetalipoproteinemia: The importance of aetiology. *Clin. Endocrinol.* **2013**, *79*, 49–54. [CrossRef] [PubMed]

20. Thelwall, P.E.; Smith, F.E.; Leavitt, M.C.; Canty, D.; Hu, W.; Hollingsworth, K.G.; Thoma, C.; Trenell, M.I.; Taylor, R.; Rutkowski, J.V.; *et al.* Hepatic cholesteryl ester accumulation in lysosomal acid lipase deficiency: Non-invasive identification and treatment monitoring by magnetic resonance. *J. Hepatol.* **2013**, *59*, 543–549. [CrossRef] [PubMed]

21. Muntoni, S.; Wiebusch, H.; Jansen-Rust, M.; Rust, S.; Schulte, H.; Berger, K.; Pisciotta, L.; Bertolini, S.; Funke, H.; Seedorf, U.; *et al.* Heterozygosity for lysosomal acid lipase E8SJM mutation and serum lipid concentrations. *Nutr. Metab. Cardiovasc. Dis.* **2013**, *23*, 732–736. [CrossRef] [PubMed]

22. Pisciotta, L.; Fresa, R.; Bellocchio, A.; Pino, E.; Guido, V.; Cantafora, A.; di Rocco, M.; Calandra, S.; Bertolini, S. Cholesteryl ester storage disease (CESD) due to novel mutations in the LIPA gene. *Mol. Genet. Metab.* **2009**, *97*, 143–148. [CrossRef] [PubMed]

23. Bernstein, D.L.; Hulkova, H.; Bialer, M.G.; Desnick, R.J. Cholesteryl ester storage disease: Review of the findings in 135 reported patients with an underdiagnosed disease. *J. Hepatol.* **2013**, *58*, 1230–1243. [CrossRef] [PubMed]

24. Reiner, Z.; Guardamagna, O.; Nair, D.; Soran, H.; Hovingh, K.; Bertolini, S.; Jones, S.; Coric, M.; Calandra, S.; Hamilton, J.; *et al.* Lysosomal acid lipase deficiency—An under-recognized cause of dyslipidaemia and liver dysfunction. *Atherosclerosis* **2014**, *235*, 21–30. [CrossRef] [PubMed]

25. Hulkova, H.; Elleder, M. Distinctive histopathological features that support a diagnosis of cholesterol ester storage disease in liver biopsy specimens. *Histopathology* **2012**, *60*, 1107–1113. [CrossRef] [PubMed]

26. Fasano, T.; Pisciotta, L.; Bocchi, L.; Guardamagna, O.; Assandro, P.; Rabacchi, C.; Zanoni, P.; Filocamo, M.; Bertolini, S.; Calandra, S. Lysosomal lipase deficiency: Molecular characterization of eleven patients with wolman or cholesteryl ester storage disease. *Mol. Genet. Metab.* **2012**, *105*, 450–456. [CrossRef] [PubMed]

27. Dubland, J.A.; Francis, G.A. Lysosomal acid lipase: At the crossroads of normal and atherogenic cholesterol metabolism. *Front. Cell Dev. Biol.* **2015**, *3*, 3. [CrossRef] [PubMed]

28. Stocker, R.; Keaney, J.F., Jr. Role of oxidative modifications in atherosclerosis. *Physiol. Rev.* **2004**, *84*, 1381–1478. [CrossRef] [PubMed]

29. Hakala, J.K.; Oksjoki, R.; Laine, P.; Du, H.; Grabowski, G.A.; Kovanen, P.T.; Pentikainen, M.O. Lysosomal enzymes are released from cultured human macrophages, hydrolyze LDL *in vitro*, and are present extracellularly in human atherosclerotic lesions. *Arterioscler. Thromb. Vasc. Biol.* **2003**, *23*, 1430–1436. [CrossRef] [PubMed]

30. Hamilton, J.; Jones, I.; Srivastava, R.; Galloway, P. A new method for the measurement of lysosomal acid lipase in dried blood spots using the inhibitor lalistat 2. *Clin. Chim. Acta* **2012**, *413*, 1207–1210. [CrossRef] [PubMed]

31. Zschenker, O.; Illies, T.; Ameis, D. Overexpression of lysosomal acid lipase and other proteins in atherosclerosis. *J. Biochem.* **2006**, *140*, 23–38. [CrossRef] [PubMed]

32. Baratta, F.; Pastori, D.; del Ben, M.; Polimeni, L.; Labbadia, G.; di Santo, S.; Piemonte, F.; Tozzi, G.; Violi, F.; Angelico, F. Reduced lysosomal acid lipase activity in adult patients with non-alcoholic fatty liver disease. *EBioMedicine* **2015**, *2*, 750–754. [CrossRef] [PubMed]

33. Burton, B.K.; Balwani, M.; Feillet, F.; Baric, I.; Burrow, T.A.; Camarena Grande, C.; Coker, M.; Deegan, P.; Consuelo-Sanchez, A.; di Rocco, M.; *et al.* A phase 3 trial of sebelipase alfa in lysosomal acid lipase deficiency. *N. Engl. J. Med.* **2015**, *373*, 1010–1020. [CrossRef] [PubMed]

6

Nonalcoholic Fatty Liver Disease: Pros and Cons of Histologic Systems of Evaluation

Elizabeth M. Brunt

Department of Pathology and Immunology, Washington University School of Medicine, Campus Box 8118, St. Louis, MO 63110, USA; ebrunt@wustl.edu

Academic Editors: Amedeo Lonardo and Giovanni Targher

Abstract: The diagnostic phenotype of nonalcoholic fatty liver disease (NAFLD)—in particular, the most significant form in terms of prognosis, nonalcoholic steatohepatitis (NASH)—continues to rely on liver tissue evaluation, in spite of remarkable advances in non-invasive algorithms developed from serum-based tests and imaging-based or sonographically-based tests for fibrosis or liver stiffness. The most common tissue evaluation remains percutaneous liver biopsy; considerations given to the needle size and the location of the biopsy have the potential to yield the most representative tissue for evaluation. The pathologist's efforts are directed to not only global diagnosis, but also assessment of severity of injury. Just as in other forms of chronic liver disease, these assessments can be divided into necroinflammatory activity, and fibrosis with parenchymal remodeling, in order to separately analyze potentially reversible (grade) and non-reversible (stage) lesions. These concepts formed the bases for current methods of evaluating the lesions that collectively comprise the phenotypic spectra of NAFLD. Four extant methods have specific applications; there are pros and cons to each, and this forms the basis of the review.

Keywords: nonalcoholic fatty liver disease; nonalcoholic steatohepatitis; pathology

1. Introduction

The value of liver biopsy evaluation for diagnosis in clinical care and effectiveness of intervention in clinical research in the field of nonalcoholic fatty liver disease (NAFLD) has remained unquestioned as knowledge in the field has continued to grow over the course of the last three and a half decades since the publication attributed as one of the early descriptions in humans [1]. Currently several clinical algorithms based on serum-based tests can be used to predict the likelihood of NAFLD, nonalcoholic steatohepatitis (NASH) or presence or severity of fibrosis, reviewed [2]. As well, sonographically-based tests of liver "stiffness" and imaging-based tests for presence of hepatic fat are variably validated and becoming more available [3]. The unquestioned value of all non-invasive testing is for patient follow-up; in sophisticated hands, these tests also play a role in determination of need for liver biopsy, as the latter, an invasive test with known low but potential risk of morbidity cannot be utilized as a screening test [4]. The best noninvasive tests have been developed and validated against the "gold-standard" of liver biopsy in order to produce equivalent information regarding the state of the liver parenchyma.

Liver biopsy cannot be considered a "perfect" test, however, but the short-comings of this can largely be overcome once understood. For instance, the consideration of sampling "error" [5] was detailed in a study in 2005 that demonstrated differences in grade and stage by the blinded pathologist even when biopsies were obtained from the identical location. However, as in most chronic liver diseases, this "error" is likely a reflection of the disease heterogeneity of NAFLD, and must be accounted for by providing sufficient numbers of subjects in clinical trials. Another less well-known short-coming of liver biopsy, particularly when done by radiologists, or in the setting of bariatric surgery, is the use of appropriately sized (*i.e.*, large-bore) needles, [6], and potential differences between the right and left lobes of the liver. For instance, the subcapsular portal tracts in the left lobe are larger and closer to the capsule than in the right lobe; if not aware of this, a pathologist can misinterpret the seemingly enlarged portal structures from a left lobe biopsy for fibrotic portal structures, particularly if a small bore needle has been used to obtain the biopsy. Determining histologic inflammation in the liver parenchyma will not lead to valid results from a biopsy obtained in a surgical procedure, as anesthesia alone will lead to parenchymal and perivenular collections of polymorphonuclear leukocytes, collectively known as "surgical hepatitis". Discerning which foci were present prior to anesthesia, and which are due to surgical hepatitis is not possible. Further, if a study protocol includes biopsy, agreement of exact location should be made in advance with all investigators so that pre and post intervention biopsies are truly comparable. Finally, the interpreting pathologist's expertise and familiarity with the spectra of lesions in the disease process are factors to be considered in NAFLD, as in any other form of liver disease [7,8].

Once the decision for liver biopsy has been made, whether for clinical (*i.e.*, diagnostic or prognostic) purposes, or for clinical trial protocol, the next steps involve the histopathologic interpretation for diagnosis, and for semi-quantitative lesion evaluations, if requested, for protocol or study purposes. Methods for these are the subjects of the remainder of this review.

2. Diagnosing Fatty Liver Disease in Liver Biopsy

Before any form of assessment of severity of injury or fibrosis can be applied, the pathologist must be certain that the biopsy actually is diagnostic of the clinically presumptive disease; this basic exercise applies to all forms of liver disease. NAFLD is an umbrella term applied to a range of histopathologic phenotypes in adults, adolescents and children. It is important that the pathologist report is limited to the findings noted, and count on the clinical team to put these together with all information regarding possible etiologies that may present in a similar manner, including, for instance, Wilson disease, other inborn errors of metabolism, and alcoholic liver disease. Discussed in detail in recent reviews [9], they will be briefly summarized herein. In adults, prior to advanced fibrosis and parenchymal remodeling (nodularity), the parenchyma shows varying degrees of steatosis within the zone 3 hepatocytes (those around the terminal hepatic venule). The large and small droplet steatosis is termed macrovesicular due to the fact it is either a single large droplet or several droplets readily separable to the microscopic eye. Often, the two are co-existent in the same hepatocyte. Thus, the term, "large and small droplet macrovesicular steatosis" is applied. When only steatosis is present in the biopsy, the diagnostic term, NAFL, is given. For this, >5% of hepatocytes within the biopsy must be occupied by this type of visible fat droplets. In a minority of cases, non-zonal clusters of hepatocytes also have true microvesicular steatosis; an association was noted with greater severity of disease in these cases in a large series from the NASH Clinical Research Network (CRN) [10]. The terminal "D" of NAFLD is removed by convention, as steatosis is considered non-progressive, although exceptions have been noted in subjects, most of whom subsequently gain weight or the metabolic status changed [11,12].

The second component of NAFLD is inflammatory cells; these may be seen within the acini (aka lobules), or in portal tracts, or both. The inflammatory components of this disease are quite complex, but with the routine hematoxylin and eosin stain to the pathologist's view microscopically, can be divided into mononuclear cells (lymphocytes, monocytes), eosinophils, polymorphonuclear cells (pmn's), and Kupffer cells. Even occasional plasma cells can be noted. Kupffer cells are pigmented, enlarged and either singly or in clusters surrounding an apoptotic hepatocyte (microgranuloma) or a fat droplet (lipogranuloma). Lipogranulomas often have an associated eosinophilic leukocyte, and when adjacent to a terminal hepatic venule or within a portal tract, may also have collagen. Epithelioid or caseating granulomatous inflammation are not features of NAFLD, and deserve further attention. Pmn's surrounding individual hepatocytes, referred to as "satellitosis", are indicative of alcoholic hepatitis; clusters of pmn's signify possible sepsis or may occur if the biopsy is obtained during a surgical procedure when the patient is under anesthesia. Thus, caution is warranted when pmn clusters are easily noted; attempting to "count" inflammatory foci in such a specimen is not advisable.

Portal inflammation consists of similar cell types as described above (except the macrophages are not Kupffer cells) in varying degrees, including lipogranulomas. Other types of granulomatous inflammation should be further evaluated. Bile duct injury may be seen, but should be further evaluated. Marked portal inflammation and lymphoid aggregates, diffuse interface activity, and plasma-cell rich infiltrates are all lesions that deserve further investigation. Numerous polymorphonuclear leukocytes, when present, are typically present as cholangitis, cholangiolitis/pericholangitis and indicate an extra-hepatic biliary process such as obstruction or pancreatitis, or alcoholic liver disease. Canalicular bile plugs in zone 3 correlate with these findings and warrant further investigation. Cholangiolar bile is indicative of sepsis. The combination of macrovesicular steatosis and inflammation has been termed steatosis with inflammation; this is not, however, diagnostic of steatohepatitis.

2.1. Nonalcoholic Steatohepatitis (NASH)

For the diagnosis of NASH, the most recognized form of injury in NAFLD with potential to progress to fibrosis and cirrhosis and its complications, there is a requirement not only for the steatosis and inflammation as described above, but also for a particular form of hepatocyte injury known as ballooning. While some authorities have stated that steatosis with inflammation and perisinusoidal fibrosis are adequate for a diagnosis of steatohepatitis, it is not clear that this group of findings represents a lesion with actual potential of progression, or represents a step in regression of steatohepatitis (i.e., loss of ballooning). The NASH CRN Pathology Committee categorizes this within a set of lesions as "Borderline, Zone 3", and specifies that hepatocellular ballooning must be present for a diagnosis of steatohepatitis. NASH can be diagnosed in the absence of fibrosis. The initial collagen deposition in adult NASH is in the perisinusoidal spaces in zone 3; with progression, fibrosis is additionally noted in periportal spaces, often associated with a ductular reaction. More advanced fibrosis is indicated by bridging between vascular structures: central veins to central veins (via perisinusoidal spaces); central–portal; portal–portal; with nodularity of the intervening parenchyma. Cirrhosis is the final outcome of advanced fibrosis and remodeling. Residual perisinusoidal fibrosis may or may not remain.

An intriguing and important concept in NASH is that with advanced disease, i.e., fibrosis and architectural remodeling with bridging fibrosis and nodularity, and ultimately the vascular remodeling of cirrhosis, the lesions of activity described above may or may not continue to be present. Investigators have used this information to justify a correlation with the assignment of the diagnosis of "cryptogenic cirrhosis" to cases in which no identifying lesions of active liver disease can be found. In a strict sense, however, without a prior biopsy diagnosis of NASH, this may not be correct in all cases. Many cases of cryptogenic cirrhosis, in fact, may be burned-out cirrhosis from other causes such as prior alcohol abuse, autoimmune hepatitis, heterozygous α-1-antitrypsin liver disease, or even more rare processes (e.g., keratin mutations). However, there are bona fide cases of burned-out NASH in which there remain histologic "hints": e.g., foci of perisinusoidal fibrosis, occasional ballooned hepatocytes, rare Mallory–Denk bodies in a non-alcohol user. If there is a prior biopsy with NASH, the "burned-out" cirrhosis is no longer "cryptogenic", but is cirrhosis secondary to prior NASH.

2.2. Pediatric Nonalcoholic Fatty Liver Disease (NAFLD)

Pediatric NAFLD is known to be unique in its pre-cirrhotic histopathologic features. This has been accepted since the seminal descriptions of Schwimmer et al. in 2005 [13], and validated subsequently by others. Interestingly, as of yet, there is no accepted diagnosis of "steatohepatitis" in children, although clearly the end results, cirrhosis and hepatocellular carcinoma, do occur. The initial findings in children are of large droplet macrovesicular steatosis either in a periportal or panacinar distribution and when inflammation is present, it is more common in the portal collagen than in the lobules. Ballooned hepatocytes are few if any. Portal expansion by fibrosis occurs initially, and perisinusoidal fibrosis may or may never be seen. The categorization of Borderline, Zone 1 has been utilized by the NASH CRN for the above-described lesions.

3. Grading and Staging the Lesions of NAFLD

Four current methods of semi-quantitatively evaluating histologic lesions of NAFLD are summarized in Table 1; they include a proposal referred to as the "Brunt" system [14], the NASH CRN Pathology Committee system for NAFLD Activity Score (NAS) and fibrosis score [15], the "Fatty Liver Inhibition of Progression (FLIP)" algorithm [16,17] and a pediatric score based on weighted values for the features of NAFLD, the Pediatric NAFLD Histologic Score [18]. The first was restricted to adults and to NASH; the middle two can apply to the full range of NAFLD; the NASH CRN system alone applies to adults and children.

3.1. Brunt Proposal for Grading and Staging

The proposal for grading and staging the lesions of NASH was made when the disease itself was still being questioned as an entity other than surreptitious alcoholism; it was clear that further work would not progress until a systematic method of analyzing the pathology was in place. Thus, this proposal was just that: a first proposed method to separately analyze grade and stage, similarly to what was being done with other forms of chronic hepatitis, but with adjustments for the lesions of fatty liver disease [14]. There was systematic review of 52 adult biopsies from 51 clinically diagnosed subjects with NASH with semi-quantitative assessment and notation of location of steatosis, and ballooning; semi-quantitative assessment for lobular and portal inflammation and Periodic Acid Schiff after diastase digestion (PASd) Kupffer cells, Mallory–Denk bodies, acidophil bodies, iron, and glycogenated nuclei, lipogranulomas and locations of fibrosis, zone 3 perisinusoidal, portal/periportal, and bridging. "Gestalt" diagnosis of severity of each case (mild, moderate, severe) then followed. The "global grade" was based on review of the semi-quantitative lesions and impression-based grades, and focused in particular on steatosis, hepatocellular ballooning, zone 3 accentuation of injury. It was noted that the initial, and often persistent form of fibrosis is perisinusoidal; this differs from the distinctly portal-based fibrosis of chronic hepatitis and biliary fibrosis. The so-called "Brunt" method continued the paradigm of maintaining separation of grade (lesions of activity) and stage (lesions of fibrosis and parenchymal remodeling), as had been established by the systems for evaluation in chronic hepatitis [19]. The method of grading and staging was written to be applied after the diagnosis of NASH had been rendered, and was considered a "global" assessment such that grades 1–3, mild, moderate and severe, were evaluations of combinations of steatosis, lobular and portal inflammation and ballooning. Hepatocyte ballooning was noted as the major determinant of severity and steatosis amount was the least determinant; inflammation increased with each grade. Fibrosis was scored according to the observed location and extent of collagen deposition as described above. Grade and stage were noted to be disparate, as in chronic hepatitis although none of the low stage biopsies showed severe steatohepatitis. Higher grade did correlate with higher mean aspartate aminotransferase (AST), but not with alanine aminotransferase (ALT). This system was created for NASH, and thus did not take into account the full spectrum of NAFLD, nor did the system address lesions of pediatric NAFLD. Although the system has been widely utilized and applied, it was never formally validated. It is, however, a useful benchmark for diagnosing NASH as it highlighted the increasing severity of ballooning with increased severity of grade. This proposal also documented the characteristic fibrosis of adult NASH.

Table 1. Histologic methods of semi-quantitative evaluation of nonalcoholic fatty liver disease (NAFLD).

System/Characteristics	Brunt System [14]	NASH CRN [15]	*SAF/** FLIP Algorithm [16,17]	Pediatric NAFLD Histologic Score [18]
Patient Population	Adults only	Adults + Children	Adults	Children
Applicable to	NASH	All NAFLD	All NAFLD	Peds NAFLD
Grade	Mild, Moderate, Severe; S + LI, PI + B; Unweighted but steatosis does not affect score; LI + PI, ballooning increase incrementally with score	NAFLD Activity Score (NAS): S + LI + B = 0–8; Unweighted scores for each lesion	Steatosis is not a component of activity Activity: LI + B; * SAF: Steatosis + Activity + Fibrosis = $S_x A_x F_x$; ** FLIP: Fatty Liver Inhibition of Progression algorithm for diagnosis	Weighted sums of S + LI + PI + B, see text
	Steatosis 0: 0 1: 0%–33% 2: 34%–66% 3: >66%	Steatosis 0: <5% 1: 5%–33% 2: 34%–66% 3: >67%	Steatosis 0: <5% 1: 5%–33% 2: 34%–66% 3: >67%	
	LI 0:0 1: 1–2/20x 2: 2–4/20X 3: >4/20x	LI 0:0 1: <2/20x 2: 2–4/20X 3: >4/20X	LI 0: 0 1: <2/20x 2: 2/20x –	Same as NASH CRN plus Portal Inflammation 0–2
Details of Scoring	PI: 0: none 1: mild 2: moderate 3: severe	Ballooning; 0: None 1: Few 2: Many –	Ballooning; 0–2 0: 0 1: clusters, reticulated cytoplasm 2: enlarged hepatocytes –	
	Ballooning	Prominent	–	
	Acinar location	–	–	
	Mild	–	–	
	Marked	–	–	
	Fibrosis Stage 0: none 1: zone 3 perisinusoidal 2: 1 + periportal 3: bridging 4: cirrhosis	Fibrosis Stage 0: none 1a: zone 3 perisinusoidal, delicate 1b: zone 3 perisinusoidal, dense 1c: portal only 2: 1a or 1b + periportal 3: bridging 4: cirrhosis	Fibrosis Stage F0: 0 F1: zone 3 perisinusoidal (all), or portal only F2: zone 3 + periportal F3: bridging F4: cirrhosis	Fibrosis Stage: As with NASH CRN

Table 1. *Cont.*

System/Characteristics	Brunt System [14]	NASH CRN [15]	* SAF/** FLIP Algorithm [16,17]	Pediatric NAFLD Histologic Score [18]
Fibrosis Stages	0–4	0–4; # 1a, 1b, 1c	0–4; # 1a, 1b, 1c	0–4
Scoring Method Used for diagnosis	Minimal criteria for dx	Correlates but does not replace; used in clinical trials for feature comparisons	Yes, for diagnosis	Yes, for diagnosis
Clinical Associations	Grade: AST	ALT, AST	AST, ALT	WC, MetSynd, TG, Fibrosis in biopsy

S = steatosis amount; LI = lobular inflammation; PI = portal inflammation; B = ballooning; # 1a, 1b, 1c: see text. ALT = alanine aminotransferase; AST = aspartate aminotransferase; WC = Waist circumference; MetSynd = Metabolic Syndrome; TG = triglyceride levels.

3.2. NASH Clinical Research Network (CRN) Scoring System

The National Institute of Digestive Diseases and Kidney (NIDDK) of the National Institutes of Health (NIH) established the NASH Clinical Research Network (CRN) in order to undertake multicenter observational and interventional trials. The Pathology Committee was tasked with developing and validating a method for semi-quantitatively evaluating changes in histologic features in these studies. The result was a feature-based system referred to commonly as the NAFLD Activity Score (NAS) [15]. This is a score for lesions of activity based on carefully analyzed results of 32 twice-reviewed biopsies of adults and 18 once reviewed biopsies of children by a group of 9 liver pathologists. The review consisted of 14 lesions of NAFLD (the same as above in similar fashion, plus presence of foci of microvesicular steatosis, megamitochondria, and microgranulomas) and three diagnostic categories: NASH, not NASH and borderline. The lesions that ultimately comprised the NAS were determined by multiple logistic regression to correspond with the separately derived diagnoses of NASH: macrovesicular steatosis, lobular inflammation and ballooning. The final NAS was based on unweighted scores of each, and ranged from 0 to 8. As noted in Table 1, although the lesion scores are unweighted, the fact that steatosis and lobular inflammation range from 0 to 3 whereas ballooning range from 0 to 2, gives steatosis more weight in the NAS. The separately derived diagnoses of NASH mostly correlated with scores ⩾5; NAS < 3 had been diagnosed as not NASH. Fibrosis stage was a modification of the Brunt system in order to account for pediatric portal-only fibrosis (stage 1c); zone 3 delicate (1a) or dense (1b) fibrosis were created for the purpose of clinical trials. The manuscript that presented the NAS described other observations of importance that remain relevant today: the diagnosis does not rest solely on the presence of particular lesions; the score was not created to replace a pathologist's diagnosis or as a severity scale or to measure rapidity of progression, but rather as a method of analysis in assessing overall histologic change. A subsequent study of 976 centrally reviewed adult biopsies from the NASH CRN highlighted the significance of separating the pattern-based pathologists' activity of diagnosis from the feature-based score [20]. Although there was significant overlap between the diagnosis and the NAS, some details are worth re-iterating. While 75% of definite steatohepatitis cases had NAS ⩾ 5, 28% of borderline diagnoses and 7% of "not NASH" also had NAS ⩾ 5. Thus, for clinical trial entry, or for clinical management, if the NAS were the basis of decision making, the latter and last cases would be "mis-categorized". Further, and of most importance, in a regression model, while both the diagnosis of steatohepatitis and the NAS were statistically strongly associated with liver enzymes (ALT and AST) in both the one variable (either NAS or NASH diagnosis) and two variable (both NAS and NASH diagnosis) models, and features of Metabolic Syndrome, diabetes, and measures of insulin resistance, the homeostatic model assessment of insulin resistance and the quantitative insulin sensitivity check index (HOMA-IR and QUICKI) were associated with both in the one variable model, these latter features only remained statistically associated with the diagnosis of steatohepatitis in the two variable model. Thus, the implication is strong that not only are the particular histologic features of steatohepatitis important, but the overall pattern of those features (*i.e.*, the determination of diagnosis) is important in correlation with liver injury, as well as underlying factors of the disease process.

3.3. Fatty Liver Inhibition of Progression (FLIP) Algorithm

A third approach to adult NAFLD scoring has been proposed and validated by Bedossa *et al.* [17]; the score was developed in 679 liver biopsies from morbidly obese patients undergoing bariatric surgery with at least one metabolic complication (*i.e.*, diabetes, hypertension, dyslipidemia or obstructive sleep apnea), and validated in 60 liver biopsies of subjects with metabolic syndrome, but not morbid obesity. The algorithm, subsequently tested for observer variability by two groups of pathologists, a European study group, the Fatty Liver Inhibition of Progression (FLIP) pathology group, and a pathology group of general pathologists with varying amounts of liver pathology training [16]. The score is based on two now recognized concepts; even though large droplet macrovesicular steatosis is an obviously recognized, and required, feature of non-cirrhotic NAFLD, it is likely not a driver in progression of disease, thus, the feature should not carry much weight, if any at all, in a histologic score. However, ballooning and lobular inflammation have been noted in several studies to be significant features in progressive disease, thus, these should be more weighted as determinants of progression. Thus, the "activity score" is derived from the combination of the semi-quantitative values of the two [17]. The details for semi-quantitative scores differ slightly from prior methods: lobular inflammation ranges from 0 to 2 (instead of 0–3), ballooning 0–2 (with descriptions of ballooning as detailed in Table 1). As the final score is meant to represent a diagnosis, steatosis (S_x) must be >0, activity (ballooning plus lobular inflammation (A_x) must be $\geqslant$2, in which ballooning is at least 1. Fibrosis is based on the NASH CRN scale, and reported as "F". One of the primary advantages of this score is the manner of reporting: by giving a subscore for each component of the SAF (Steatosis + Activity + Fibrosis), the amount of steatosis and fibrosis are communicated and one may make comparisons for the features with other biopsies from the same patient. Activity, the most important of the scores is an additive score, so, similar to the NAS, one cannot determine how much is ballooning and how much is lobular inflammation, thus, as with the NAS, improvement in either would not be visible by the SAF alone. Increased values of the SAF correlated well with increased values of serum AST and ALT. Correlations with known metabolic features of NAFLD/NASH, such as markers of insulin resistance, were not reported for the different activity scores that discriminate NAFLD and NASH.

The second study done by the FLIP pathologists and a group of community pathologists [16] was done to test the validity of the SAF algorithm in non-bariatric subjects as well as to test the usefulness of such an algorithm for practical use. Both groups of pathologists' diagnoses improved when the SAF was utilized and both groups had high kappa values when utilizing the SAF. One of the discussed concepts was the challenge for pathologists to make the distinction(s) of NASH and non-NASH in liver biopsy material, whereas use of an algorithm such as the SAF could mitigate against the necessity of such. An example given was a case of steatosis with only fibrosis, but no other features. Additionally, the graphic of the SAF score showed that it could be possible to have $S > 0\ A_{1(B1 + L0)}$ (i.e., steatosis > 0, activity score of 1 because of ballooning score of 1 but no lobular inflammation) with a final diagnosis of "steatosis". Both of these examples are troublesome and highlight the oversimplification of the SAF on its own. The former could potentially fit into a "borderline" category of either zone 1 or zone 3 depending on where the fibrosis is located and the latter could fit into borderline zone 3, also depending if the ballooning and steatosis were in zone 3. Alternatively, both could fit into examples of resolution of prior NASH, and one would want to compare them with prior biopsies. Although both of the studies that proposed and discussed the values of the SAF reiterated that it was not meant to replace a written pathology report, neither mentioned the authors' concepts of fundamentals of NASH diagnosis other than the presence of the lesions in the SAF. Zonal localization and accentuation of lesions in adults and children were not assessed, nor can they be, by the algorithm proposed.

3.4. Pediatric NAFLD Histologic Score

The final scoring system proposed is specifically for the pediatric group by Alkhouri et al. [18]. The score proposed was developed from 203 biopsies of children with NASH or "notNASH" according to the pathologist's diagnosis, and given NAS and fibrosis scores according to the NIDDK NASH CRN system with the exception of adding a portal inflammation score of 0–2 for none, mild or moderate portal inflammation. After logistic regression, each feature was weighted and a final Pediatric NAFLD Histologic Score (PNHS) was developed that can be calculated by entering their values into the website [21]. Both the training and validation sets had high area under receiver operating curve (AUROC) values. Interestingly, 65.9% of NASH biopsies had ballooning, as did 4.4% of notNASH biopsies, but 34.1% of NASH biopsies also were diagnosed as such without ballooning. The NAS was greater in NASH biopsies than in notNASH biopsies (mean values 4.5 ± 1.4 vs. 2.2 ± 0.59, $p < 0.001$), as expected, as was fibrosis >0 ($p < 0.001$). The score was developed in order to better reflect pediatric "NASH" than the term "borderline" steatohepatitis for both clinical care and clinical trials. Whether it has been in use long enough to accomplish this goal or not cannot be clearly stated at this time. The need to utilize a website for determination of a score and therefore a diagnostic category is interesting and the goal worthwhile, but the concept is somewhat worrisome to diagnostic pathologists as the suggestion that a calculated algorithm can actually replace the interpretative experience that is involved in deriving a final diagnosis is not something one accepts with certainty. The "art" of interpretation continues to play a role in all fields of medicine, regardless of the rigor with which it is applied.

4. Conclusions

It is apparent that NAFLD and NASH are complex entities, not only for clinicians, basic scientists, but also for diagnostic pathologists. Even though much progress has been made, it is worthwhile to remember that scoring methods are measures of injury, but not replacements of diagnostic assessment, and thus, pathologists need to first be trained to recognize patterns of disease, and then to apply appropriate scoring systems. There are pros and cons to any scoring system for all disease processes, as discussed above for NAFLD and NASH. As continued work is done, however, the expectations for more "pros" and fewers "cons" remain.

Acknowledgments: The author would like to thank Amedeo Lonardo and Giovanni Targher for the honor of the invitation to write this review.

Author Contributions: The author has written the text alone.

References

1.   Ludwig, J.; Viggiano, T.R.; McGill, D.B.; Oh, B.J. Nonalcoholic steatohepatitis: Mayo Clinic experiences with a hitherto unnamed disease. *Mayo Clin. Proc.* **1980**, *55*, 434–438. [PubMed]

2.   Brunt, E.M.; Neuschwander-Tetri, B.A.; Burt, A.D. Fatty Liver Disease: Alcoholic and Nonalcoholic. In *MacSween's Pathology of the Liver*, 6th ed.; Burt, A.D., Portmann, B., Ferrell, L., Eds.; Churchill Livingstone/Elsevier: Edinburgh, UK, 2012; pp. 293–359.

3.   Brunt, E.M.; Wong, V.W.-S.; Nobili, V.; Day, C.P.; Sookoian, S.; Maher, J.J.; Sirlin, C.; Neuschwander-Tetri, B.A.; Rinella, M.E. Nonalcoholic fatty liver disease. *Nat. Rev. Prim.* **2015**. in press. [CrossRef]

4.   Torres, D.M.; Williams, C.D.; Harrison, S.A. Features, diagnosis, and treatment of nonalcoholic fatty liver disease. *Clin. Gastroenterol. Hepatol.* **2012**, *10*, 837–858. [CrossRef] [PubMed]

5.   Ratziu, V.; Charlotte, F.; Heurtier, A.; Gombert, S.; Giral, P.; Bruckert, E.; Grimaldi, A.; Capron, F.; Poynard, T. Sampling variability of liver biopsy in nonalcoholic fatty liver disease. *Gastroenterology* **2005**, *128*, 1898–1906. [CrossRef] [PubMed]

6.   Larson, S.P.; Bowers, S.P.; Palekar, N.A.; Ward, J.A.; Pulcini, J.P.; Harrison, S.A. Histopathologic variability between the right and left lobes of the liver in morbidly obese patients undergoing Roux-en-Y bypass. *Clin. Gastroenterol. Hepatol.* **2007**, *5*, 1329–1332. [CrossRef] [PubMed]

7.   Vuppalanchi, R.; Unalp, A.; van Natta, M.L.; Cummings, O.W.; Sandrasegaran, K.E.; Hameed, T.; Tonascia, J.; Chalasani, N. Effects of liver biopsy sample length and number of readings on histologic yield for nonalcoholic fatty liver disease. *Clin. Gastroenterol. Hepatol.* **2009**, *7*, 481–486. [CrossRef] [PubMed]

8.   Bedossa, P.; Bioulacsage, P.; Callard, P.; Chevallier, M.; Degott, C.; Deugnier, Y.; Fabre, M.; Reynes, M.; Voigt, J.J.; Zafrani, E.S.; *et al.* Intraobserver and interobserver variations in liver biopsy interpretation in patients with chronic hepatitis c. *Hepatology* **1994**, *20*, 15–20.

9.   Kleiner, D.E.; Brunt, E.M. Nonalcoholic fatty liver disease: Pathologic patterns and biopsy evaluation in clinical research. *Semin. Liver Dis.* **2012**, *32*, 3–13. [CrossRef] [PubMed]

10.   Tandra, S.; Yeh, M.M.; Brunt, E.M.; Vuppalanchi, R.; Cummings, O.W.; Unalp-Arida, A.; Wilson, L.A.; Chalasani, N. Presence and significance of microvesicular steatosis in nonalcoholic fatty liver disease. *J. Hepatol.* **2011**, *55*, 654–659. [CrossRef] [PubMed]

11. Pais, R.; Charlotte, F.; Fedchuk, L.; Bedossa, P.; Lebray, P.; Poynard, T.; Ratziu, V. A systematic review of follow-up biopsies reveals disease progression in patients with non-alcoholic fatty liver. *J. Hepatol.* **2013**, *59*, 550–556. [CrossRef] [PubMed]

12. McPherson, S.; Hardy, T.; Henderson, E.; Burt, A.D.; Day, C.P.; Anstee, Q.M. Evidence of NAFLD progression from steatosis to fibrosing-steatohepatitis using paired biopsies: Implications for prognosis and clinical management. *J. Hepatol.* **2015**, *62*, 1148–1155. [CrossRef] [PubMed]

13. Schwimmer, J.B.; Behling, C.; Newbury, R.; Deutsch, R.; Nievergelt, C.; Schork, N.J.; Lavine, J.E. Histopathology of pediatric nonalcoholic fatty liver disease. *Hepatology* **2005**, *42*, 641–649. [CrossRef] [PubMed]

14. Brunt, E.M.; Janney, C.G.; di Bisceglie, A.M.; Neuschwander-Tetri, B.A.; Bacon, B.R. Nonalcoholic steatohepatitis: A proposal for grading and staging the histological lesions. *Am. J. Gastroenterol.* **1999**, *94*, 2467–2474. [CrossRef] [PubMed]

15. Kleiner, D.E.; Brunt, E.M.; van Natta, M.; Behling, C.; Contos, M.J.; Cummings, O.W.; Ferrell, L.D.; Liu, Y.C.; Torbenson, M.S.; Unalp-Arida, A.; *et al.* Design and validation of a histological scoring system for nonalcoholic fatty liver disease. *Hepatology* **2005**, *41*, 1313–1321. [CrossRef] [PubMed]

16. Bedossa, P. Utility and appropriateness of the fatty liver inhibition of progression (FLIP) algorithm and steatosis, activity, and fibrosis (SAF) score in the evaluation of biopsies of nonalcoholic fatty liver disease. *Hepatology* **2014**, *60*, 565–575. [CrossRef] [PubMed]

17. Bedossa, P.; Poitou, C.; Veyrie, N.; Bouillot, J.-L.; Basdevant, A.; Paradis, V.; Tordjman, J.; Clement, K. Histopathological algorithm and scoring system for evaluation of liver lesions in morbidly obese patients. *Hepatology* **2012**, *56*, 1751–1759. [CrossRef] [PubMed]

18. Alkhouri, N.; de Vito, R.; Alisi, A.; Yerian, L.; Lopez, R.; Feldstein, A.E.; Nobili, V. Development and validation of a new histological score for pediatric non-alcoholic fatty liver disease. *J. Hepatol.* **2012**, *57*, 1312–1318. [CrossRef] [PubMed]

19. Brunt, E.M. Grading and staging the histopathological lesions of chronic hepatitis: The Knodell histology activity index and beyond. *Hepatology* **2000**, *31*, 241–246. [CrossRef] [PubMed]

20. Brunt, E.M.; Kleiner, D.E.; Wilson, L.; Belt, P.; Neuschwander-Tetri, B.A. NASH Clinical Research Network (CRN). The NAS and the histopathologic diagnosis of NASH: Distinct clinicopathologic meanings. *Hepatology* **2011**, *53*, 810–820. [CrossRef] [PubMed]

21. Pediatric NAFLD Histologic Score. Available online: http://rcc.simpal.com/RCEval.cgi?RCID=RPCxtv#RESULT (accessed on 15 November 2015).

7

Mitochondrial Molecular Pathophysiology of Nonalcoholic Fatty Liver Disease: A Proteomics Approach

Natalia Nuño-Lámbarri [1,†], **Varenka J. Barbero-Becerra** [1,†], **Misael Uribe** [2] **and Norberto C. Chávez-Tapia** [1,2,*]

[1]   Traslational Research Unit, Médica Sur Clinic & Foundation, Mexico City 14050, Mexico; nnunol@medicasur.org.mx (N.N.-L.); vbarberob@medicasur.org.mx (V.J.B.-B.)

[2]   Obesity and Digestive Diseases Unit, Médica Sur Clinic & Foundation, Mexico City 14050, Mexico; muribe@medicasur.org.mx

*   Correspondence: nchavezt@medicasur.org.mx

†   These authors contributed equally to this work.

Academic Editor: Amedeo Lonardo

Abstract: Nonalcoholic fatty liver disease (NAFLD) is a chronic liver condition that can progress to nonalcoholic steatohepatitis, cirrhosis and cancer. It is considered an emerging health problem due to malnourishment or a high-fat diet (HFD) intake, which is observed worldwide. It is well known that the hepatocytes' apoptosis phenomenon is one of the most important features of NAFLD. Thus, this review focuses on revealing, through a proteomics approach, the complex network of protein interactions that promote fibrosis, liver cell stress, and apoptosis. According to different types of *in vitro* and murine models, it has been found that oxidative/nitrative protein stress leads to mitochondrial dysfunction, which plays a major role in stimulating NAFLD damage. Human studies have revealed the importance of novel biomarkers, such as retinol-binding protein 4, lumican, transgelin 2 and hemoglobin, which have a significant role in the disease. The post-genome era has brought proteomics technology, which allows the determination of molecular pathogenesis in NAFLD. This has led to the search for biomarkers which improve early diagnosis and optimal treatment and which may effectively prevent fatal consequences such as cirrhosis or cancer.

Keywords: proteomics; NAFLD; mitochondrial dysfunction

1. Introduction

Non-alcoholic fatty liver disease (NAFLD) is a clinicopathological condition that is commonly associated with dyslipidemia, insulin resistance, cardiovascular disease, obesity metabolic syndrome and type 2 diabetes mellitus (T2DM) [1]. Moreover, the liver is targeted by signals from other tissues, including adipose tissue, the gut and its microbiota [2], comprising a wide spectrum of liver damage, ranging from simple steatosis to steatohepatitis [3], which is a major health problem affecting an estimated 25% of the adult population worldwide. Although NAFLD is highly prevalent on all continents, the highest prevalence rates were reported in South America (31%) and the Middle East (32%) while the lowest prevalence was reported in Africa (14%). Also, the prevalence between the United States and Europe is similar, and an interesting finding was the relatively high prevalence found in the Asian population (27%) [4].

NAFLD can progress to nonalcoholic steatohepatitis (NASH) in 12%–40% of cases. NASH can be distinguished by the presence of hepatocyte ballooning, apoptosis, inflammatory infiltrates, and collagen deposition. Over a period of 10–15 years, 15% of patients with NASH will exhibit progression to liver cirrhosis. Annually, 4% of hepatic decompensation is generated by cirrhosis that has not been caused by viral hepatitis, while the overall risk of generating cancer in 10 years is 10% [5].

Currently, proteomics are an essential approach that have improved the study of the complex pathogenesis of NAFLD, becoming more outstanding since they have been applied in the health sciences and industry [6] and being useful in the determination of pathophysiology and identifying new markers for disease diagnosis [7].

Proteomics provide essential information of the biologically active entity named protein, which includes its post-translational modifications and interactions with other proteins [8]. Proteomic techniques are primarily based on electrophoresis and mass spectrometry [9]. In recent years, genomics, proteomics, and bioinformatic techniques have been developed synergistically and have experienced a surprising development, which has brought about major advances in medicine.

1.1. Identification of Specific Proteins through in Vitro Studies

In vitro models are necessary for elucidating the mechanisms of liver damage in NAFLD, as they are for understanding the complex network of cellular interactions, apoptosis and oxidative stress, the mechanisms that lead to mitochondrial damage which promotes fibrosis.

Hepatic oxidative stress and injury are mechanisms associated with polyploidy, which is one of the most dramatic changes that can occur in the genome [10]. A hepatocyte NAFLD model has shown that oxidative stress triggers the activation of a G2/M DNA damage checkpoint, preventing the activation of the cyclin B1/CDK1 complex, which causes an inefficient progression through the S/G2 phases, suggesting that polyploidy in mononuclear cell populations is an early event in NAFLD development [11].

During liver injury, perpetuation of the insult induces progressive deterioration of hepatic damage with the production of extracellular matrix (ECM) remodeling components, which contribute to uncontrolled ECM turnover [12], leading to an excessive accumulation of extracellular proteins, proteoglycans, and carbohydrates that ends in a pathological state that is called fibrosis [13]. Components of the fibrotic liver ECM had been previously cataloged by sodium dodecyl sulfate polyacrylamide gel electrophoresis (SDS–PAGE) separation and mass spectrometry (GeLC-MS)–based proteomics approaches [14]. An *in vitro* liver fibrosis model using mass spectrometry analysis in cell-derived ECM identified 61 structural or secreted ECM proteins (48 proteins for a hepatic stellate cell line, LX-2, and 31 proteins for human foreskin fibroblasts) [14]. Several proteins identified in this study have been linked with fibrotic processes that occur in the liver and other organs; fibrillin, which was previously implicated in the activation of transforming growth factor β (TGF-β) storage, was among those proteins [15]. Furthermore, two new fibrotic constituent proteins identified in this study, CYR61 and Wnt-5a, were also validated in the fibrotic liver [14]. GELC-MS–based proteomics coupled to an ECM-enrichment strategy in an *in vitro* model of liver fibrosis may be a valuable tool for determining the mechanisms underlying fibrosis and for the identification of novel therapeutic targets or biomarkers.

Fibrosis is not the only mechanism of liver damage; apoptosis has also been studied since it is one of the most important features of NAFLD [16]. The participation of certain proteins, such as cytochrome b5, annexin A5 and A6, and protein disulfide isomerase fragments, has been confirmed in murine and human cell apoptosis models [17]. On the other hand, it has been reported that cholesterol induces Bax and caspase-3 [18], which may be important proteins for apoptosis; however, cholesterol did not increase the expression of p53 and Bcl-2 in steatotic cells, suggesting an important role for cell death mechanisms in hepatocytes [19].

Furthermore, proteomic techniques could be useful in other scenarios such as liver regeneration; an analysis was performed through label-free quantitative mass spectrometry in which human embryonic stem cells were differentiated into hepatocyte-like cells to investigate the effects of the cell secretome, which demonstrated that hepatocyte-like cells derived from stem cells contribute to the recovery from injured liver tissue in mice by delivering trophic factors that support liver regeneration [20].

The application of this strategy to different *in vitro* disease models may therefore significantly improve identifying specific proteins, and provide the first step toward elucidating the mechanisms which underlie fibrosis and novel therapeutic targets or biomarkers.

1.2. In Vivo NAFLD Studies

Obesity is related to several diseases, such as NAFLD and NASH, being linked to mitochondrial dysfunction and deficiency of nitric oxide (NO). Chronic consumption of a high-fat diet (HFD) in a murine model induces NASH, and it is accompanied by profound changes in mitochondrial bioenergetics. Conversely, HFD decreased the activity of cytochrome c oxidase and increased sensitivity to the NO-dependent inhibition of mitochondrial respiration [21]. According to HFD intake, a densitometry analysis revealed that 22 proteins were significantly altered, whereas 67 proteins remained unchanged. The last events are a bit far from proposing a mechanism; however, this response could be considered as a regulatory mechanism according to the microenvironment where it develops (Figure 1) [21].

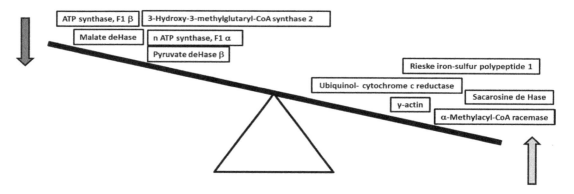

Figure 1. Mitochondrial proteins altered by high-fat diet.

Chronic exposure of mice to a HFD induces hepatic steatosis, modifying the liver mitochondrial proteome, including changes in proteins related to oxidative phosphorylation, protein folding, and lipid and sulfur amino acid metabolism [21]. Mitochondrial dysfunction may be generated by high concentrations of reactive oxygen species (ROS) which inhibit the respiratory chain and integrity of mitochondrial DNA and also contribute to organelle toxicity, the suppression of fatty acid oxidation and the rise in lipid peroxidation [22].

Liver steatosis may be due to an excess of fatty acids (FA), glucose, lipotoxicity, or insulin resistance (IR), and it induces *de novo* lipid synthesis by the activation of nuclear receptors such as sterol regulatory element-binding protein 1 (SREBP-1), carbohydrate-responsive element-binding protein (ChREBP-1), and peroxisome proliferator-activated receptor γ (PPARγ) [23]. Moreover, PPARγ activation increased cellular free FA uptake, exceeding the adaptive pathways of hepatic lipid export and catabolism, suggesting an adipogenic transformation of hepatocytes [24]. The presence of steatosis is tightly associated with chronic hepatic inflammation, an effect mediated in part by activation of the Ikκ-b/NF-κB signaling pathway.

A murine model of steatosis induced with a HFD increases NF-κB activity, which is associated with the elevated hepatic expression of pro-inflammatory cytokines such as TNF-α and IL-1 which are activated by ROS created by lipid peroxidation, responsible not only for promoting insulin resistance and Kupffer cell activation, but also for mediating cholesterol and triglyceride metabolism [25,26].

TNF-α act upon leukocyte infiltration in the liver, contributing to intracellular oxidative stress and mitochondrial dysfunction; in fact, TNF receptor adaptor proteins initiate the phosphorylation of mitogen-activated protein kinases (MAPK 1), which in turn activate c-Jun N-terminal kinases

(JNK) [27]. Prolonged activation of the downstream signaling molecule JNK was found to promote inflammation and apoptosis [28], amplifying hepatocyte damage [29].

Studies in JNK2 knockout mice indicated that this protein might be important for caspase 8 activation and apoptosis mitochondrial pathways in response to TNF-α [30]. Treatment with anti-TNF-α antibodies improved mitochondrial respiration and inflammation, and alleviated hepatic steatosis in mouse models of NASH [31]. Also, it has been seen that Gegenqinlian decoction (GGQLD), a Chinese herbal medicine, can decrease serum elevated TNF-α levels, being an optimal approach for managing lipid metabolic, inflammatory, and histological abnormalities via the PPARγ/TNF-α pathway in NAFLD [26].

Mitochondria adjust to lipid accumulation in hepatocytes raising the levels of β-oxidation; nevertheless, increased substrate transfer to the mitochondrial electron transport chain leads to a rise in ROS production and finally insulin resistance, playing an important role in hepatic lipid metabolism [32]. In a murine model study, with the use of gel electrophoresis (DIGE) and MALDI-TOF techniques, 95 proteins were identified to exhibit significant changes during the development of NAFLD, whereas protein down-regulation was observed for enoyl coenzyme A hydratase (ECHS1), which catalyzes the second step of the mitochondrial β-oxidation of fatty acids, probably because of HFD-related hepatic steatosis [33]. These findings suggest an important role for ECHS1 in lipid accumulation in *in vivo* NAFLD models [34].

Furthermore, the HFD-mediated decrease in ATP synthase subunits (F1α and β) may also compromise mitochondrial energy conservation; these findings, together with a decrease in the content of malate and pyruvate dehydrogenase, which are key mitochondrial metabolism enzymes, provide strong evidence supporting the occurrence of bioenergetics dysfunction in response to chronic exposure to a HFD, which can be linked to NAFLD liver proteome changes [35]. Moreover, some proteins associated with acetyl-CoA intake and oxidative stress are molecular markers of hepatic steatosis in ob/ob mice that have been identified by liver mitochondrial 2D-DIGE proteomics [36]. Also, a comparative study of liver mitochondrial proteomics, using Ingenuity Pathway Analysis software (IPA; Ingenuity Systems, Mountain View, Redwood City, CA, USA), found that among the 1100 protein analyzed, aldehyde dehydrogenase 2 (ALDH2), and 3-hydroxy-3-methylglutaryl-CoA synthase 2 (HMGCS2) were altered [37]. In summary, analysis of sub-mitochondrial and cellular proteomes indicates that metabolic adaptations occurring in hypertriglyceridemic mice hepatocytes induce an enhanced acetyl-CoA, glycerol-3-phosphate, ATP and Nicotinamide adenine dinucleotide phosphate (NADPH) availability for *de novo* triglyceride (TG) biosynthesis. They also strongly suggest that the cytosol of HuApoC-III mouse hepatocytes is the subject of an important oxidative stress, probably as a result of free fatty acid (FFA) over-accumulation, iron overload and enhanced activity of some ROS-producing catabolic enzymes [38].

Also, the increase of intracellular triacylglycerols may be promoted by the inhibition of lipoprotein assembly and secretion [23]. Recently it has been found that fetuin A is an adaptor protein for saturated fatty acid–induced activation of Toll-like receptor 4 signaling, promoting lipid-induced insulin resistance; also, fetuin B secretion from the liver is increased by steatosis and diminishes glucose lowering through insulin-independent mechanisms [39].

It is important to study alcoholic fatty liver disease (AFLD) since it shares some hepatocyte injury mechanisms with NAFLD. AFLD appears in 90% of people who consume ⩾60 mg per day of alcohol; however, both have the deterioration of mitochondrial functions because of protein nitration in common [40]. Under normal conditions, these function capacity alterations can be managed by properly using the antioxidant host defense system and by the removal of nitrated proteins, which can serve as a defense mechanism against nitroxidative stress–related harmful consequences [35].

Peroxynitrite and protein nitration were suggested to be the main causes of acute and chronic AFLD injury models [41]. Also, several mouse models have been used to evaluate the effect of protein nitration on nitroxidative stress [42]. For instance, the role of protein nitration has been studied in mouse strains with ablated genes that are involved in the regulation of superoxide and NO levels [43] in which the identification of peptides that originate from nitrated proteins can be performed using matrix-assisted laser desorption/ionization time-of-flight mass spectrometry (MALDI-TOF MS) [44,45].

Moreover, knockout inducible nitric oxide synthase (iNOS) mice with a Lieber–De Carli ethanol liquid diet exhibit a markedly decreased level of nitrated proteins, which confers resistance to AFLD and, together with protein nitration, inhibits complex I (NADH ubiquinone oxidoreductase) and complex V (ATP synthase) activities in models of acute and chronic alcohol exposure [46,47].

The authors suggest that these damaging effects are probably caused by protein nitration, as the administration of iNOS inhibitors and peroxynitrite scavengers, such as uric acid, ameliorated the ethanol-induced nitration and the inhibition of activity and mitochondrial depletion of ATP synthase. In addition, the deletion of superoxide dismutase 2 (SOD2) would scavenge superoxide and block peroxynitrite formation, yielding the extension of mitochondrial DNA depletion, whereas SOD2 over-expression yielded opposite outcomes [47].

On the other hand, cytosolic SOD1 also exhibits a protective role against ethanol-mediated hepatic damage [48]. In SOD1-deficient mice, the levels of protective hepatic ATP content and SOD2 expression were decreased, whereas oxidative damage and nitro-Tyr formation were elevated in response to ethanol feeding, thus leading to greater hepatic injury [41]. Up to this point, evidence suggests that hepatic mitochondria from ethanol-fed murine models are more sensitive to NO and reactive nitrogen species. It seems that after ethanol exposure, mitochondrial liver dysfunction might develop a cytosolic antioxidant defense, which could be an important feature of chronic hepatotoxicity damaging the proteome and genome [49].

In regards to the inflammatory response, it is important to mention that ethanol hepatotoxicity was significantly prevented through a mechanism that involves a decrease in tumor necrosis factor α (TNF-α) formation, in hepatocytes isolated from alcohol-fed rats, through the SDS–PAGE technique [50]. It was not surprising that TNF-α knockout mice exhibited a significantly less severe ethanol-mediated hepatotoxicity, markedly accompanied by lower levels of protein Tyr nitration [51].

The Fernandez-Checa group have shown that mitochondrial free cholesterol loading in steatohepatitis sensitizes to TNF and Fas through mitochondrial glutathione (GSH) depletion [31]. Protein Tyr nitration and its functional consequences might explain the role of protein nitration in promoting many forms of liver disease, including AFLD and NAFLD [52]. The levels of protein nitration are correlated with the increased levels of hepatic transaminases, steatosis, and necrosis [43]. It is also very important to study the NO bioavailability throughout the course of NAFLD. In an HFD mouse model, it was shown that NO contents were initially increased, causing mitochondrial damage accompanied by alterations in mitochondrial proteins, such as thiolase, complex I (NADH ubiquinone oxidoreductase), aldehyde dehydrogenase 2 (ALDH2), and complex V (ATP synthase); in contrast, NO levels decreased at later stages of NAFLD [43]. NO might be an encouraging inflammatory regulatory marker according to the NAFLD damage stage.

1.3. Human Studies

Based on the hypothesis that liver injury in NAFLD and NASH is caused by protein effectors, as described for the *in vitro* and *in vivo* models, human studies are critical because they may help establish biomarkers that can be used for an earlier diagnosis and more effective treatments.

Dr. Feldstein's group reported that extracellular vesicle (EV) proteomes carry a selective antigenic composition that might be used to diagnose NAFLD non-invasively. They analyzed cell death, inflammation, and antioxidant and pathological angiogenesis in steatotic mice, finding that some functional activities of oxidoreductase, hydrolase, endopeptidase inhibitors, signal transducers and lipid binding proteins were abundantly expressed in EVs [53]. Another study in patients with simple steatosis showed that a group of cytochrome P450 family proteins, such as CYP2E1, CYP4A11, and CYP2C9, are upregulated, being associated with lipid droplets (LDs). On the other hand, mitochondrial proteins were found to be downregulated, suggesting that these enzymes are involved in NAFLD development and mitochondrial dysfunction. Increased adipose differentiation-related protein

(ADRP) and fatty acid synthase (FAS) mRNA and protein expression were found to be upregulated in the LD fractions of patients with steatosis. It has been recently recognized that in fatty liver disease, the LD-associated protein 17β-HSD13 expression was upregulated [54].

There are several molecules that have been associated with liver damage progression. For instance, two important proteomic studies in adult patients using liver tissue and serum respectively, with and without NAFLD, revealed an increased expression of lumican (a keratan sulphate proteoglycan involved in collagen cross-linking and epithelial–mesenchymal transition) [55]. The expression of lumican was similarly abundant in obese patients with normal liver histology and in obese patients with simple steatosis; however, it was over-expressed in mild progressive NASH patients [56]. Thus, lumican is expressed differentially across the progressive stages of NAFLD, and not just in patients with moderate to advanced fibrosis, raising the possibility of over-expressed hepatic lumican as an early marker of a profibrotic state in patients with NAFLD [57]. Also, fatty acid-binding protein 1 (FABP-1) is another protein involved in multiple biological functions, such as intracellular fatty acid transport, cholesterol and phospholipid metabolism, which plays an important facilitative role in hepatic fatty acid oxidation [58,59]. FABP-1 is relatively over-expressed in patients with simple steatosis compared with those with obesity; however, throughout the NAFLD stages, it was observed that FABP-1 was significantly under-expressed in patients with mild and progressive NASH [60].

A novel analysis of hepatic peptides performed on an electrospray ionization mass spectrometry (ESI-MS) biosystem (an analytical technique that can provide both qualitative (structure) and quantitative (molecular mass or concentration) information on analyte molecules after their conversion to ions) [61] was conducted on several phenotypes of fatty liver disease, where 1362 hepatic proteins were assessed. Several proteins were consistently abundant among study groups, whereas albumin, hemoglobinβ, hemoglobinα, dihydropyrimidinase, enolase, the metal-transport protein ATX1, and HSP gp96 were likely differentially abundant because of the biological effects of increased hepatic lipid content or inflammation [56]. Furthermore, it has been observed that serum and hepatic TNF-α levels are elevated in patients with NAFLD, correlating with the animal models which had already been studied. Conversely, inhibition of TNF-α signaling improves insulin resistance (IR) and histological parameters of NAFLD [26].

In another study which involved NAFLD patients who underwent bariatric surgery, quantified protein peak intensity levels were selected from SELDI-TOF mass spectrometry [62]; the results revealed that fibrinogen γ was elevated, playing a role in blood clotting and serving as a depot for active fibroblast growth factor receptor 2 (FGF2) in the blood, and it may be connected to liver fibrosis [63]. However, the role of fibrinogen γ in NAFLD remains speculative and needs to be well defined. Moreover, this study involves patients with varying stages of NAFLD. Several protein biomarkers were identified and classified from priority 1 to 4, according to quality identification (ID); priority 1 proteins have the greatest likelihood of correct ID (multiple unique sequences identified), such as transgelin 2, retinol-binding protein 4, lumican, and paraoxonase 1, among others [62].

Importantly, it seems that each protein may have biological significance in the microenvironment in which it is expressed. For instance, the fibrinogen β chain, retinol-binding protein 4 (RBP4), serum amyloid P component, lumican, transgelin 2, and CD5 antigen-like exhibit differential levels of expression among patient groups and present a global success rate of 76%, whereas complement component C7, the insulin-like growth factor acid labile subunit, and transgelin 2 present a global success rate of 90% wherein they are characterized by simple steatosis and NASH and are able to accurately differentiate between control subjects and patients with all forms of NAFLD [62]. RBP4 is an important protein synthesized by the liver and adipose tissue, carrying vitamin A in the blood; it has been involved in the development of IR and has been related to increased NAFLD severity [64].

NAFLD development has been associated with elevated serum hemoglobin levels, being independent of body mass index, type 2 diabetes, and other metabolic diseases [29,65]. One of the potential explanations for the observed associations between increased hemoglobin and NAFLD may be related to oxidative stress, catalyzed by iron excess accumulation and probably causing thrombosis, leading to hepatocyte injury [66,67]. The relationship between serum hemoglobin and NAFLD may be partially modulated by haptoglobin levels, which act as an antioxidant binding to free hemoglobin and inhibiting the hemoglobin-induced oxidative damage [65]. Furthermore, excessive erythrocytosis increased hemoglobin in NAFLD subjects without a diagnosis of metabolic syndrome (MS), and this should be considered in the selection of cases for histological assessment of disease severity and progression [68]. On the other hand, Lixin Zhu *et al.* showed that in NASH, hemoglobin is highly expressed and synthesized in hepatocytes, being released into the circulatory system and providing a possible explanation for serum free hemoglobin [69]. Therefore, hemoglobin measurements should be considered part of the clinical evaluation markers for severity of liver damage in patients with NAFLD [67,70].

Finding clinical biomarkers that have arisen from proteomic technologies, which reveal biological reactions and could distinguish NAFLD from NASH, is of great importance (Table 1). However, accurate human studies which involved protein analysis related to mitochondrial dysfunction are lacking. Oxidative-nitrated stress proteins play a major role in stimulating damage in various hepatic diseases, including AFLD and NAFLD mediated by ethanol. As these proteins are essential for normal mitochondrial function, protein nitration might lead to irreversible modification of the respiratory-chain proteins [29].

2. Conclusions

In vitro studies are the basis for elucidating the pathogenic network that is involved in NAFLD, which is interesting because of the recognition of some proteins involved in liver fibrosis. Conversely, *in vivo* studies have focused on the bioenergetics dysfunction caused by chronic exposure to HFD, which can be linked to changes in protein interactions in the liver proteome between NAFLD and NASH (Figure 2) [14]. Human studies have revealed the importance of novel proteins that were identified as having a high rate of confidence in the presence of NAFLD and NASH and seem to emerge as good marker candidates (Table 1). Deeper and more accurate human studies will be required to identify the network of complex proteomes that underlies the pathogenesis related to mitochondrial dysfunction, where its functional consequences might explain the pathophysiological mechanism which follows many forms of liver diseases.

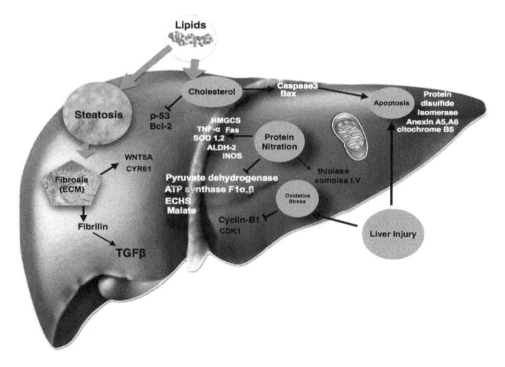

Figure 2. Activation and inhibition of different proteins in NAFLD.

Table 1. Proteins involved in NAFLD and potential markers for NAFLD.

Research Context	Protein	Implications and Findings	Study	Year
Cell Cycle	Cyclin B1 CDK1	Polyploidy in mononuclear cell populations is an early event in NAFLD development.	Gentric, Maillet et al. [11]	2015
Fibrosis	Fibrillin TGF-β CYR61 Wnt-5a Lumican Fibrinogeny FGF2	Mechanisms underlying fibrotic processes. Early marker of a profibrotic state in patients with NAFLD.	Lorena, Darby et al. [15]	2004
			Rashid, Humphries et al. [14]	2012
			Fitzpatrick and Dhawan [57]	2014
			Younossi, Baranova et al. [63]	2005
Apoptosis	Cytochrome b5 Annexin A5 Annexin A6 Bax Caspase 3 Caspase 8	Important role for cell death mechanisms in hepatocytes.	Jayaraman, Roberts et al. [17]	2005
			Yamaguchi, Chen et al. [18]	2004
			Zhu, Xie et al. [19]	2014
			Sabapathy, Hochedlinger et al. [30]	2004
Lipid synthesis	SREBP-1 ChREBP-1 PPARγ Acetyl-CoA Glycerol-3-phosphate Fetuin A Fetuin B	Adaptive pathways of hepatic lipid export and catabolism. Hepatocytes are subjected to an important oxidative stress. Promote lipid-induced insulin resistance.	Anderson and Borlak [23]	2008
			Al Sharif, Alov et al. [24]	2014
			Ehx, Gerin et al. [38]	2014
Inflammation	NF-κB TNF-α IL-1 MAPK1 JNK	Promote insulin resistance, Kupffer cells activation, cholesterol and triglyceride metabolism, intracellular oxidative stress.	Cai, Yuan et al. [25]	2005
			Wang, Liu et al. [26]	2015
			Lim, Dillon et al. [29]	2014
β-Oxidation	ECHS1	Lipid accumulation in NAFLD.	Zhang, Yang et al. [33]	2010
			Lewis, Hagstrom et al. [34]	2002
Oxidative stress	ALDH2 HMGCS2 Hemoglobin Haptoglobin	Acetyl-CoA consumption and oxidative stress as molecular markers of hepatic steatosis. Catalyze the accumulation of iron in excess.	Douette, Navet et al. [36]	2005
			Peinado, Diaz-Ruiz et al. [37]	2014
Antioxidants	SOD2 SOD1	Protective role in mitochondrial DNA depletion, and hepatic ATP content.	Mansouri, Tarhuni et al. [47]	2010
			Kessova, et al. [48]	2003
Lipid droplets	CYP2E1 CYP4A11 CYP2C9	Enzymes involved in mitochondrial dysfunction and the development of NAFLD.	Su, Wang et al. [54]	2014
Lipid metabolism	FABP-1	Intracellular fatty acid transport, cholesterol and phospholipid metabolism, and plays an important facilitative role in hepatic fatty acid oxidation.	Binas and Erol Higuchi [58]	2007
			Kato et al. [59]	2011

Cyclin-dependent kinase 1 (CDK1), Transforming growth factor beta (TGFβ), Cysteine-rich angiogenic inducer 61 (CYR61), Wingless-Type MMTV Integration Site Family, Member 5A (Wnt-5a), Fibroblast Growth Factor 2 (FGF2), BCL2-Associated X Protein (Bax), Sterol regulatory element-binding protein 1 (SREBP-1), Carbohydrate-responsive element-binding protein 1 (ChREBP-1), Peroxisome proliferator-activated receptor gamma (PPARγ), Nuclear factor κB (NF-κB), Tumor necrosis factor α (TNF-α), Interleukin 1 (IL-1), Mitogen-activated protein kinase 1 (MAPK1), c-Jun N-terminal kinase (JNK), Enoyl-CoA hydratase short chain 1 (ECHS1), Aldehyde dehydrogenase 2 (ALDH2), 3-hydroxy-3-methylglutaryl-CoA synthase 2 (HMGCS2), Superoxide dismutase 1 (SOD1), Superoxide dismutase 2 (SOD2), Cytochrome P450 family 2 subfamily E member 1 (CYP2E1), Cytochrome P450 family 4 subfamily A member 11 (CYP4A11), Cytochrome P450 family 2 subfamily C member 9 (CYP2C9) and Fatty acid binding protein 1 (FABP-1).

Acknowledgments: This study was supported by the Médica Sur Clinic and Foundation. It is it appreciated the assistance received by Victor Medina Lopez in the correction and improvement of this article.

Author Contributions: Natalia Nuño-Lámbarri and Varenka J. Barbero-Becerra wrote the article; Misael Uribe and Norberto C. Chávez-Tapia revised and corrected the final version of the manuscript.

References

1.   Ballestri, S.; Zona, S.; Targher, G.; Romagnoli, D.; Baldelli, E.; Nascimbeni, F.; Roverato, A.; Guaraldi, G.; Lonardo, A. Nonalcoholic fatty liver disease is associated with an almost two-fold increased risk of incident type 2 diabetes and metabolic syndrome. Evidence from a systematic review and meta-analysis. *J. Gastroenterol. Hepatol.* **2015**. [CrossRef]

2.   Petta, S.; Valenti, L.; Bugianesi, E.; Targher, G.; Bellentani, S.; Bonino, F.; Special Interest Group on Personalised Hepatology of the Italian Association for the Study of the Liver (AISF). A "systems medicine" approach to the study of non-alcoholic fatty liver disease. *Dig. Liver Dis.* **2016**, *48*, 333–342. [PubMed]

3.   Lomonaco, R.; Sunny, N.E.; Bril, F.; Cusi, K. Nonalcoholic fatty liver disease: Current issues and novel treatment approaches. *Drugs* **2013**, *73*, 1–14. [CrossRef] [PubMed]

4.   Younossi, Z.M.; Koenig, A.B.; Abdelatif, D.; Fazel, Y.; Henry, L.; Wymer, M. Global epidemiology of non-alcoholic fatty liver disease-meta-analytic assessment of prevalence, incidence and outcomes. *Hepatology* **2015**. [CrossRef] [PubMed]

5.   Fuchs, M. Non-alcoholic Fatty liver disease: The bile Acid-activated farnesoid x receptor as an emerging treatment target. *J. Lipids* **2012**, *2012*, 934396. [CrossRef] [PubMed]

6.   Enriquez, J. Genomics and the world's economy. *Science* **1998**, *281*, 925–926. [CrossRef] [PubMed]

7.   Blackstock, W.P.; Weir, M.P. Proteomics: Quantitative and physical mapping of cellular proteins. *Trends Biotechnol.* **1999**, *17*, 121–127. [CrossRef]

8.   Gerold, G.; Bruening, J.; Pietschmann, T. Decoding protein networks during virus entry by quantitative proteomics. *Virus Res.* **2015**. [CrossRef] [PubMed]

9.   Larbi, N.B.; Jefferies, C. 2D-DIGE: Comparative proteomics of cellular signalling pathways. *Methods Mol. Biol.* **2009**, *517*, 105–132. [PubMed]

10.   Celton-Morizur, S.; Desdouets, C. Polyploidization of liver cells. *Adv. Exp. Med. Biol.* **2010**, *676*, 123–135. [PubMed]

11.   Gentric, G.; Maillet, V.; Paradis, V.; Couton, D.; L'Hermitte, A.; Panasyuk, G.; Fromenty, B.; Celton-Morizur, S.; Desdouets, C. Oxidative stress promotes pathologic polyploidization in nonalcoholic fatty liver disease. *J. Clin. Investig.* **2015**, *125*, 981–992. [CrossRef] [PubMed]

12.   Mormone, E.; George, J.; Nieto, N. Molecular pathogenesis of hepatic fibrosis and current therapeutic approaches. *Chem. Biol. Interact.* **2011**, *193*, 225–231. [CrossRef] [PubMed]

13.   Riedman, S.L. Mechanisms of hepatic fibrogenesis. *Gastroenterology* **2008**, *134*, 1655–1669. [CrossRef] [PubMed]

14.   Rashid, S.T.; Humphries, J.D.; Byron, A.; Dhar, A.; Askari, J.A.; Selley, J.N.; Knight, D.; Goldin, R.D.; Thursz, M.; Humphries, M.J. Proteomic analysis of extracellular matrix from the hepatic stellate cell line LX-2 identifies CYR61 and Wnt-5a as novel constituents of fibrotic liver. *J. Proteome Res.* **2012**, *11*, 4052–4064. [CrossRef] [PubMed]

15.   Lorena, D.; Darby, I.A.; Reinhardt, D.P.; Sapin, V.; Rosenbaum, J.; Desmoulière, A. Fibrillin-1 expression in normal and fibrotic rat liver and in cultured hepatic fibroblastic cells: Modulation by mechanical stress and role in cell adhesion. *Lab. Investig.* **2004**, *84*, 203–212. [CrossRef] [PubMed]

16.   Williams, K.H.; Vieira De Ribeiro, A.J.; Prakoso, E.; Veillard, A.S.; Shackel, N.A.; Brooks, B.; Bu, Y.; Cavanagh, E.; Raleigh, J.; McLennan, S.V.; *et al.* Circulating dipeptidyl peptidase-4 activity correlates with measures of hepatocyte apoptosis and fibrosis in non-alcoholic fatty liver disease in type 2 diabetes mellitus and obesity: A dual cohort cross-sectional study. *J. Diabetes* **2015**, *7*, 809–819. [CrossRef] [PubMed]

17.   Jayaraman, A.; Roberts, K.A.; Yoon, J.; Yarmush, D.M.; Duan, X.; Lee, K.; Yarmush, M.L. Identification of neutrophil gelatinase-associated lipocalin (NGAL) as a discriminatory marker of the hepatocyte-secreted protein response to IL-1β: A proteomic analysis. *Biotechnol. Bioeng.* **2005**, *91*, 502–515. [CrossRef] [PubMed]

18.   Yamaguchi, H.; Chen, J.; Bhalla, K.; Wang, H.-G. Regulation of Bax activation and apoptotic response to microtubule-damaging agents by p53 transcription-dependent and -independent pathways. *J. Biol. Chem.* **2004**, *279*, 39431–39437. [CrossRef] [PubMed]

19.   Zhu, C.; Xie, P.; Zhao, F.; Zhang, L.; An, W.; Zhan, Y. Mechanism of the promotion of steatotic HepG2 cell apoptosis by cholesterol. *Int. J. Clin. Exp. Pathol.* **2014**, *7*, 6807–6813.

20.   Woo, D.H.; Kim, S.K.; Lim, H.J.; Heo, J.; Park, H.S.; Kang, G.Y.; Kim, S.E.; You, H.J.; Hoeppner, D.J.; Kim, Y.; *et al.* Direct and indirect contribution of human embryonic stem cell-derived hepatocyte-like cells to liver repair in mice. *Gastroenterology* **2012**, *142*, 602–611. [CrossRef] [PubMed]

21.   Eccleston, H.B.; Andringa, K.A.; Betancourt, A.M.; Betancourt, A.L.; Mantena, S.K.; Swain, T.M.; Tinsley, H.N.; Nolte, R.N.; Nagy, T.R.; Nagy, G.A.; *et al.* Chronic exposure to a high-fat diet induces hepatic steatosis, impairs nitric oxide bioavailability, and modifies the mitochondrial proteome in mice. *Antioxid. Redox Signal.* **2011**, *15*, 447–459.

22. Garcia-Ruiz, C.; Fernandez-Checa, J.C. Mitochondrial glutathione: Hepatocellular survival-death switch. *J. Gastroenterol. Hepatol.* **2006**, *21*, S3–S6. [CrossRef] [PubMed]

23. Anderson, N.; Borlak, J. Molecular mechanisms and therapeutic targets in steatosis and steatohepatitis. *Pharmacol. Rev.* **2008**, *60*, 311–357. [CrossRef] [PubMed]

24. Al Sharif, M.; Alov, P.; Vitcheva, V.; Pajeva, I.; Tsakovska, I. Modes-of-action related to repeated dose toxicity: Tissue-specific biological roles of PPARγ ligand-dependent dysregulation in nonalcoholic fatty liver disease. *PPAR Res.* **2014**, *2014*, 432647. [CrossRef] [PubMed]

25. Cai, D.; Yuan, M.; Frantz, D.F.; Melendez, P.A.; Hansen, L.; Lee, J.; Shoelson, S.E. Local and systemic insulin resistance resulting from hepatic activation of IKK-β and NF-κB. *Nat. Med.* **2005**, *11*, 183–190. [CrossRef] [PubMed]

26. Wang, Y.L.; Liu, L.J.; Zhao, W.J.; Li, J.X. Intervening TNF-α via PPARγ with gegenqinlian decoction in experimental nonalcoholic fatty liver disease. *Evid. Based Complement. Altern. Med.* **2015**, *2015*, 715638. [CrossRef] [PubMed]

27. Schwabe, R.F.; Brenner, D.A. Mechanisms of Liver Injury. I. TNF-α-induced liver injury: Role of IKK, JNK, and ROS pathways. *Am. J. Physiol. Gastrointest. Liver Physiol.* **2006**, *290*, G583–G589. [CrossRef] [PubMed]

28. Chen, Y.R.; Wang, X.; Templeton, D.; Davis, R.J.; Tan, T.H. The role of c-Jun N-terminal kinase (JNK) in apoptosis induced by ultraviolet C and γ radiation. Duration of JNK activation may determine cell death and proliferation. *J. Biol. Chem.* **1996**, *271*, 31929–31936. [CrossRef] [PubMed]

29. Lim, J.W.; Dillon, J.; Miller, M. Proteomic and genomic studies of non-alcoholic fatty liver disease—Clues in the pathogenesis. *World J. Gastroenterol.* **2014**, *20*, 8325–8340. [CrossRef] [PubMed]

30. Sabapathy, K.; Hochedlinger, K.; Nam, S.Y.; Bauer, A.; Karin, M.; Wagner, E.F. Distinct roles for JNK1 and JNK2 in regulating JNK activity and c-Jun-dependent cell proliferation. *Mol. Cell* **2004**, *15*, 713–725. [CrossRef] [PubMed]

31. Mari, M.; Caballero, F.; Colell, A.; Morales, A.; Caballeria, J.; Fernandez, A.; Enrich, C.; Fernandez-Checa, J.C.; García-Ruiz, C. Mitochondrial free cholesterol loading sensitizes to TNF- and Fas-mediated steatohepatitis. *Cell Metab.* **2006**, *4*, 185–198. [CrossRef] [PubMed]

32. Gusdon, A.M.; Song, K.X.; Qu, S. Nonalcoholic fatty liver disease: Pathogenesis and therapeutics from a mitochondria-centric perspective. *Oxid. Med. Cell. Longev.* **2014**, *2014*, 637027. [CrossRef] [PubMed]

33. Zhang, X.; Yang, J.; Guo, Y.; Ye, H.; Yu, C.; Xu, C.; Xu, L.; Wu, S.; Sun, W.; Wei, H.; *et al.* Functional proteomic analysis of nonalcoholic fatty liver disease in rat models: Enoyl-coenzyme a hydratase down-regulation exacerbates hepatic steatosis. *Hepatology* **2010**, *51*, 1190–1199. [CrossRef] [PubMed]

34. Lewis, D.L.; Hagstrom, J.E.; Loomis, A.G.; Wolff, J.A.; Herweijer, H. Efficient delivery of siRNA for inhibition of gene expression in postnatal mice. *Nat. Genet.* **2002**, *32*, 107–108. [CrossRef] [PubMed]

35. Pessayre, D.; Mansouri, A.; Fromenty, B. Nonalcoholic steatosis and steatohepatitis. V. Mitochondrial dysfunction in steatohepatitis. *Am. J. Physiol. Gastrointest. Liver Physiol.* **2002**, *282*, G193–G199. [CrossRef] [PubMed]

36. Douette, P.; Navet, R.; Gerkens, P.; de Pauw, E.; Leprince, P.; Sluse-Goffart, C.; Sluse, F.E. Steatosis-induced proteomic changes in liver mitochondria evidenced by two-dimensional differential in-gel electrophoresis. *J. Proteome Res.* **2005**, *4*, 2024–2031. [CrossRef] [PubMed]

37. Peinado, J.R.; Diaz-Ruiz, A.; Frühbeck, G.; Malagon, M.M. Mitochondria in metabolic disease: Getting clues from proteomic studies. *Proteomics* **2014**, *14*, 452–466. [CrossRef] [PubMed]

38. Ehx, G.; Gérin, S.; Mathy, G.; Franck, F.; Oliveira, H.C.; Vercesi, A.E.; Sluse, F.E. Liver proteomic response to hypertriglyceridemia in human-apolipoprotein C-III transgenic mice at cellular and mitochondrial compartment levels. *Lipids Health Dis.* **2014**, *13*, 116. [CrossRef] [PubMed]

39. Meex, R.C.; Hoy, A.J.; Morris, A.; Brown, R.D.; Lo, J.C.Y.; Burke, M.; Goode, R.J.A.; Kingwell, B.A.; Kraakman, M.J.; Febbraio, M.A.; *et al.* Fetuin B is a secreted hepatocyte factor linking steatosis to impaired glucose metabolism. *Cell Metab.* **2015**, *22*, 1078–1089. [CrossRef] [PubMed]

40. Ray, S.; Khanra, D.; Sonthalia, N.; Kundu, S.; Biswas, K.; Talukdar, A.; Saha, M.; Bera, H. Clinico-biochemical correlation to histological findings in alcoholic liver disease: A single centre study from eastern India. *J. Clin. Diagn. Res.* **2014**, *8*, MC01–MC05. [CrossRef] [PubMed]

41. Larosche, I.; Lettéron, P.; Berson, A.; Fromenty, B.; Huang, T.T.; Moreau, R.; Pessayre, D.; Mansouri, A. Hepatic mitochondrial DNA depletion after an alcohol binge in mice: Probable role of peroxynitrite and modulation by manganese superoxide dismutase. *J. Pharmacol. Exp. Ther.* **2010**, *332*, 886–897. [CrossRef] [PubMed]

42. McKim, S.E.; Gäbele, E.; Isayama, F.; Lambert, J.C.; Tucker, L.M.; Wheeler, M.D.; Connor, H.D.; Mason, R.P.; Doll, M.A.; Hein, D.W.; *et al.* Inducible nitric oxide synthase is required in alcohol-induced liver injury: Studies with knockout mice. *Gastroenterology* **2003**, *125*, 1834–1844. [CrossRef] [PubMed]

43. Abdelmegeed, M.A.; Song, B.J. Functional roles of protein nitration in acute and chronic liver diseases. *Oxid. Med. Cell. Longev.* **2014**, *2014*, 149627. [CrossRef] [PubMed]

44. Sanyal, A.J.; Campbell-Sargent, C.; Mirshahi, F.; Rizzo, W.B.; Contos, M.J.; Sterling, R.K.; Luketic, V.A.; Shiffman, M.L.; Clore, J.N. Nonalcoholic steatohepatitis: Association of insulin resistance and mitochondrial abnormalities. *Gastroenterology* **2001**, *120*, 1183–1192. [CrossRef] [PubMed]

45. Rodriguez-Suarez, E.; Mato, J.M.; Elortza, F. Proteomics analysis of human nonalcoholic fatty liver. *Methods Mol. Biol.* **2012**, *909*, 241–258. [PubMed]

46. Venkatraman, A.; Shiva, S.; Wigley, A.; Ulasova, E.; Chhieng, D.; Bailey, S.M.; Darley-Usmar, V.M. The role of iNOS in alcohol-dependent hepatotoxicity and mitochondrial dysfunction in mice. *Hepatology* **2004**, *40*, 565–573. [CrossRef] [PubMed]

47. Mansouri, A.; Tarhuni, A.; Larosche, I.; Reyl-Desmars, F.; Demeilliers, C.; Degoul, F.; Nahon, P.; Sutton, A.; Moreau, R.; Fromenty, B.; *et al.* MnSOD overexpression prevents liver mitochondrial DNA depletion after an alcohol binge but worsens this effect after prolonged alcohol consumption in mice. *Dig. Dis.* **2010**, *28*, 756–775. [CrossRef] [PubMed]

48. Kessova, I.G.; Ho, Y.S.; Thung, S.; Cederbaum, A.I. Alcohol-induced liver injury in mice lacking Cu, Zn-superoxide dismutase. *Hepatology* **2003**, *38*, 1136–1145. [CrossRef] [PubMed]

49. Venkatraman, A.; Landar, A.; Davis, A.J.; Chamlee, L.; Sanderson, T.; Kim, H.; Page, G.; Pompilius, M.; Ballinger, S.; Darley-Usmar, V.; *et al.* Modification of the mitochondrial proteome in response to the stress of ethanol-dependent hepatotoxicity. *J. Biol. Chem.* **2004**, *279*, 22092–22101. [CrossRef] [PubMed]

50. Zelickson, B.R.; Benavides, G.A.; Johnson, M.S.; Chacko, B.K.; Venkatraman, A.; Landar, A.; Betancourt, A.M.; Bailey, S.M.; Darley-Usmar, V.M. Nitric oxide and hypoxia exacerbate alcohol-induced mitochondrial dysfunction in hepatocytes. *Biochim. Biophys. Acta* **2011**, *1807*, 1573–1582. [CrossRef] [PubMed]

51. Smathers, R.L.; Galligan, J.J.; Stewart, B.J.; Petersen, D.R. Overview of lipid peroxidation products and hepatic protein modification in alcoholic liver disease. *Chem. Biol. Interact.* **2011**, *192*, 107–112. [CrossRef] [PubMed]

52. Charbonneau, A.; Marette, A. Inducible nitric oxide synthase induction underlies lipid-induced hepatic insulin resistance in mice: Potential role of tyrosine nitration of insulin signaling proteins. *Diabetes* **2010**, *59*, 861–871. [CrossRef] [PubMed]

53. Povero, D.; Eguchi, A.; Li, H.; Johnson, C.D.; Papouchado, B.G.; Wree, A.; Messer, K.; Feldstein, A.E. Circulating extracellular vesicles with specific proteome and liver microRNAs are potential biomarkers for liver injury in experimental fatty liver disease. *PLoS ONE* **2014**, *9*, e113651. [CrossRef] [PubMed]

54. Su, W.; Wang, Y.; Jia, X.; Wu, W.; Li, L.; Tian, X.; Li, S.; Wang, C.; Xu, H.; Cao, J.; *et al.* Comparative proteomic study reveals 17β-HSD13 as a pathogenic protein in nonalcoholic fatty liver disease. *Proc. Natl. Acad. Sci. USA* **2014**, *111*, 11437–11442. [CrossRef] [PubMed]

55. Krishnan, A.; Li, X.; Kao, W.Y.; Viker, K.; Butters, K.; Masuoka, H.; Knudsen, B.; Gores, G.; Charlton, M. Lumican, an extracellular matrix proteoglycan, is a novel requisite for hepatic fibrosis. *Lab. Investig.* **2012**, *92*, 1712–1725. [CrossRef] [PubMed]

56. Charlton, M.; Viker, K.; Krishnan, A.; Sanderson, S.; Veldt, B.; Kaalsbeek, A.J.; Kendrick, M.; Thompson, G.; Que, F.; Swain, J.; *et al.* Differential expression of lumican and fatty acid binding protein-1: New insights into the histologic spectrum of nonalcoholic fatty liver disease. *Hepatology* **2009**, *49*, 1375–1384. [CrossRef] [PubMed]

57. Fitzpatrick, E.; Dhawan, A. Noninvasive biomarkers in non-alcoholic fatty liver disease: Current status and a glimpse of the future. *World J. Gastroenterol.* **2014**, *20*, 10851–10863. [CrossRef] [PubMed]

58. Binas, B.; Erol, E. FABPs as determinants of myocellular and hepatic fuel metabolism. *Mol. Cell. Biochem.* **2007**, *299*, 75–84. [CrossRef] [PubMed]

59. Higuchi, N.; Kato, M.; Tanaka, M.; Miyazaki, M.; Takao, S.; Kohjima, M.; Kotoh, K.; Enjoji, M.; Nakamuta, M.; Takayanagi, R. Effects of insulin resistance and hepatic lipid accumulation on hepatic mRNA expression levels of apoB, MTP and L-FABP in non-alcoholic fatty liver disease. *Exp. Ther. Med.* **2011**, *2*, 1077–1081. [PubMed]

60. Veerkamp, J.H.; van Moerkerk, H.T. Fatty acid-binding protein and its relation to fatty acid oxidation. *Mol. Cell. Biochem.* **1993**, *123*, 101–106. [CrossRef] [PubMed]

61. Ho, C.S.; Lam, C.W.; Chan, M.H.; Cheung, R.C.; Law, L.K.; Lit, L.C.; Ng, K.F.; Suen, M.W.; Tai, H.L. Electrospray ionisation mass spectrometry: Principles and clinical applications. *Clin. Biochem. Rev.* **2003**, *24*, 3–12. [PubMed]

62. Bell, L.N.; Theodorakis, J.L.; Vuppalanchi, R.; Saxena, R.; Bemis, K.G.; Wang, M.; Chalasani, N. Serum proteomics and biomarker discovery across the spectrum of nonalcoholic fatty liver disease. *Hepatology* **2010**, *51*, 111–120. [CrossRef] [PubMed]

63. Younossi, Z.M.; Baranova, A.; Ziegler, K.; del Giacco, L.; Schlauch, K.; Born, T.L.; Elariny, H.; Gorreta, F.; VanMeter, A.; Younoszai, A. A genomic and proteomic study of the spectrum of nonalcoholic fatty liver disease. *Hepatology* **2005**, *42*, 665–674. [CrossRef] [PubMed]

64. Janke, J.; Engeli, S.; Boschmann, M.; Adams, F.; Böhnke, J.; Luft, F.C.; Sharma, A.M.; Jordan, J. Retinol-binding protein 4 in human obesity. *Diabetes* **2006**, *55*, 2805–2810. [CrossRef] [PubMed]

65. Yu, C.; Xu, C.; Xu, L.; Yu, J.; Miao, M.; Li, Y. Serum proteomic analysis revealed diagnostic value of hemoglobin for nonalcoholic fatty liver disease. *J. Hepatol.* **2012**, *56*, 241–247. [CrossRef] [PubMed]

66. Jiang, Y.; Zeng, J.; Chen, B. Hemoglobin combined with triglyceride and ferritin in predicting non-alcoholic fatty liver. *J. Gastroenterol. Hepatol.* **2014**, *29*, 1508–1514. [CrossRef] [PubMed]

67. Akyuz, U.; Yesil, A.; Yilmaz, Y. Characterization of lean patients with nonalcoholic fatty liver disease: Potential role of high hemoglobin levels. *Scand. J. Gastroenterol.* **2015**, *50*, 341–346. [CrossRef] [PubMed]

68. Yilmaz, Y.; Senates, E.; Ayyildiz, T.; Colak, Y.; Tuncer, I.; Ovunc, A.O.; Dolar, E.; Kalayci, C. Characterization of nonalcoholic fatty liver disease unrelated to the metabolic syndrome. *Eur. J. Clin. Investig.* **2012**, *42*, 411–418. [CrossRef] [PubMed]

69. Liu, W.; Baker, S.S.; Baker, R.D.; Nowak, N.J.; Zhu, L. Upregulation of hemoglobin expression by oxidative stress in hepatocytes and its implication in nonalcoholic steatohepatitis. *PLoS ONE* **2011**, *6*, e24363. [CrossRef] [PubMed]

70. Trak-Smayra, V.; Dargere, D.; Noun, R.; Albuquerque, M.; Yaghi, C.; Gannagé-Yared, M.H.; Bedossa, P.; Paradis, V. Serum proteomic profiling of obese patients: Correlation with liver pathology and evolution after bariatric surgery. *Gut* **2009**, *58*, 825–832. [CrossRef] [PubMed]

8

Diet, Microbiota, Obesity and NAFLD: A Dangerous Quartet

Mariana Verdelho Machado [1,2] **and Helena Cortez-Pinto** [1,2,*]

1   Departamento de Gastrenterologia, Hospital de Santa Maria, Centro Hospitalar Lisboa Norte (CHLN),
     1649-035 Lisbon, Portugal; mverdelhomachado@gmail.com
2   Laboratório de Nutrição, Faculdade de Medicina de Lisboa, Universidade de Lisboa,
     Alameda da Universidade, 1649-004 Lisboa, Portugal
*   Correspondence: hlcortezpinto@netcabo.pt

Academic Editors: Amedeo Lonardo and Giovanni Targher

Abstract: Recently, the importance of the gut-liver-adipose tissue axis has become evident. Nonalcoholic fatty liver disease (NAFLD) is the hepatic disease of a systemic metabolic disorder that radiates from energy-surplus induced adiposopathy. The gut microbiota has tremendous influences in our whole-body metabolism, and is crucial for our well-being and health. Microorganisms precede humans in more than 400 million years and our guest flora evolved with us in order to help us face aggressor microorganisms, to help us maximize the energy that can be extracted from nutrients, and to produce essential nutrients/vitamins that we are not equipped to produce. However, our gut microbiota can be disturbed, dysbiota, and become itself a source of stress and injury. Dysbiota may adversely impact metabolism and immune responses favoring obesity and obesity-related disorders such as insulin resistance/diabetes mellitus and NAFLD. In this review, we will summarize the latest evidence of the role of microbiota/dysbiota in diet-induced obesity and NAFLD, as well as the potential therapeutic role of targeting the microbiota in this set.

Keywords: nonalcoholic fatty liver disease; microbiota; diet; obesity; dysbiota; probiotics

1. Introduction

Nonalcoholic fatty liver disease (NAFLD) refers to the ectopic accumulation of fat in the liver. In its primary form, NAFLD is the hepatic manifestation of metabolic dysfunction associated with energy surplus-induced adiposopathy. The term adiposopathy has only recently been introduced in the medical lexicon and translates the adipose tissue dysfunction that occurs, in susceptible individuals, as a consequence of chronic positive caloric balance and sedentary lifestyle [1]. The true significance of hepatic steatosis as a contributing player in obesity-induced dysmetabolism and global metabolic and cardiovascular health is still unclear [2]. Regarding liver health, although most patients will present stable, non-progressive disease, the high prevalence of this condition explains why NAFLD is the number one cause of chronic liver disease in Western world and will predictably be the number one cause of end-stage liver disease in the near future [3].

Little more than a decade ago, a major breakthrough linked the gut microbiota to the pathogenesis of obesity and NAFLD [4]. Since then, medical research in the field has flourished exponentially. However, huge gaps in knowledge still preclude us to have effective therapeutic strategies for obesity and NAFLD that act through modulation of gut microbiota.

The gut microbiota comprises 10 to 100 trillion microbes. The gut microbiota is composed by bacteria, archea, virus, and fungi, being dominated by four main phyla of bacteria: Firmicutes, Bacterioidetes, Actinobacteria, and Proteobacteria, which represent more than 95% [5,6]. The collective genome of the gut microbiota, referred to as a microbiome, contains at least 100 times more genes than the human genome [6]. Those extra genes are crucial to maintain our homeostasis. In fact, the gut microbiome is enriched in several genes important for glycans and aminoacids metabolism, xenobiotics metabolism, methanogenesis, and biosynthesis of vitamins [6]. This explains why the gut microbiota contributes to host nutrition, bone mineral density, modulation of the immune system, xenobiotics metabolism, intestinal cell development and proliferation, and protection against pathogens [7].

One important question still not fully answered is if there is a core microbiota common to humans. In fact, although culture-based studies suggest that healthy humans would share the same gut bacterial species, culture-independent studies showed that each individual harbors a unique collection of bacterial strains and species [7,8]. Not only gut microbiota is specific to individual, it is also highly resilient, promptly returning to baseline after perturbation [7,9–11]. However, recovery may be impaired with recurrent perturbation [12]. Interestingly, despite the unique individual gut microbiota, humans share similar functional gene profiles, implying a core functional microbiome [8].

The composition of the gut microbiota is regulated by (a) external factors such as vaginal *versus* cesarean section delivery, breast feeding, antibiotics, pre/probiotics, diet, hygienic habits, and random chance resulting in a colonization cascade; (b) interaction with the host such as genetics, Paneth cell function, mucus composition, secretion of antimicrobial peptides; and (c) interaction between microbes, which can result in competition or cooperation [5,13,14].

In this review, we will summarize the latest research on the interplay between diet, gut microbiota, obesity, and fatty liver disease. We will also discuss the evidence of microbiota-targeting approaches in the treatment of NAFLD.

2. Microbiota and Obesity

The first clue on the role of the microbiota in the pathogenesis of obesity came from Backhed *et al.* [4] studies. They compared body weight gain in germ free mice and conventionally raised mice, and found that the latter gained more weight, with increased adipose tissue and body fat percentage, which could not be explained by different diet intake. Importantly, metabolic status was worse in conventionally raised mice, with higher leptin levels, lower insulin sensitivity and greater fat accumulation in the liver. Further supporting the concept that body weight was regulated by gut microbiota, transplantation of microbiota harvested from conventionally raised mice into germ free mice resulted in an increase in body weight and decrease in insulin sensitivity [4]. Moreover, the same group showed that, not only germ-free mice were leaner than conventionally raised mice, they were also resistant to western-type high-fat diet induced obesity [15]. Lastly, studies on animal models showed us that not all microbiota has the same effect on metabolism, and raised the possibility of an obesity-specific microbiota. In fact, transplantation of microbiota harvested by either genetically-obese ob/ob mice [16] or high-fat diet induced obese mice [17] into germ free mice mimicked the obese insulin resistant phenotype. Supporting the animal data, a small human study in male patients with the metabolic syndrome submitted to autologous or allogenic (from a lean donor) intestinal microbiota via duodenal tube, showed improvement in insulin sensitivity when the donor was lean [18].

Since then, several groups tried to characterize the obese-associated microbiota. Studies in either genetically or diet-induced obese mice showed differences in the microbiota when comparing with lean mice. Obese mice consistently showed a decrease in Bacterioidetes and an increase in Firmicutes (particularly from the class Millicutes) [19–21]. This increase in Firmicutes associated with an increase in enzymes able to breakdown indigestible polysaccharides from diet and producing short chain fatty acids (SCFA) [19]. Obese mice also presented an increase in methanogenic Archea, which associates with a lower hydrogen partial pressure and optimization of bacterial fermentation [19].

Studies in human obesity showed lower microbial diversity and similar differences in the intestinal microbiota as suggested by animal studies [22–24].

In summary, there is an obesity-associated gut microbiota, and obesity can be infectiously transmitted by transplant of that microbiome, suggesting that it is the microbiota itself that promotes obesity. Supporting this concept, a prospective study in children showed that the risk of being overweight at seven years old could be predicted by the composition of gut microbiota at six months old, which associated with lower prevalence of *Bifidobacterium* and higher of *Staphylococcus aureus* [25].

Obese mice waste less energy in the stools as compared to lean mice, and as little as a 20% decrease in fecal Bacterioidetes associates with 150 Kcal decrease in energy harvest from the diet [26]. The microbiota can modulate body weight through several mechanisms. One such mechanism is the differential fermentation of indigestible carbohydrates in SCFA: butyrate, propionate, and acetate [27]. Overall, colonic-derived SCFA account for 10% of harvested energy from the diet, with acetate being the main source of energy [28]. Butyrate and propionate are considered anti-obesogenic, and acetate mainly obesogenic. Interestingly, while acetate and propionate are mainly produced by the phylum Bacterioidetes, butyrate is mainly produced by Firmicutes (the most important belonging to clostridial lusters IV and XIVa: *Faecalibacterium prausnitzii*, *Eubacterium rectale*, and *Rosuberia intestinalis*) [29,30]. Butyrate is a major source of energy for colonocytes, increasing intestinal health and potentially decreasing gut permeability and preventing metabolic endotoxemia [31]. Butyrate also seems to positively affect insulin sensitivity through stimulation of the release of the incretins glucagon-like peptide-1 (GLP-1) and gastric inhibitory polypeptide (GIP) [32]. Both butyrate and propionate can increase the expression of the anorexigenic adipokine leptin [33]. Other beneficial effects of propionate are inhibition of resistin expression by the adipose tissue [34] and inhibition of cholesterol synthesis through inhibition of acetyl-CoA synthetase and via buffering fatty acids to gluconeogenesis in detriment of cholesterol synthesis [27]. On the other hand, acetate is the most substantially absorbed SCFA, and is a substrate for lipogenesis and cholesterol synthesis in the liver and adipose tissue [27]. Finally, SCFA bind to specific receptors in the gut, liver, and adipose tissue, GRP43 and GRP41, which seem to have anti-inflammatory and metabolic actions that protect from obesity [28]. Interestingly, supplementation of oral butyrate in mice fed a Western diet, partially prevented liver steatosis and inflammation, while having no effect on obesity [35].

Gut microbiota can also decrease the intestinal expression of the adipose tissue lipoprotein lipase inhibitor fasting induced adipose factor (Fiaf), also known as angiopoietin-like factor IV (ANGPTL4). The net result is increased uptake of fatty acids in the adipose tissue and liver, favoring expansion of the adipose tissue and hepatic steatosis. Microbiota also prevents the beneficial action of Fiaf in the expression of peroxisome proliferator-activated receptor (PPAR)-1α coactivator (PGC) and fatty acids oxidation [15,36]. Other mechanisms by which gut microbiota promote obesity are an increase in mucosal gut blood flow enhancing nutrients absorption [37]; inhibition of adenosine monophosphate-activated protein kinase AMPK in the liver and muscle, and consequently inhibiting peripheral fatty acids oxidation and insulin resistance [15]; and modulation of the pattern of conjugated bile acids and its function in lipid absorption [38].

Obesity itself may also change the microbiota, independently of the diet. For example, leptin, an adipokine whose levels are increased in obesity, has a direct role regulating the gut microbiota composition, through the modulation of antimicrobial peptides secretion by Paneth cells in the gut [39]. As such, a vicious circle between microbiota and adiposity promotes further worsening of obesity.

3. Microbiota and Nonalcoholic Fatty Liver Disease (NAFLD)/Nonalcoholic Steatohepatitis (NASH)

NAFLD strongly associates with obesity. The aggregate data suggests that the gut microbiota may play a significant role in the pathogenesis of obesity, as such it would be logical to think that the gut microbiota also plays a role in the development of NAFLD and its progressive form, nonalcoholic steatohepatitis (NASH). Indeed, that seems to be the case. Transplanting harvested microbiota from conventionally raised mice to germ free mice, besides increasing body weight, it also increases the fat content in the liver [4]. Furthermore, treatment with antibiotics protected from hepatic steatosis in different dietary and genetic obese rodent models [40,41]. However, the association between gut microbiota and NAFLD goes beyond the association with obesity.

Several studies in animal models and patients with NAFLD or NASH showed an association with small bowel overgrowth and increased intestinal permeability [42–49]. Brun *et al.* [45], compared two strains of genetically obese mice, leptin deficient ob/ob and leptin-resistant db/db, with lean control mice. They found that obese mice had increased intestinal permeability with lower intestinal resistance and profound changes in the cytoskeleton of cells in the intestinal mucosa. In association with increased gut permeability, obese mice, as compared to lean mice, had higher circulating levels of inflammatory cytokines and portal endotoxemia. Finally, hepatic stellate cells from obese mice expressed higher levels of the lipopolysaccharide (LPS) co-receptor CD14, and responded with a more inflammatory and fibrogenic phenotype after stimulation with LPS [45]. Furthermore, a study compared NAFLD patients with healthy subjects, and found that patients with NAFLD had an increased susceptibility to develop increased intestinal permeability after a minor challenge with low dose aspirin [46]. Concordant with those observations, obesity and NAFLD associates with metabolic endotoxemia, *i.e.*, increased blood levels of lipopolysaccharide (LPS), a component of the wall of Gram-negative bacteria that binds to specific receptors, toll like receptor-4 (TLR-4), and can promote hepatic and systemic inflammation [47,49,50]. Verdam *et al.* [51] also showed an increase in plasma antibodies against LPS in patients with NASH as compared to healthy controls, which progressively increased with increased severity of liver disease. The role of LPS is highlighted by the study by Cani *et al.* [50] in which LPS injections in mice simulated the effects of a high-fat diet, in terms of weight gain, insulin resistance, and development of NAFLD. Furthermore, mice deficient in TLR-4 are not only protected from LPS-induced obesity and NAFLD, but also from high-fat diet-induced obesity and NAFLD [50], as well as NAFLD and NASH in different rodent models [47,52–54].

Perturbations in the metabolism of bile acids seem to have a prominent role in the pathogenesis of NAFLD [55]. Bile acids are not only critical in the absorption of fat, they are also signaling molecules with actions in their own metabolism, as well as energy, lipoproteins, and glucose metabolism, through its receptors farsenoid X receptor FXR and TGR5. There is a known mutual influence between bile acids and gut microbiota. Bile acids have potent antimicrobial properties [56]. On the other hand, the gut microbiota increases the diversity of bile acids through the deconjugation, dehydrogenation, and dehydroxylation of primary bile acids. In fact, conventionally raised mice, as compared to germ free mice presented a decrease in tauro-conjugates (which are potent FXR antagonists and hence positive regulators of bile acids synthesis), while maintaining levels of the more toxic cholic acid [57].

Recently, two studies elegantly demonstrated that NAFLD could be a transmissible disease, through gut microbiota. Le Roy *et al.* [58] fed mice with high fat diet for 16 weeks, and while most of the animals developed NAFLD, insulin resistance, and systemic inflammation (dubbed responders), some mice did not develop NAFLD or insulin resistance (dubbed non-responders). When they transplanted germ free mice with microbiota harvested from those animals, they obtained a metabolic and liver phenotype only if the donors were responders. Furthermore, mice with a genetic deficiency of the inflammasome in the gut exhibited a perturbed gut-innate immunity and an abnormal gut microbiota with increased Bacterioidetes (particularly from the family Porphyromondaceae) and decreased Firmicutes. Those mice developed worse liver damage when fed NASH-inducing diets, with increased steatosis, inflammation, and aminotransferases levels, as compared to their wild type counterparts. Interestingly, co-housing those transgenic mice with wild type mice turned the latter more sensitive to the diet-inducing NASH, effect that was abrogated by concomitant treatment with antibiotics [59]. Lastly, de Minicis *et al.* [60] modulated gut microbiota through high-fat diet (which induced an increase in Proteobacteria), before submitting mice to bile duct ligation. Those mice developed worse fibrosis than chow diet fed mice. They simulated the increased susceptibility to fibrosis by transplanting gut microbiota from high-fat diet fed mice, which was even worse when they selectively transplanted Gram-negative bacteria.

The gut microbiota also seems to have a role in NAFLD-associated hepatocarcinogenesis. Yoshimoto *et al.* [61] showed that, in different animal models of obesity, dysbiota associates with increased deoxycholic acid reaching the liver through the enterohepatic circulation. This bile acid was able to produce a senescence phenotype in hepatic stellate cells that induced a secretory profile able to promote inflammation and tumorigenesis.

Several studies in adult patients, have tried to evaluate if the presence of NAFLD associates with a specific dysbiota [62–67] (Table 1). Those are small studies, with different populations and controls and often without histological diagnosis. Furthermore, statistical significance was achieved in different categories in the taxonomic hierarchy. Though NAFLD/NASH seems to share some of the microbiota specificities associated with obesity, at the phylum level, only one study found NASH to be associated with a decreased percentage of Bacterioidetes [63]. The two studies that compared patients with NAFLD with healthy controls found an increase of the genus *Lactobacillus*, and a decrease in the family Ruminococcaceae in NAFLD patients [64,67]. Regarding the association with *Lactobacillus*, it is surprising, since several species from this genus are frequently used as probiotics. *Lactobacillus* are lactic acid bacteria that can inhibit pathogens, enhance the epithelial barrier function, and modulate immune responses [68], actions that would seem protective in the pathogenesis of NAFLD/NASH. However, *Lactobacillus* may associate with the production of volatile organic compounds such as acetate and ethanol [69], which may be important in the pathogenesis of obesity and NAFLD [64]. In fact, the genus *Lactobacillus* comprises over 180 species and a wide variety of organisms; while some can only produce lactic acid from the fermentation of sugars (e.g., *L. acidophilus* and *L. salivarius*), other can also produce ethanol (e.g., *L. casei*, *L. brevis* and *L. plantarum*). Again, the decrease of Ruminococcaceae may also translate to a decrease in the production of SCFA such as butyrate, since many bacteria from that family produce butyrate [70]. A decrease in butyrate-producing bacteria, such as the genus *Faecalibacterium* [70] has also been associated with NASH, as compared to healthy controls [65]. As compared to healthy subjects, patients with NAFLD also showed increased percentage of bacteria from the genera *Escherichia* and pathogenic *Streptococcus*, both known to potentially induce persistent inflammation in the intestinal mucosa, and to be associated with inflammatory bowel disease [71,72]. In accordance, patients with NAFLD exhibited higher expression of proinflammatory cytokines in the intestinal mucosa [67]. Some *Escherichia* species also produce ethanol, which can further increase gut permeability. In fact, children with NASH also displayed increased levels of *Escherichia* bacteria in their stools [73].

Spencer *et al.* [62] evaluated an interaction between choline metabolism and microbiota in the development of NAFLD. They studied 15 inpatient women and submitted them to depletion of choline. They found that differences in two classes of bacteria (decrease in Gammaproteobacteria and increase in Erysipelotrichi), in association with genetic polymorphisms in phosphatidylethanolamine N-methyltransferase (PEMT, a key enzyme in the choline metabolism), could predict the susceptibility to develop NAFLD with choline depletion. This is highly relevant, because the median choline intake in the United States is half the recommended dose (recommended dose: 550 mg per day) [74]. Gut microbiota can further promote choline depletion by hydrolyzing choline to trimethylamine, which can be further metabolized in the liver into the toxic compound trimethylamine N-oxide (TMAO). Interestingly, feeding mice with high fat diet is known to shift the gut microbiota into a choline degradation profile [75].

In patients with NAFLD, the presence of NASH associated with an increase in the genus *Bacteroides* [66]. This skew in favor of *Bacteroides* may translate to an increase in the toxic bile deoxycholic acid, which is known to induce apoptosis in hepatocytes and to be increased in patients with NASH [76,77]. Furthermore, *Bacteroides* has been associated with an increase in branched-chain fatty acids derived from aminoacids fermentation, which have diabetogenic potential [78]. Lastly, in patients with NAFLD, the presence of significant fibrosis also associated with increased content of the genus *Ruminococcus*, which is difficult to interpret, since it is a highly heterogeneous genus including both potentially beneficial and detrimental species [66]. Nevertheless, some species from the *Ruminococcus* genus are pro-inflammatory and able to produce ethanol [79–81], two potential pathogenic mechanisms in the progression of NAFLD.

Table 1. Studies evaluating microbiota in human NAFLD/NASH.

Study	Population	Phyla	Class	Order	Family	Genera	Species
Spencer, M.D., 2011 [62]	15 women with a choline deficient diet and risk for NAFLD	Firmicutes	↑**Erysipelotrichi**			↑*Clostridium*	↑*C. coccoide*
		Proteobacteriaceae	→**Gammaproteobacteria**				
Mouzaki, H., 2013 [63]	17 controls biopsy proven: 11 SS 22 NASH	↓**Bacteroidetes**					
Raman, H., 2013 [64]	30 obese with NAFLD 30 healthy controls	Firmicutes	Clostridia	Clostridiales	Clostridiaceae	*Clostridium*	
			Bacilli	Lactobacillales	Lactobacillaceae	↑*Lactobacillus*	
			Clostridia	Clostridiales	↑**Lachnospiraceae**	↑*Robinsoniella* ↑*Roseburia* ↑*Dorea*	
					↓**Ruminococcecae**	↓*Oscillibacter*	
		Bacterioidetes	Bacterioidia	Bacteroidales	↑**Porphyromonadaceae**	↑*Parabacteroides*	
Wong, V.W.S., 2013 [65]	16 NASH 22 healthy controls	↓**Firmicutes**	Clostridia	↓**Clostridiales**	Clostridiaceae	↓*Faecalibacterium* ↓*Anaesporobacter*	
			Negativicutes	Selenomonadales	Veillonellaceae	↑*Allisonela*	
		Proteobacteria	Gammaproteobacteria	↑**Aeromonadales**	↑**Succinivibrionaceae**		
Boursier, J., 2015 [66]	57 patients with NAFLD: 30 F0/F1 27 > F1	Bacterioidetes	Bacterioidia	↑**Bacterioidales** (NASH)			
		Firmicutes	Clostridia	Clostridiales	Rumminococcecae	↑**Ruminococcus** (>F1)	
Jiang, W., 2015 [67]	53 NAFLD 32 healthy controls	Bacterioidetes	Bacterioidia	Bacteroidales	**Porphyromonadaceae**	↓*Odoribacter*	
					Rikenellaceae	↓*Alistipes*	
					Prevotellaceae	↓*Prevotella*	
			Bacilli	Lactobacillales	Lactobacillaceae	↑*Lactobacillus*	
					Streptococcaceae	↑*Streptococcus*	
		Firmicutes	Clostridia	Clostridiales	Clostridiaceae	↑*Clostridium*	
					↓**Ruminococcecae**	↓*Oscillibacter*	
						↓*Flavonitractor*	
		Proteobacteriaceae	Gammaproteobacteria	Enterobacteriales	Enterobactereaceae	↑*Escherichia*	
		↓**Lentisphaerae**					

In bold are the associations described. NAFLD, nonalcoholic fatty liver disease; NASH, nonalcoholic steatohepatitis, F0/F1, no or mild fibrosis, >F1, significant fibrosis. Arrows indicate the differences in the studied group as compared to the control group.

NAFLD and particularly NASH also seem to associate with specific changes in the oral microbiota. Yoneda *et al.* [82] studied 150 patients with NAFLD (of those 102 with NASH) and 60 healthy controls, and found that infection with *Porphyromonas gingivalis* (the major cause of periodontitis) tripled the risk for NAFLD and quadrupled the risk for NASH, independent of ge and metabolic syndrome. In 10 patients with NAFLD, treatment of periodontitis prompted an improvement in liver enzymes [82]. Furthermore, in patients with NASH, positive immunohistochemistry for *P. gingivalis* associated with increased fibrosis [83]. In mice fed high-fat diet, infection with *P. gingivalis* associated with endotoxemia and increased blood levels of proinflammatory cytokines, as well as worse liver disease, including worse fibrosis [82,83].

In summary, gut microbiota can contribute to the development and progression of NAFLD via several mechanisms: (a) modulation of energy homeostasis and energy harvested from diet with associated obesity and dysmetabolism [4,26]; (b) modulation of intestinal permeability promoting endotoxemia as well as other microbe products that promote systemic and hepatic inflammation [50]; (c) modulation of the choline metabolism (required for very low density lipoproteins VLDL synthesis and export of lipids from the liver) [75]; (d) generation of endogenous ethanol as well as other toxic products such as TMAO [73,84–86]; and (e) modulation of bile acids homeostasis and FXR function [87,88] (Figure 1).

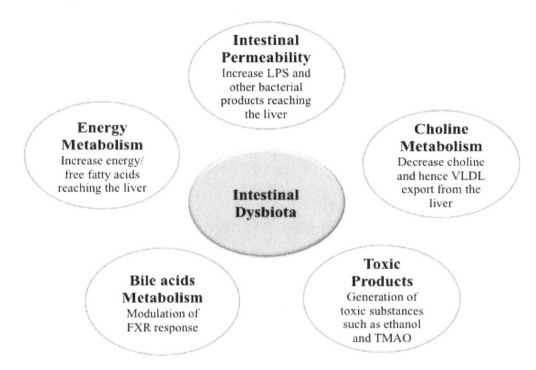

Figure 1. Nonalcoholic fatty liver disease (NAFLD) associated mechanisms of intestinal dysbiota.

4. Diet and Microbiota

Both the quality and quantity of our diet strongly modulate the gut microbiota. Different diets associate with different compositions of the microbiota. De Fillipo *et al.*'s [89] work beautifully translates this concept. They compared the fecal microbiota of European children (who ate a modern Western diet) with children from a rural African village of Burkina Faso (which ate a high-fiber diet, similar to the ancient diet soon after the birth of agriculture). Children from Burkina Faso had a decreased Firmicutes/Bacterioidetes ratio, a higher percentage of bacteria from the genera *Prevotella* and *Xylanibacter* (known to be equipped with enzymes in the degradation of indigestible carbohydrates), and a decrease in the proinflammatory Enterobacteriaceae, *Shigella* and *Escherichia*.

They also had higher amounts of SCFA in the stools. This study suggests that gut microbiota coevolved with the polysaccharide rich diet in order to maximize energy intake from fibers [89].

How quickly can a change in the diet induce differences in the microbiome? In mice, we can induce changes in the gut microbiome after just one single day on a different diet [17]. Studies in humans also showed diet-driven changes in the intestinal microbiota occurring as early as in three to four days [90]. In a clinical study, David *et al.* [91] were able to induce differences in microbiota, that would be metabolically more fit to the type of diet administered, entirely animal or entirely plant products, in just five days. Furthermore, volunteers placed on a three-day high or low-calorie diet, showed that even this short-term increase in energy intake, associated with an increased Firmicutes/Bacterioidetes ratio, correlated with a decrease in the proportion of energy loss in the stools [26]. Indeed, diets enriched in fibers associate with an increase in the fecal loss of energy [92]. However, after stopping the diet, microbiota quickly returned to the basal state, translating the high resilience of our gut flora. Similarly, a dietary intervention in obese or overweight subjects, consisting of administering an energy-restricted high protein diet during six weeks, increased the diversity of species in the gut, along with decreased adiposity, which reverted to basal levels after the diet was stopped [93]. In contrast, long-term diets were able to induce more profound changes in the microbiota than short-term ones [94].

Chronic high-fat diet feeding in mice is known to change gut microbiota with progressive increase in Firmicutes and decrease in Bacterioidetes [20,21]. One important question regarding diet-induced changes in the microbiota is whether it is the composition of the diet or the number of calories ingested that has an effect on gut flora. Also, is diet or obesity itself the important factor for our gut health? Several lines of evidence suggest that both quantity and quality of the diet modulate gut microbiota. Mice deficient in resistin-like molecule β are resistant to high-fat diet induced obesity, however they still shift their gut microbiota with a decrease in Bacterioidetes and increase in Firmicutes as well as Proteobacteria, in response to those diets, in a similar way as their wild type counterparts [95]. This suggests that it is diet and not obesity, the critical factor determining the gut microbiota. On the other hand, when genetically obese leptin resistant mice were pair-fed with wild type mice, they still maintained the same differences in gut microbiota as genetically obese leptin resistant mice fed *ad libitum* [39]. This suggests that leptin itself (and hence the obesity state) may modulate gut microbiota independently of the diet.

Suggesting a critical effect on the composition of the diet, different formulations of high-fat diet, with different percentages of saturated and polyunsaturated fatty acids, seem to have different effects on the gut microbiota. Feeding mice with diets with higher percentage of saturated fatty acids not only seemed to associate with worse weight gain and hepatic steatosis, it also induced more profound changes in the microbiome, with a decrease in diversity and an increase in the Firmicutes/Bacterioidetes ratio [96]. Concordant with the concept of diet composition and gut microbiota crosstalk, mice were fed with either low-fat diet for 35 weeks (remaining lean), high-fat diet for 35 weeks (becoming and remaining obese), low-fat diet for 12 weeks followed by restricted intake of low-fat diet for 23 weeks (to maintain a 20% reduction in body weight), or high-fat diet for 12 weeks followed by restricted intake of high-fat diet for 23 weeks (in order to gain weight and then maintain a 20% reduction in body weight) [97]. The authors found that, regardless of weight status, low-fat diets induced the higher abundance of Firmicutes due to two species from the genus *Allobaculum'* and the high-fat diets induced the higher abundance of non-*Allobaculum* Firmicutes, Bacterioidetes and Mucispirillum. The aggregate animal data suggest a contribution of the quality of the diet *versus* the caloric intake in the composition of the gut microbiota.

Similar conclusions regarding the importance of quality *versus* quantity of the diet, can be taken from a study on obese volunteers that ate one of two isocaloric diets: low carbohydrates/high fat or high carbohydrates/low fat [98]. While the former diet associated with a decrease in fecal SCFA and *Bifidobacterium*, the latter associated with an increase in total anaerobes in fecal samples.

Fava *et al.* [99] studied subjects at increased risk for the metabolic syndrome. Those subjects were given a high saturated fat diet for four weeks and, subsequently, randomized for one of the following diets: high saturated fat diet, high monosaturated fat (MUFA)/high glycemic index diet, high MUFA/low glycemic index diet, high carbohydrate/high glycemic index diet and high carbohydrate/low glycemic index diet. They found that high carbohydrate diets (low fat) increased fecal *Bifidobacterium* and improved glucose metabolism, however if the diet had high glycemic index, it associated with an increase in fecal Bacteroides (which were associated with NASH in patients with NAFLD [66]), and if the glycemic index were lower, it associated with an increase in *Faecalibacterium prausnitzii* (which seems beneficial in protecting from NASH [65]). Furthermore, high saturated fat diets associated with increased fecal SCFA content. In conclusion, the Fava *et al.* [99] study beautifully translates that different compositions of isocaloric diets can modulate the gut microbiota, with potential impact in the risk for the development of the metabolic syndrome and NASH.

Studies in mice showed that high-fat diets could increase fecal content of hydrogen sulfide producing bacteria such as from the family Desulfovibrionaceae. This is a relevant effect since hydrogen sulfide is toxic to colonocytes, perturbing intestinal barrier function and increasing endotoxemia [100]. Another important association was made with *Akkermansia muciniphila*, a specific type of mucin-degrading bacteria that improves intestinal barrier. *Akkermansia muciniphila* levels were shown to decrease after high fat diet [101].

Recently, different groups showed that bariatric surgery might induce weight loss not necessarily by a decrease in food intake and through malabsorption, but also by modulating the gut microbiota. Obese patients submitted to bariatric surgery experienced profound changes in the gut microbiota that correlated with weight loss, including: an increase in diversity, decrease in Firmicutes and methanogenic Archea, with concurrent increases in Bacterioidetes and Gammaproteobacteria, as well as a decrease in lactic acid bacteria such as *Lactobacillus* and *Bifidobacterium* [102–104]. Indeed, causality between modulation of gut microbiota and weight loss was proved by Liou *et al.* [105] Transfering the gut microbiota from mice that underwent bariatric surgery into non-operated germ-free mice, resulted in weight loss, decreased body and liver fat, as compared to germ-free mice receiving gut microbiota from mice submitted to sham surgery.

More recently, bile acids entered the equation between bariatric surgery, altered microbiota and weight loss. In fact, bariatric surgery is known to associate with increased circulating levels of bile acids and FXR signaling [106–109]. Suggesting a role of bile acids through FXR signaling, FXR deficient mice submitted to high-fat diet induced obesity and subsequent bariatric surgery (vertical sleeve gastrectomy), were less prone to sustained weight loss after surgery, with compensatory increase in food intake within three to five weeks [110]. Also, they did not improve glycemic control after surgery. Interestingly, as compared to wild type mice, in FXR deficient mice, bariatric surgery had an attenuated ability to modulate the gut microbiota, with no inhibition of Bacteroides and maintaining a decrease in *Roseburia* (known to also be decreased in human type 2 diabetes mellitus).

5. Microbiota as a Therapeutic Target

We can intervene in order to modulate our gut microbiota either giving commensal organisms known to improve our health status (dubbed probiotics), giving carbohydrates that stimulate the growth of potential beneficial commensals (dubbed prebiotics), or by giving a mix of both (dubbed symbiotics). In this review we will focus on the evidence on probiotics and symbiotics, since data on prebiotics alone are less robust.

Probiotics can potentially be beneficial in the treatment of NAFLD/NASH through several mechanisms: (a) competition with pathogenic species and antimicrobial effect modulating IgA secretion; (b) anti-inflammatory effect with inhibition of pro-inflammatory cytokines production; (c) increased gut satiety signals such as induction of YY peptide and inhibition of orexigenic ghrelin; (d) promotion of intestinal epithelium integrity and improvement of intestinal barrier; (e) decreased harvesting of energy from non-digestible carbohydrates; (f) decreased production of ethanol and other volatile organic compounds; (g) increased production of Fiaf; (h) decreased fatty acid oxidation in the liver; (i) insulin-sensitizing effect via synthesis of GLP-1; (j) modulation of bile acids and cholesterol metabolism; as well as (k) modulation of choline metabolism [13,111,112].

Due to the high resilience of our gut microbiota that easily tends to return to baseline after perturbation, interventions aimed to modulate the gut microbiota are deemed to early relapse to the initial dysbiota state after stopping the intervention, unless long-term approaches are used.

Several pre-clinical studies evaluated the role of probiotics in protecting from obesity and/or the metabolic syndrome, in different rodent models of obesity [113–117]. The studies are difficult to compare because not only are the models used different, the probiotics used are also different. While not all studies achieved a decrease in body weight and adiposity [117], all showed some metabolic benefit. Similarly, clinical studies in obese patients used different probiotics [118–122]. Those studies had small sample sizes and many of them were uncontrolled interventions [118,120,121]. Not all interventions achieved an improvement in body weight [118] or in metabolic profile [119,121]. While small pilot studies on prebiotics applied to obese patients did modify the gut microbiota [123] and improved lipid profile, in general those interventions failed to achieve weight loss or improvement in the glucose metabolism [124–126].

Probiotics have also been studied as a therapeutic tool for NAFLD/NASH. Three preclinical studies in mouse models of NAFLD associated with genetic and/or diet-induced obesity evaluated the role of a probiotic preparation, VSL#3. VSL#3 contains eight bacterial species from the genera *Bifidobacterium*, *Lactobacillus*, and *Streptococcus salivarius* subsp. thermophilus. This intervention improved steatosis, aminotransferases levels, serum lipids and insulin resistance [127–129]. Additionally, mice fed methionine-choline diet, a model of severe NASH not associated with obesity or the metabolic syndrome, developed less liver fibrosis when treated with VSL#3 [130]. Other probiotics also showed beneficial effects in animal models of NAFLD/NASH [131–139].

In humans, only small short-term pilot studies evaluated different probiotic/symbiotic preparations as a therapeutic approach for NAFLD (Table 2) [140–147]. However, the expectations on probiotics as a therapeutic tool in NAFLD are so high, that there are more systematic reviews and meta-analysis [13,112,148–154] on the topic than primary studies itself. Most studies did find a decrease in aminotransferases levels and hepatic steatosis after a short-term intervention. However, in terms of dysmetabolism, these studies failed to show benefit in anthropometric parameters and effect on lipid and glucose metabolism was not consistent among studies. Eslamparast *et al.* [146] noninvasively assessed liver fibrosis with transient elastography, pre- and post-intervention. They performed a randomized clinical trial, compared to placebo in 26 patients with NAFLD in each arm. They used a probiotic mixture that included different species from *Lactobacillus*, *Bifidobacterium*, and *Streptococcus* genera, as well as two different yeasts. After seven months of therapy, they did achieve a difference between probiotic and placebo arms in liver fibrosis, favoring the probiotic arm. One randomized clinical trial, with 36 patients with NASH in the probiotic group and 36 in the control group, performed liver biopsy pre and post-intervention [143]. After six months of treatment with Zirfos (a symbiotic with *B. longum*), patients in the symbiotic group, as compared to the placebo group, profited in terms of hepatic steatosis, but had no advantage in hepatocellular ballooning, liver inflammation, or liver fibrosis.

In summary, though promising, the evidence for the use of probiotics in the treatment of NAFLD/NASH is still insufficient. Studies are small, with short-term interventions, different formulations, different compositions of probiotics/symbiotics, and different durations of treatment. Also, most studies lack liver biopsy. The one study that systematically performed liver biopsy pre- and post-intervention failed to demonstrate significant differences between probiotics and placebo in important histological endpoints such as hepatic inflammation and fibrosis [143].

Table 2. Studies evaluating the therapeutic role of probiotics in human NAFLD/NASH.

Study	Design	Probiotic Composition	Results
Loguercio, C., 2002 [140]	10 patients with NASH No control group Two months intervention	LAB: *L. acidophilus, L, rhamnosus, L plantarum, L. salivarius, L. casei, L. bulgaricus, B. lactis, B. bifidus, B. breve,* FOS, vitamins	↓ liver enzymes: ALT and γGT ↓ TNF-α levels and oxidative stress Relapse after stopping the intervention
Loguercio, C., 2005 [141]	22 patients with NASH No control group Three months intervention	VSL#3: *B. breve, B. longum, B. infantis, L. acidophilus, L. plantarum, L. paracasei, L. bulgaricus, S. Thermophilus* (2 capsules, twice a day)	↓ liver enzymes ↓ oxidative stress
Aller, R., 2011 [142]	Patients with NAFLD: probiotic group *n* = 15 and control group *n* = 15 Three months intervention	Mixture of 500 million *L. bulgaricus + S. thermophiles*	↓ liver enzymes: ALT no difference in anthropometric metrics no difference in lipid / glucose metabolism no difference in IL-6 or TNF-α levels
Malaguarnera, M., 2012 [143]	Patients with NASH: Probiotic group *n* = 34 and control group *n* = 29 Biopsy pre and post-intervention Six months intervention	Zirfos: FOS, *B. longum*, vitamins	↓ liver enzymes: AST ↓ LDL-cholesterol and insulin resistance ↓ TNF-α levels and endotoxemia no difference in anthropometric metrics ↓ steatosis and NAS score no difference in ballooning, inflammation or fibrosis
Wong, V.WS., 2013 [144]	Patients with NASH: probiotic group *n* = 10 and control group *n* = 10 Six months intervention	Lepicol: *L. deslbrueckii, L. acidophilus, L. rhamnosus, B. bifidum*	↓ liver steatosis by H-MRS ↓ liver enzymes: AST no difference in anthropometric metrics no difference in lipid / glucose metabolism
Nabavi, S., 2014 [145]	Patients with NAFLD: probiotic group *n* = 36 and control group *n* = 36 Two months intervention	Probiotic yogurt containing *L. acidophilus* La5 and *B. lactis* Bb12	↓ liver enzymes: ALT and AST ↓ total cholesterol and LDL-cholesterol
Eslamparast, T., 2014 [146]	Patients with NAFLD: Probiotic group *n* = 26 and control group *n* = 26 Fibroscan© pre and post-intervention Seven months intervention	Protexin: *L. plantarum, L. bulgaricus, L. acidophilus, L. casei, B. bifidum, S. thermophilus, S. faecium, Torulopsis* spp, *Aspergillus oryzae*	↓ liver enzymes: AST, ALT and γGT ↓ TNF-α levels ↓ fibrosis assessed by transient elastography
Sepideh, A., 2015 [147]	Patients with NAFLD: probiotic group *n* = 21 and control group *n* = 21 Two months intervention	Lactocare: *L. casei, L. acidophilus, L. rhamnosus, L. bulgaricus, B. breve, B. longum, S. Thermophilus* (2 capsules per day)	↓ insulin resistance and IL-6 no difference in anthropometric metrics no difference in TNF-α levels

ALT, alanine aminotransferase; AST, aspartate aminotransferase; FOS, fructooligosaccharides; γGT, γ-glutamyl transpeptidase; H-MRS, proton magnetic resonance spectroscopy; IL-6, interleukin-6; LDL, low density lipoprotein; NAFLD, nonalcoholic fatty liver disease; NASH, nonalcoholic steatohepatitis; TNF-α, tumor necrosis factor α. Arrows indicate the differences in the intervention group as compared to the control group.

6. Conclusions

Obesity-associated NAFLD is the hepatic pandemic of our century. The gut microbiota has a huge impact in the pathogenesis of obesity and its metabolic complications, as well as in the development and progression of NAFLD. Gut dysbiosis promotes obesity through modulation of the energy harvested from the diet, as well as through direct modulation of adipose tissue and hepatic metabolism. Bacterial products may be toxic, two examples being ethanol and TMAO. Dysbiota may also perturb choline and bile acid metabolism, with detrimental effects in the liver. Furthermore, gut dysbiota can perturb the intestinal barrier, and bacterial products may induce systemic toxicity, including hepatic toxicity, that favors proinflammatory states and liver injury.

Several lines of evidence link NAFLD to dysbiosis; for example NAFLD associates with small bowel bacterial overgrowth, increased intestinal permeability, and endotoxemia. Also, in animal models of NAFLD/NASH, as well as in patients, the composition of the gut microbiota tends to be different from healthy subjects. Lastly, in animal models, NAFLD can be a transmissible disease by fecal microbiota transplantation from donors prone to develop NAFLD.

Taken into consideration the acknowledged role of gut dysbiosis in the pathogenesis of NAFLD/NASH, there are huge expectations on the role of probiotics/symbiotics in modulating the gut microbiota and hence having a therapeutic role in NAFLD. Despite the enthusiasm on the field, the available studies are small, heterogeneous, short-term, and do not properly address hepatic histology/risk for progressive liver disease. Hence, the lack of solid evidence, still precludes us implementing probiotics in the management of NAFLD/NASH. Extensive pre-clinical studies comparing different approaches in different animal models of NASH would be important to better delineate large multicentric well-designed, well-powered studies in patients with NASH. Other strategies for modulating the gut microbiota, such as fecal microbiota transplantation may merit further study.

References

1. Bays, H. Adiposopathy, "sick fat", ockham's razor, and resolution of the obesity paradox. *Curr. Atheroscler. Rep.* **2014**, *16*, 409. [CrossRef] [PubMed]
2. Byrne, C.D.; Targher, G. NAFLD: A multisystem disease. *J. Hepatol.* **2015**, *62*, S47–S64. [CrossRef] [PubMed]
3. Charlton, M.R.; Burns, J.M.; Pedersen, R.A.; Watt, K.D.; Heimbach, J.K.; Dierkhising, R.A. Frequency and outcomes of liver transplantation for nonalcoholic steatohepatitis in the United States. *Gastroenterology* **2011**, *141*, 1249–1253. [CrossRef] [PubMed]
4. Backhed, F.; Ding, H.; Wang, T.; Hooper, L.V.; Koh, G.Y.; Nagy, A.; Semenkovich, C.F.; Gordon, J.I. The gut microbiota as an environmental factor that regulates fat storage. *Proc. Natl. Acad. Sci. USA* **2004**, *101*, 15718–15723. [CrossRef] [PubMed]
5. Lagier, J.C.; Million, M.; Hugon, P.; Armougom, F.; Raoult, D. Human gut microbiota: Repertoire and variations. *Front. Cell. Infect. Microbiol.* **2012**, *2*, 136. [CrossRef] [PubMed]
6. Gill, S.R.; Pop, M.; Deboy, R.T.; Eckburg, P.B.; Turnbaugh, P.J.; Samuel, B.S.; Gordon, J.I.; Relman, D.A.; Fraser-Liggett, C.M.; Nelson, K.E. Metagenomic analysis of the human distal gut microbiome. *Science* **2006**, *312*, 1355–1359. [CrossRef] [PubMed]
7. Seksik, P.; Landman, C. Understanding microbiome data: A primer for clinicians. *Dig. Dis.* **2015**, *33*, 11–16. [CrossRef] [PubMed]
8. Lozupone, C.A.; Stombaugh, J.I.; Gordon, J.I.; Jansson, J.K.; Knight, R. Diversity, stability and resilience of the human gut microbiota. *Nature* **2012**, *489*, 220–230. [CrossRef] [PubMed]
9. Imajo, K.; Yoneda, M.; Ogawa, Y.; Wada, K.; Nakajima, A. Microbiota and nonalcoholic steatohepatitis. *Semin. Immunopathol.* **2014**, *36*, 115–132. [CrossRef] [PubMed]
10. Martinez, I.; Muller, C.E.; Walter, J. Long-term temporal analysis of the human fecal microbiota revealed a stable core of dominant bacterial species. *PLoS ONE* **2013**, *8*, e69621. [CrossRef] [PubMed]

11. Faith, J.J.; Guruge, J.L.; Charbonneau, M.; Subramanian, S.; Seedorf, H.; Goodman, A.L.; Clemente, J.C.; Knight, R.; Heath, A.C.; Leibel, R.L.; *et al.* The long-term stability of the human gut microbiota. *Science* **2013**, *341*, 1237439. [CrossRef] [PubMed]

12. Dethlefsen, L.; Relman, D.A. Incomplete recovery and individualized responses of the human distal gut microbiota to repeated antibiotic perturbation. *Proc. Natl. Acad. Sci. USA* **2011**, *108*, 4554–4561. [CrossRef] [PubMed]

13. Tarantino, G.; Finelli, C. Systematic review on intervention with prebiotics/probiotics in patients with obesity-related nonalcoholic fatty liver disease. *Future Microbiol.* **2015**, *10*, 889–902. [CrossRef] [PubMed]

14. Donaldson, G.P.; Lee, S.M.; Mazmanian, S.K. Gut biogeography of the bacterial microbiota. *Nat. Rev. Microbiol.* **2016**, *14*, 20–32. [CrossRef] [PubMed]

15. Backhed, F.; Manchester, J.K.; Semenkovich, C.F.; Gordon, J.I. Mechanisms underlying the resistance to diet-induced obesity in germ-free mice. *Proc. Natl. Acad. Sci. USA* **2007**, *104*, 979–984. [CrossRef] [PubMed]

16. Turnbaugh, P.J.; Ley, R.E.; Mahowald, M.A.; Magrini, V.; Mardis, E.R.; Gordon, J.I. An obesity-associated gut microbiome with increased capacity for energy harvest. *Nature* **2006**, *444*, 1027–1031. [CrossRef] [PubMed]

17. Turnbaugh, P.J.; Ridaura, V.K.; Faith, J.J.; Rey, F.E.; Knight, R.; Gordon, J.I. The effect of diet on the human gut microbiome: A metagenomic analysis in humanized gnotobiotic mice. *Sci. Transl. Med.* **2009**, *1*, 6ra14. [CrossRef] [PubMed]

18. Vrieze, A.; van Nood, E.; Holleman, F.; Salojarvi, J.; Kootte, R.S.; Bartelsman, J.F.; Dallinga-Thie, G.M.; Ackermans, M.T.; Serlie, M.J.; Oozeer, R.; *et al.* Transfer of intestinal microbiota from lean donors increases insulin sensitivity in individuals with metabolic syndrome. *Gastroenterology* **2012**, *143*, 913–916. [CrossRef] [PubMed]

19. Ley, R.E.; Backhed, F.; Turnbaugh, P.; Lozupone, C.A.; Knight, R.D.; Gordon, J.I. Obesity alters gut microbial ecology. *Proc. Natl. Acad. Sci. USA* **2005**, *102*, 11070–11075. [CrossRef] [PubMed]

20. Murphy, E.F.; Cotter, P.D.; Healy, S.; Marques, T.M.; O'Sullivan, O.; Fouhy, F.; Clarke, S.F.; O'Toole, P.W.; Quigley, E.M.; Stanton, C.; *et al.* Composition and energy harvesting capacity of the gut microbiota: Relationship to diet, obesity and time in mouse models. *Gut* **2010**, *59*, 1635–1642. [CrossRef] [PubMed]

21. Turnbaugh, P.J.; Backhed, F.; Fulton, L.; Gordon, J.I. Diet-induced obesity is linked to marked but reversible alterations in the mouse distal gut microbiome. *Cell Host Microbe* **2008**, *3*, 213–223. [CrossRef] [PubMed]

22. Turnbaugh, P.J.; Hamady, M.; Yatsunenko, T.; Cantarel, B.L.; Duncan, A.; Ley, R.E.; Sogin, M.L.; Jones, W.J.; Roe, B.A.; Affourtit, J.P.; *et al.* A core gut microbiome in obese and lean twins. *Nature* **2009**, *457*, 480–484. [CrossRef] [PubMed]

23. Patil, D.P.; Dhotre, D.P.; Chavan, S.G.; Sultan, A.; Jain, D.S.; Lanjekar, V.B.; Gangawani, J.; Shah, P.S.; Todkar, J.S.; Shah, S.; *et al.* Molecular analysis of gut microbiota in obesity among indian individuals. *J. Biosci.* **2012**, *37*, 647–657. [CrossRef] [PubMed]

24. Ferrer, M.; Ruiz, A.; Lanza, F.; Haange, S.B.; Oberbach, A.; Till, H.; Bargiela, R.; Campoy, C.; Segura, M.T.; Richter, M.; *et al.* Microbiota from the distal guts of lean and obese adolescents exhibit partial functional redundancy besides clear differences in community structure. *Environ. Microbiol.* **2013**, *15*, 211–226. [CrossRef] [PubMed]

25. Kalliomaki, M.; Collado, M.C.; Salminen, S.; Isolauri, E. Early differences in fecal microbiota composition in children may predict overweight. *Am. J. Clin. Nutr.* **2008**, *87*, 534–538. [PubMed]

26. Jumpertz, R.; Le, D.S.; Turnbaugh, P.J.; Trinidad, C.; Bogardus, C.; Gordon, J.I.; Krakoff, J. Energy-balance studies reveal associations between gut microbes, caloric load, and nutrient absorption in humans. *Am. J. Clin. Nutr.* **2011**, *94*, 58–65. [CrossRef] [PubMed]

27. Chakraborti, C.K. New-found link between microbiota and obesity. *World J. Gastrointest. Pathophysiol.* **2015**, *6*, 110–119. [CrossRef] [PubMed]

28. Brahe, L.K.; Astrup, A.; Larsen, L.H. Is butyrate the link between diet, intestinal microbiota and obesity-related metabolic diseases? *Obes. Rev.* **2013**, *14*, 950–959. [CrossRef] [PubMed]

29. Louis, P.; Flint, H.J. Diversity, metabolism and microbial ecology of butyrate-producing bacteria from the human large intestine. *FEMS Microbiol. Lett.* **2009**, *294*, 1–8. [CrossRef] [PubMed]

30. Abdallah Ismail, N.; Ragab, S.H.; Abd Elbaky, A.; Shoeib, A.R.; Alhosary, Y.; Fekry, D. Frequency of firmicutes and bacteroidetes in gut microbiota in obese and normal weight egyptian children and adults. *Arch. Med. Sci.* **2011**, *7*, 501–507. [CrossRef] [PubMed]

31. Roy, C.C.; Kien, C.L.; Bouthillier, L.; Levy, E. Short-chain fatty acids: Ready for prime time? *Nutr. Clin. Pract.* **2006**, *21*, 351–366. [CrossRef] [PubMed]

32. Lin, H.V.; Frassetto, A.; Kowalik, E.J., Jr.; Nawrocki, A.R.; Lu, M.M.; Kosinski, J.R.; Hubert, J.A.; Szeto, D.; Yao, X.; Forrest, G.; *et al.* Butyrate and propionate protect against diet-induced obesity and regulate gut hormones via free fatty acid receptor 3-independent mechanisms. *PLoS ONE* **2012**, *7*, e35240.

33. Xiong, Y.; Miyamoto, N.; Shibata, K.; Valasek, M.A.; Motoike, T.; Kedzierski, R.M.; Yanagisawa, M. Short-chain fatty acids stimulate leptin production in adipocytes through the G protein-coupled receptor GPR41. *Proc. Natl. Acad. Sci. USA* **2004**, *101*, 1045–1050. [CrossRef] [PubMed]

34. Al-Lahham, S.H.; Roelofsen, H.; Priebe, M.; Weening, D.; Dijkstra, M.; Hoek, A.; Rezaee, F.; Venema, K.; Vonk, R.J. Regulation of adipokine production in human adipose tissue by propionic acid. *Eur. J. Clin. Investig.* **2010**, *40*, 401–407. [CrossRef] [PubMed]

35. Jin, C.J.; Sellmann, C.; Engstler, A.J.; Ziegenhardt, D.; Bergheim, I. Supplementation of sodium butyrate protects mice from the development of non-alcoholic steatohepatitis (NASH). *Br. J. Nutr.* **2015**, *114*, 1745–1755. [CrossRef] [PubMed]

36. Aronsson, L.; Huang, Y.; Parini, P.; Korach-Andre, M.; Hakansson, J.; Gustafsson, J.A.; Pettersson, S.; Arulampalam, V.; Rafter, J. Decreased fat storage by lactobacillus paracasei is associated with increased levels of angiopoietin-like 4 protein (ANGPTL4). *PLoS ONE* **2010**, *5*, e13087. [CrossRef] [PubMed]

37. Ding, S.; Chi, M.M.; Scull, B.P.; Rigby, R.; Schwerbrock, N.M.; Magness, S.; Jobin, C.; Lund, P.K. High-fat diet: Bacteria interactions promote intestinal inflammation which precedes and correlates with obesity and insulin resistance in mouse. *PLoS ONE* **2010**, *5*, e12191. [CrossRef] [PubMed]

38. Claus, S.P.; Ellero, S.L.; Berger, B.; Krause, L.; Bruttin, A.; Molina, J.; Paris, A.; Want, E.J.; de Waziers, I.; Cloarec, O.; *et al.* Colonization-induced host-gut microbial metabolic interaction. *MBio* **2011**, *2*, e00271–e00210. [CrossRef] [PubMed]

39. Rajala, M.W.; Patterson, C.M.; Opp, J.S.; Foltin, S.K.; Young, V.B.; Myers, M.G., Jr. Leptin acts independently of food intake to modulate gut microbial composition in male mice. *Endocrinology* **2014**, *155*, 748–757. [CrossRef] [PubMed]

40. Bergheim, I.; Weber, S.; Vos, M.; Kramer, S.; Volynets, V.; Kaserouni, S.; McClain, C.J.; Bischoff, S.C. Antibiotics protect against fructose-induced hepatic lipid accumulation in mice: Role of endotoxin. *J. Hepatol.* **2008**, *48*, 983–992. [CrossRef] [PubMed]

41. Membrez, M.; Blancher, F.; Jaquet, M.; Bibiloni, R.; Cani, P.D.; Burcelin, R.G.; Corthesy, I.; Mace, K.; Chou, C.J. Gut microbiota modulation with norfloxacin and ampicillin enhances glucose tolerance in mice. *FASEB J.* **2008**, *22*, 2416–2426. [CrossRef] [PubMed]

42. Drenick, E.J.; Fisler, J.; Johnson, D. Hepatic steatosis after intestinal bypass—Prevention and reversal by metronidazole, irrespective of protein-calorie malnutrition. *Gastroenterology* **1982**, *82*, 535–548. [PubMed]

43. Nazim, M.; Stamp, G.; Hodgson, H.J. Non-alcoholic steatohepatitis associated with small intestinal diverticulosis and bacterial overgrowth. *Hepatogastroenterology* **1989**, *36*, 349–351. [PubMed]

44. Wigg, A.J.; Roberts-Thomson, I.C.; Dymock, R.B.; McCarthy, P.J.; Grose, R.H.; Cummins, A.G. The role of small intestinal bacterial overgrowth, intestinal permeability, endotoxaemia, and tumour necrosis factor α in the pathogenesis of non-alcoholic steatohepatitis. *Gut* **2001**, *48*, 206–211. [CrossRef] [PubMed]

45. Brun, P.; Castagliuolo, I.; di Leo, V.; Buda, A.; Pinzani, M.; Palu, G.; Martines, D. Increased intestinal permeability in obese mice: New evidence in the pathogenesis of nonalcoholic steatohepatitis. *Am. J. Physiol. Gastrointest. Liver Physiol.* **2007**, *292*, G518–G525. [CrossRef] [PubMed]

46. Farhadi, A.; Gundlapalli, S.; Shaikh, M.; Frantzides, C.; Harrell, L.; Kwasny, M.M.; Keshavarzian, A. Susceptibility to gut leakiness: A possible mechanism for endotoxaemia in non-alcoholic steatohepatitis. *Liver Int.* **2008**, *28*, 1026–1033. [CrossRef] [PubMed]

47. Spruss, A.; Kanuri, G.; Wagnerberger, S.; Haub, S.; Bischoff, S.C.; Bergheim, I. Toll-like receptor 4 is involved in the development of fructose-induced hepatic steatosis in mice. *Hepatology* **2009**, *50*, 1094–1104. [CrossRef] [PubMed]

48. Miele, L.; Valenza, V.; la Torre, G.; Montalto, M.; Cammarota, G.; Ricci, R.; Masciana, R.; Forgione, A.; Gabrieli, M.L.; Perotti, G.; *et al.* Increased intestinal permeability and tight junction alterations in nonalcoholic fatty liver disease. *Hepatology* **2009**, *49*, 1877–1887. [CrossRef] [PubMed]

49.   Shanab, A.A.; Scully, P.; Crosbie, O.; Buckley, M.; O'Mahony, L.; Shanahan, F.; Gazareen, S.; Murphy, E.; Quigley, E.M. Small intestinal bacterial overgrowth in nonalcoholic steatohepatitis: Association with toll-like receptor 4 expression and plasma levels of interleukin 8. *Dig. Dis. Sci.* **2011**, *56*, 1524–1534. [CrossRef] [PubMed]

50.   Cani, P.D.; Amar, J.; Iglesias, M.A.; Poggi, M.; Knauf, C.; Bastelica, D.; Neyrinck, A.M.; Fava, F.; Tuohy, K.M.; Chabo, C.; *et al.* Metabolic endotoxemia initiates obesity and insulin resistance. *Diabetes* **2007**, *56*, 1761–1772. [CrossRef] [PubMed]

51.   Verdam, F.J.; Rensen, S.S.; Driessen, A.; Greve, J.W.; Buurman, W.A. Novel evidence for chronic exposure to endotoxin in human nonalcoholic steatohepatitis. *J. Clin. Gastroenterol.* **2011**, *45*, 149–152. [CrossRef] [PubMed]

52.   Poggi, M.; Bastelica, D.; Gual, P.; Iglesias, M.A.; Gremeaux, T.; Knauf, C.; Peiretti, F.; Verdier, M.; Juhan-Vague, I.; Tanti, J.F.; *et al.* C3H/HEJ mice carrying a toll-like receptor 4 mutation are protected against the development of insulin resistance in white adipose tissue in response to a high-fat diet. *Diabetologia* **2007**, *50*, 1267–1276. [CrossRef] [PubMed]

53.   Csak, T.; Velayudham, A.; Hritz, I.; Petrasek, J.; Levin, I.; Lippai, D.; Catalano, D.; Mandrekar, P.; Dolganiuc, A.; Kurt-Jones, E.; *et al.* Deficiency in myeloid differentiation factor-2 and toll-like receptor 4 expression attenuates nonalcoholic steatohepatitis and fibrosis in mice. *Am. J. Physiol. Gastrointest. Liver Physiol.* **2011**, *300*, G433–G441. [CrossRef] [PubMed]

54.   Ye, D.; Li, F.Y.; Lam, K.S.; Li, H.; Jia, W.; Wang, Y.; Man, K.; Lo, C.M.; Li, X.; Xu, A. Toll-like receptor-4 mediates obesity-induced non-alcoholic steatohepatitis through activation of X-box binding protein-1 in mice. *Gut* **2012**, *61*, 1058–1067. [CrossRef] [PubMed]

55.   Yuan, L.; Bambha, K. Bile acid receptors and nonalcoholic fatty liver disease. *World J. Hepatol.* **2015**, *7*, 2811–2818. [CrossRef] [PubMed]

56.   Stacey, M.; Webb, M. Studies on the antibacterial properties of the bile acids and some compounds derived from cholanic acid. *Proc. R. Soc. Med.* **1947**, *134*, 523–537. [CrossRef] [PubMed]

57.   Sayin, S.I.; Wahlstrom, A.; Felin, J.; Jantti, S.; Marschall, H.U.; Bamberg, K.; Angelin, B.; Hyotylainen, T.; Oresic, M.; Backhed, F. Gut microbiota regulates bile acid metabolism by reducing the levels of tauro-β-muricholic acid, a naturally occurring fxr antagonist. *Cell Metab.* **2013**, *17*, 225–235. [CrossRef] [PubMed]

58.   Le Roy, T.; Llopis, M.; Lepage, P.; Bruneau, A.; Rabot, S.; Bevilacqua, C.; Martin, P.; Philippe, C.; Walker, F.; Bado, A.; *et al.* Intestinal microbiota determines development of non-alcoholic fatty liver disease in mice. *Gut* **2013**, *62*, 1787–1794. [CrossRef] [PubMed]

59.   Henao-Mejia, J.; Elinav, E.; Jin, C.; Hao, L.; Mehal, W.Z.; Strowig, T.; Thaiss, C.A.; Kau, A.L.; Eisenbarth, S.C.; Jurczak, M.J.; *et al.* Inflammasome-mediated dysbiosis regulates progression of NAFLD and obesity. *Nature* **2012**, *482*, 179–185. [CrossRef] [PubMed]

60.   De Minicis, S.; Rychlicki, C.; Agostinelli, L.; Saccomanno, S.; Candelaresi, C.; Trozzi, L.; Mingarelli, E.; Facinelli, B.; Magi, G.; Palmieri, C.; *et al.* Dysbiosis contributes to fibrogenesis in the course of chronic liver injury in mice. *Hepatology* **2014**, *59*, 1738–1749. [CrossRef] [PubMed]

61.   Yoshimoto, S.; Loo, T.M.; Atarashi, K.; Kanda, H.; Sato, S.; Oyadomari, S.; Iwakura, Y.; Oshima, K.; Morita, H.; Hattori, M.; *et al.* Obesity-induced gut microbial metabolite promotes liver cancer through senescence secretome. *Nature* **2013**, *499*, 97–101. [CrossRef] [PubMed]

62.   Spencer, M.D.; Hamp, T.J.; Reid, R.W.; Fischer, L.M.; Zeisel, S.H.; Fodor, A.A. Association between composition of the human gastrointestinal microbiome and development of fatty liver with choline deficiency. *Gastroenterology* **2011**, *140*, 976–986. [CrossRef] [PubMed]

63.   Mouzaki, M.; Comelli, E.M.; Arendt, B.M.; Bonengel, J.; Fung, S.K.; Fischer, S.E.; McGilvray, I.D.; Allard, J.P. Intestinal microbiota in patients with nonalcoholic fatty liver disease. *Hepatology* **2013**, *58*, 120–127. [CrossRef] [PubMed]

64.   Raman, M.; Ahmed, I.; Gillevet, P.M.; Probert, C.S.; Ratcliffe, N.M.; Smith, S.; Greenwood, R.; Sikaroodi, M.; Lam, V.; Crotty, P.; *et al.* Fecal microbiome and volatile organic compound metabolome in obese humans with nonalcoholic fatty liver disease. *Clin. Gastroenterol. Hepatol.* **2013**, *11*, 868–875. [CrossRef] [PubMed]

65.   Wong, V.W.; Tse, C.H.; Lam, T.T.; Wong, G.L.; Chim, A.M.; Chu, W.C.; Yeung, D.K.; Law, P.T.; Kwan, H.S.; Yu, J.; *et al.* Molecular characterization of the fecal microbiota in patients with nonalcoholic steatohepatitis—A longitudinal study. *PLoS ONE* **2013**, *8*, e62885. [CrossRef] [PubMed]

66. Boursier, J.; Mueller, O.; Barret, M.; Machado, M.; Fizanne, L.; Araujo-Perez, F.; Guy, C.D.; Seed, P.C.; Rawls, J.F.; David, L.A.; *et al.* The severity of NAFLD is associated with gut dysbiosis and shift in the metabolic function of the gut microbiota. *Hepatology* **2016**, *63*, 764–775. [CrossRef] [PubMed]

67. Jiang, W.; Wu, N.; Wang, X.; Chi, Y.; Zhang, Y.; Qiu, X.; Hu, Y.; Li, J.; Liu, Y. Dysbiosis gut microbiota associated with inflammation and impaired mucosal immune function in intestine of humans with non-alcoholic fatty liver disease. *Sci. Rep.* **2015**, *5*, 8096. [CrossRef] [PubMed]

68. Lebeer, S.; Vanderleyden, J.; de Keersmaecker, S.C. Genes and molecules of lactobacilli supporting probiotic action. *Microbiol. Mol. Biol. Rev.* **2008**, *72*, 728–764. [CrossRef] [PubMed]

69. Elshaghabee, F.M.; Bockelmann, W.; Meske, D.; de Vrese, M.; Walte, H.G.; Schrezenmeir, J.; Heller, K.J. Ethanol production by selected intestinal microorganisms and lactic acid bacteria growing under different nutritional conditions. *Front. Microbiol.* **2016**, *7*, 47. [CrossRef] [PubMed]

70. Scott, K.P.; Martin, J.C.; Duncan, S.H.; Flint, H.J. Prebiotic stimulation of human colonic butyrate-producing bacteria and bifidobacteria, *in vitro*. *FEMS Microbiol. Ecol.* **2014**, *87*, 30–40. [CrossRef] [PubMed]

71. Prorok-Hamon, M.; Friswell, M.K.; Alswied, A.; Roberts, C.L.; Song, F.; Flanagan, P.K.; Knight, P.; Codling, C.; Marchesi, J.R.; Winstanley, C.; *et al.* Colonic mucosa-associated diffusely adherent *afaC + Escherichia coli* expressing *lpfA* and *pks* are increased in inflammatory bowel disease and colon cancer. *Gut* **2014**, *63*, 761–770. [CrossRef] [PubMed]

72. Al-Jashamy, K.; Murad, A.; Zeehaida, M.; Rohaini, M.; Hasnan, J. Prevalence of colorectal cancer associated with streptococcus bovis among inflammatory bowel and chronic gastrointestinal tract disease patients. *Asian Pac. J. Cancer Prev.* **2010**, *11*, 1765–1768. [PubMed]

73. Zhu, L.; Baker, S.S.; Gill, C.; Liu, W.; Alkhouri, R.; Baker, R.D.; Gill, S.R. Characterization of gut microbiomes in nonalcoholic steatohepatitis (NASH) patients: A connection between endogenous alcohol and NASH. *Hepatology* **2013**, *57*, 601–609. [CrossRef] [PubMed]

74. Zeisel, S.H. Choline. *Adv. Nutr.* **2010**, *1*, 46–48. [CrossRef] [PubMed]

75. Dumas, M.E.; Barton, R.H.; Toye, A.; Cloarec, O.; Blancher, C.; Rothwell, A.; Fearnside, J.; Tatoud, R.; Blanc, V.; Lindon, J.C.; *et al.* Metabolic profiling reveals a contribution of gut microbiota to fatty liver phenotype in insulin-resistant mice. *Proc. Natl. Acad. Sci. USA* **2006**, *103*, 12511–12516. [CrossRef] [PubMed]

76. Ferreira, D.M.; Afonso, M.B.; Rodrigues, P.M.; Simao, A.L.; Pereira, D.M.; Borralho, P.M.; Rodrigues, C.M.; Castro, R.E. c-jun N-terminal kinase 1/c-jun activation of the p53/microRNA 34a/sirtuin 1 pathway contributes to apoptosis induced by deoxycholic acid in rat liver. *Mol. Cell. Biol.* **2014**, *34*, 1100–1120. [CrossRef] [PubMed]

77. Aranha, M.M.; Cortez-Pinto, H.; Costa, A.; da Silva, I.B.; Camilo, M.E.; de Moura, M.C.; Rodrigues, C.M. Bile acid levels are increased in the liver of patients with steatohepatitis. *Eur. J. Gastroenterol. Hepatol.* **2008**, *20*, 519–525. [CrossRef] [PubMed]

78. Newgard, C.B. Interplay between lipids and branched-chain amino acids in development of insulin resistance. *Cell Metab.* **2012**, *15*, 606–614. [CrossRef] [PubMed]

79. Png, C.W.; Linden, S.K.; Gilshenan, K.S.; Zoetendal, E.G.; McSweeney, C.S.; Sly, L.I.; McGuckin, M.A.; Florin, T.H. Mucolytic bacteria with increased prevalence in ibd mucosa augment *in vitro* utilization of mucin by other bacteria. *Am. J. Gastroenterol.* **2010**, *105*, 2420–2428. [CrossRef] [PubMed]

80. Sartor, R.B. Key questions to guide a better understanding of host-commensal microbiota interactions in intestinal inflammation. *Mucosal Immunol.* **2011**, *4*, 127–132. [CrossRef] [PubMed]

81. Christopherson, M.R.; Dawson, J.A.; Stevenson, D.M.; Cunningham, A.C.; Bramhacharya, S.; Weimer, P.J.; Kendziorski, C.; Suen, G. Unique aspects of fiber degradation by the ruminal ethanologen ruminococcus albus 7 revealed by physiological and transcriptomic analysis. *BMC Genom.* **2014**, *15*, 1066. [CrossRef] [PubMed]

82. Yoneda, M.; Naka, S.; Nakano, K.; Wada, K.; Endo, H.; Mawatari, H.; Imajo, K.; Nomura, R.; Hokamura, K.; Ono, M.; *et al.* Involvement of a periodontal pathogen, porphyromonas gingivalis on the pathogenesis of non-alcoholic fatty liver disease. *BMC Gastroenterol.* **2012**, *12*, 16. [CrossRef] [PubMed]

83. Furusho, H.; Miyauchi, M.; Hyogo, H.; Inubushi, T.; Ao, M.; Ouhara, K.; Hisatune, J.; Kurihara, H.; Sugai, M.; Hayes, C.N.; *et al.* Dental infection of porphyromonas gingivalis exacerbates high fat diet-induced steatohepatitis in mice. *J. Gastroenterol.* **2013**, *48*, 1259–1270. [CrossRef] [PubMed]

84. Cope, K.; Risby, T.; Diehl, A.M. Increased gastrointestinal ethanol production in obese mice: Implications for fatty liver disease pathogenesis. *Gastroenterology* **2000**, *119*, 1340–1347. [CrossRef] [PubMed]

85. Nair, S.; Cope, K.; Risby, T.H.; Diehl, A.M. Obesity and female gender increase breath ethanol concentration: Potential implications for the pathogenesis of nonalcoholic steatohepatitis. *Am. J. Gastroenterol.* **2001**, *96*, 1200–1204. [CrossRef] [PubMed]

86. Sajjad, A.; Mottershead, M.; Syn, W.K.; Jones, R.; Smith, S.; Nwokolo, C.U. Ciprofloxacin suppresses bacterial overgrowth, increases fasting insulin but does not correct low acylated ghrelin concentration in non-alcoholic steatohepatitis. *Aliment. Pharmacol. Ther.* **2005**, *22*, 291–299. [CrossRef] [PubMed]

87. Swann, J.R.; Want, E.J.; Geier, F.M.; Spagou, K.; Wilson, I.D.; Sidaway, J.E.; Nicholson, J.K.; Holmes, E. Systemic gut microbial modulation of bile acid metabolism in host tissue compartments. *Proc. Natl. Acad. Sci. USA* **2011**, *108*, 4523–4530. [CrossRef] [PubMed]

88. Jiang, C.; Xie, C.; Li, F.; Zhang, L.; Nichols, R.G.; Krausz, K.W.; Cai, J.; Qi, Y.; Fang, Z.Z.; Takahashi, S.; *et al.* Intestinal farnesoid X receptor signaling promotes nonalcoholic fatty liver disease. *J. Clin. Investig.* **2015**, *125*, 386–402. [CrossRef] [PubMed]

89. De Filippo, C.; Cavalieri, D.; di Paola, M.; Ramazzotti, M.; Poullet, J.B.; Massart, S.; Collini, S.; Pieraccini, G.; Lionetti, P. Impact of diet in shaping gut microbiota revealed by a comparative study in children from europe and rural africa. *Proc. Natl. Acad. Sci. USA* **2010**, *107*, 14691–14696. [CrossRef] [PubMed]

90. Walker, A.W.; Ince, J.; Duncan, S.H.; Webster, L.M.; Holtrop, G.; Ze, X.; Brown, D.; Stares, M.D.; Scott, P.; Bergerat, A.; *et al.* Dominant and diet-responsive groups of bacteria within the human colonic microbiota. *ISME J.* **2011**, *5*, 220–230. [CrossRef] [PubMed]

91. David, L.A.; Maurice, C.F.; Carmody, R.N.; Gootenberg, D.B.; Button, J.E.; Wolfe, B.E.; Ling, A.V.; Devlin, A.S.; Varma, Y.; Fischbach, M.A.; *et al.* Diet rapidly and reproducibly alters the human gut microbiome. *Nature* **2014**, *505*, 559–563. [CrossRef] [PubMed]

92. Beyer, P.L.; Flynn, M.A. Effects of high- and low-fiber diets on human feces. *J. Am. Diet. Assoc.* **1978**, *72*, 271–277. [PubMed]

93. Cotillard, A.; Kennedy, S.P.; Kong, L.C.; Prifti, E.; Pons, N.; Le Chatelier, E.; Almeida, M.; Quinquis, B.; Levenez, F.; Galleron, N.; *et al.* Dietary intervention impact on gut microbial gene richness. *Nature* **2013**, *500*, 585–588. [CrossRef] [PubMed]

94. Wu, G.D.; Chen, J.; Hoffmann, C.; Bittinger, K.; Chen, Y.Y.; Keilbaugh, S.A.; Bewtra, M.; Knights, D.; Walters, W.A.; Knight, R.; *et al.* Linking long-term dietary patterns with gut microbial enterotypes. *Science* **2011**, *334*, 105–108. [CrossRef] [PubMed]

95. Hildebrandt, M.A.; Hoffmann, C.; Sherrill-Mix, S.A.; Keilbaugh, S.A.; Hamady, M.; Chen, Y.Y.; Knight, R.; Ahima, R.S.; Bushman, F.; Wu, G.D. High-fat diet determines the composition of the murine gut microbiome independently of obesity. *Gastroenterology* **2009**, *137*, 1716–1724. [CrossRef] [PubMed]

96. De Wit, N.; Derrien, M.; Bosch-Vermeulen, H.; Oosterink, E.; Keshtkar, S.; Duval, C.; de Vogel-van den Bosch, J.; Kleerebezem, M.; Muller, M.; van der Meer, R. Saturated fat stimulates obesity and hepatic steatosis and affects gut microbiota composition by an enhanced overflow of dietary fat to the distal intestine. *Am. J. Physiol. Gastrointest. Liver Physiol.* **2012**, *303*, G589–G599. [CrossRef] [PubMed]

97. Ravussin, Y.; Koren, O.; Spor, A.; LeDuc, C.; Gutman, R.; Stombaugh, J.; Knight, R.; Ley, R.E.; Leibel, R.L. Responses of gut microbiota to diet composition and weight loss in lean and obese mice. *Obesity* **2012**, *20*, 738–747. [CrossRef] [PubMed]

98. Brinkworth, G.D.; Noakes, M.; Clifton, P.M.; Bird, A.R. Comparative effects of very low-carbohydrate, high-fat and high-carbohydrate, low-fat weight-loss diets on bowel habit and faecal short-chain fatty acids and bacterial populations. *Br. J. Nutr.* **2009**, *101*, 1493–1502. [CrossRef] [PubMed]

99. Fava, F.; Gitau, R.; Griffin, B.A.; Gibson, G.R.; Tuohy, K.M.; Lovegrove, J.A. The type and quantity of dietary fat and carbohydrate alter faecal microbiome and short-chain fatty acid excretion in a metabolic syndrome "at-risk" population. *Int. J. Obes.* **2013**, *37*, 216–223. [CrossRef] [PubMed]

100. Zhang, C.; Zhang, M.; Wang, S.; Han, R.; Cao, Y.; Hua, W.; Mao, Y.; Zhang, X.; Pang, X.; Wei, C.; *et al.* Interactions between gut microbiota, host genetics and diet relevant to development of metabolic syndromes in mice. *ISME J.* **2010**, *4*, 232–241. [CrossRef] [PubMed]

101. Everard, A.; Belzer, C.; Geurts, L.; Ouwerkerk, J.P.; Druart, C.; Bindels, L.B.; Guiot, Y.; Derrien, M.; Muccioli, G.G.; Delzenne, N.M.; *et al.* Cross-talk between akkermansia muciniphila and intestinal epithelium controls diet-induced obesity. *Proc. Natl. Acad. Sci. USA* **2013**, *110*, 9066–9071. [CrossRef] [PubMed]

102. Zhang, H.; DiBaise, J.K.; Zuccolo, A.; Kudrna, D.; Braidotti, M.; Yu, Y.; Parameswaran, P.; Crowell, M.D.; Wing, R.; Rittmann, B.E.; *et al.* Human gut microbiota in obesity and after gastric bypass. *Proc. Natl. Acad. Sci. USA* **2009**, *106*, 2365–2370. [CrossRef] [PubMed]

103. Furet, J.P.; Kong, L.C.; Tap, J.; Poitou, C.; Basdevant, A.; Bouillot, J.L.; Mariat, D.; Corthier, G.; Dore, J.; Henegar, C.; *et al.* Differential adaptation of human gut microbiota to bariatric surgery-induced weight loss: Links with metabolic and low-grade inflammation markers. *Diabetes* **2010**, *59*, 3049–3057. [CrossRef] [PubMed]

104. Kong, L.C.; Tap, J.; Aron-Wisnewsky, J.; Pelloux, V.; Basdevant, A.; Bouillot, J.L.; Zucker, J.D.; Dore, J.; Clement, K. Gut microbiota after gastric bypass in human obesity: Increased richness and associations of bacterial genera with adipose tissue genes. *Am. J. Clin. Nutr.* **2013**, *98*, 16–24. [CrossRef] [PubMed]

105. Liou, A.P.; Paziuk, M.; Luevano, J.M., Jr.; Machineni, S.; Turnbaugh, P.J.; Kaplan, L.M. Conserved shifts in the gut microbiota due to gastric bypass reduce host weight and adiposity. *Sci. Transl. Med.* **2013**, *5*, 178ra141. [CrossRef] [PubMed]

106. Patti, M.E.; Houten, S.M.; Bianco, A.C.; Bernier, R.; Larsen, P.R.; Holst, J.J.; Badman, M.K.; Maratos-Flier, E.; Mun, E.C.; Pihlajamaki, J.; *et al.* Serum bile acids are higher in humans with prior gastric bypass: Potential contribution to improved glucose and lipid metabolism. *Obesity* **2009**, *17*, 1671–1677. [CrossRef] [PubMed]

107. Kohli, R.; Bradley, D.; Setchell, K.D.; Eagon, J.C.; Abumrad, N.; Klein, S. Weight loss induced by Roux-en-Y gastric bypass but not laparoscopic adjustable gastric banding increases circulating bile acids. *J. Clin. Endocrinol. Metab.* **2013**, *98*, E708–E712. [CrossRef] [PubMed]

108. Gerhard, G.S.; Styer, A.M.; Wood, G.C.; Roesch, S.L.; Petrick, A.T.; Gabrielsen, J.; Strodel, W.E.; Still, C.D.; Argyropoulos, G. A role for fibroblast growth factor 19 and bile acids in diabetes remission after Roux-en-Y gastric bypass. *Diabetes Care* **2013**, *36*, 1859–1864. [CrossRef] [PubMed]

109. Myronovych, A.; Kirby, M.; Ryan, K.K.; Zhang, W.; Jha, P.; Setchell, K.D.; Dexheimer, P.J.; Aronow, B.; Seeley, R.J.; Kohli, R. Vertical sleeve gastrectomy reduces hepatic steatosis while increasing serum bile acids in a weight-loss-independent manner. *Obesity* **2014**, *22*, 390–400. [CrossRef] [PubMed]

110. Ryan, K.K.; Tremaroli, V.; Clemmensen, C.; Kovatcheva-Datchary, P.; Myronovych, A.; Karns, R.; Wilson-Perez, H.E.; Sandoval, D.A.; Kohli, R.; Backhed, F.; *et al.* Fxr is a molecular target for the effects of vertical sleeve gastrectomy. *Nature* **2014**, *509*, 183–188. [CrossRef] [PubMed]

111. Shen, W.; Gaskins, H.R.; McIntosh, M.K. Influence of dietary fat on intestinal microbes, inflammation, barrier function and metabolic outcomes. *J. Nutr. Biochem.* **2014**, *25*, 270–280. [CrossRef] [PubMed]

112. Ferolla, S.M.; Armiliato, G.N.; Couto, C.A.; Ferrari, T.C. Probiotics as a complementary therapeutic approach in nonalcoholic fatty liver disease. *World J. Hepatol.* **2015**, *7*, 559–565. [CrossRef] [PubMed]

113. Kang, J.H.; Yun, S.I.; Park, M.H.; Park, J.H.; Jeong, S.Y.; Park, H.O. Anti-obesity effect of lactobacillus gasseri BNR17 in high-sucrose diet-induced obese mice. *PLoS ONE* **2013**, *8*, e54617. [CrossRef] [PubMed]

114. Fak, F.; Backhed, F. Lactobacillus reuteri prevents diet-induced obesity, but not atherosclerosis, in a strain dependent fashion in Apoe$^{-/-}$ mice. *PLoS ONE* **2012**, *7*, e46837. [CrossRef] [PubMed]

115. Lee, H.Y.; Park, J.H.; Seok, S.H.; Baek, M.W.; Kim, D.J.; Lee, K.E.; Paek, K.S.; Lee, Y.; Park, J.H. Human originated bacteria, lactobacillus rhamnosus pl60, produce conjugated linoleic acid and show anti-obesity effects in diet-induced obese mice. *Biochim. Biophys. Acta* **2006**, *1761*, 736–744. [CrossRef] [PubMed]

116. An, H.M.; Park, S.Y.; Lee do, K.; Kim, J.R.; Cha, M.K.; Lee, S.W.; Lim, H.T.; Kim, K.J.; Ha, N.J. Antiobesity and lipid-lowering effects of *Bifidobacterium* spp. In high fat diet-induced obese rats. *Lipids Health Dis.* **2011**, *10*, 116. [CrossRef] [PubMed]

117. Andersson, U.; Branning, C.; Ahrne, S.; Molin, G.; Alenfall, J.; Onning, G.; Nyman, M.; Holm, C. Probiotics lower plasma glucose in the high-fat fed C57BL/6J mouse. *Benef. Microbes* **2010**, *1*, 189–196. [CrossRef] [PubMed]

118. Agerholm-Larsen, L.; Raben, A.; Haulrik, N.; Hansen, A.S.; Manders, M.; Astrup, A. Effect of 8 week intake of probiotic milk products on risk factors for cardiovascular diseases. *Eur. J. Clin. Nutr.* **2000**, *54*, 288–297. [CrossRef] [PubMed]

119. Kadooka, Y.; Sato, M.; Imaizumi, K.; Ogawa, A.; Ikuyama, K.; Akai, Y.; Okano, M.; Kagoshima, M.; Tsuchida, T. Regulation of abdominal adiposity by probiotics (*Lactobacillus gasseri* SBT2055) in adults with obese tendencies in a randomized controlled trial. *Eur. J. Clin. Nutr.* **2010**, *64*, 636–643. [CrossRef] [PubMed]

120. Mikirova, N.A.; Casciari, J.J.; Hunninghake, R.E.; Beezley, M.M. Effect of weight reduction on cardiovascular risk factors and CD34-positive cells in circulation. *Int. J. Med. Sci.* **2011**, *8*, 445–452. [CrossRef] [PubMed]

121. Kadooka, Y.; Sato, M.; Ogawa, A.; Miyoshi, M.; Uenishi, H.; Ogawa, H.; Ikuyama, K.; Kagoshima, M.; Tsuchida, T. Effect of *Lactobacillus gasseri* SBT2055 in fermented milk on abdominal adiposity in adults in a randomised controlled trial. *Br. J. Nutr.* **2013**, *110*, 1696–1703. [CrossRef] [PubMed]

122. Sanchez, M.; Darimont, C.; Drapeau, V.; Emady-Azar, S.; Lepage, M.; Rezzonico, E.; Ngom-Bru, C.; Berger, B.; Philippe, L.; Ammon-Zuffrey, C.; *et al.* Effect of lactobacillus rhamnosus cgmcc1.3724 supplementation on weight loss and maintenance in obese men and women. *Br. J. Nutr.* **2014**, *111*, 1507–1519. [CrossRef] [PubMed]

123. Dewulf, E.M.; Cani, P.D.; Claus, S.P.; Fuentes, S.; Puylaert, P.G.; Neyrinck, A.M.; Bindels, L.B.; de Vos, W.M.; Gibson, G.R.; Thissen, J.P.; *et al.* Insight into the prebiotic concept: Lessons from an exploratory, double blind intervention study with inulin-type fructans in obese women. *Gut* **2013**, *62*, 1112–1121. [CrossRef] [PubMed]

124. de Luis, D.A.; de la Fuente, B.; Izaola, O.; Conde, R.; Gutierrez, S.; Morillo, M.; Teba Torres, C. Double blind randomized clinical trial controlled by placebo with an α linoleic acid and prebiotic enriched cookie on risk cardiovascular factor in obese patients. *Nutr. Hosp.* **2011**, *26*, 827–833. [PubMed]

125. De Luis, D.A.; de la Fuente, B.; Izaola, O.; Conde, R.; Gutierrez, S.; Morillo, M.; Teba Torres, C. Randomized clinical trial with a inulin enriched cookie on risk cardiovascular factor in obese patients. *Nutr. Hosp.* **2010**, *25*, 53–59. [PubMed]

126. Balcazar-Munoz, B.R.; Martinez-Abundis, E.; Gonzalez-Ortiz, M. Effect of oral inulin administration on lipid profile and insulin sensitivity in subjects with obesity and dyslipidemia. *Rev. Med. Chile* **2003**, *131*, 597–604. [PubMed]

127. Li, Z.; Yang, S.; Lin, H.; Huang, J.; Watkins, P.A.; Moser, A.B.; Desimone, C.; Song, X.Y.; Diehl, A.M. Probiotics and antibodies to TNF inhibit inflammatory activity and improve nonalcoholic fatty liver disease. *Hepatology* **2003**, *37*, 343–350. [CrossRef] [PubMed]

128. Ma, X.; Hua, J.; Li, Z. Probiotics improve high fat diet-induced hepatic steatosis and insulin resistance by increasing hepatic NKT cells. *J. Hepatol.* **2008**, *49*, 821–830. [CrossRef] [PubMed]

129. Esposito, E.; Iacono, A.; Bianco, G.; Autore, G.; Cuzzocrea, S.; Vajro, P.; Canani, R.B.; Calignano, A.; Raso, G.M.; Meli, R. Probiotics reduce the inflammatory response induced by a high-fat diet in the liver of young rats. *J. Nutr.* **2009**, *139*, 905–911. [CrossRef] [PubMed]

130. Velayudham, A.; Dolganiuc, A.; Ellis, M.; Petrasek, J.; Kodys, K.; Mandrekar, P.; Szabo, G. Vsl#3 probiotic treatment attenuates fibrosis without changes in steatohepatitis in a diet-induced nonalcoholic steatohepatitis model in mice. *Hepatology* **2009**, *49*, 989–997. [PubMed]

131. Xu, R.Y.; Wan, Y.P.; Fang, Q.Y.; Lu, W.; Cai, W. Supplementation with probiotics modifies gut flora and attenuates liver fat accumulation in rat nonalcoholic fatty liver disease model. *J. Clin. Biochem. Nutr.* **2012**, *50*, 72–77. [CrossRef] [PubMed]

132. Bhathena, J.; Martoni, C.; Kulamarva, A.; Tomaro-Duchesneau, C.; Malhotra, M.; Paul, A.; Urbanska, A.M.; Prakash, S. Oral probiotic microcapsule formulation ameliorates non-alcoholic fatty liver disease in Bio F1B Golden Syrian hamsters. *PLoS ONE* **2013**, *8*, e58394. [CrossRef] [PubMed]

133. Endo, H.; Niioka, M.; Kobayashi, N.; Tanaka, M.; Watanabe, T. Butyrate-producing probiotics reduce nonalcoholic fatty liver disease progression in rats: New insight into the probiotics for the gut-liver axis. *PLoS ONE* **2013**, *8*, e63388.

134. Ritze, Y.; Bardos, G.; Claus, A.; Ehrmann, V.; Bergheim, I.; Schwiertz, A.; Bischoff, S.C. Lactobacillus rhamnosus GG protects against non-alcoholic fatty liver disease in mice. *PLoS ONE* **2014**, *9*, e80169.

135. Xin, J.; Zeng, D.; Wang, H.; Ni, X.; Yi, D.; Pan, K.; Jing, B. Preventing non-alcoholic fatty liver disease through lactobacillus johnsonii BS15 by attenuating inflammation and mitochondrial injury and improving gut environment in obese mice. *Appl. Microbiol. Biotechnol.* **2014**, *98*, 6817–6829. [CrossRef] [PubMed]

136. Li, C.; Nie, S.P.; Zhu, K.X.; Ding, Q.; Li, C.; Xiong, T.; Xie, M.Y. Lactobacillus plantarum ncu116 improves liver function, oxidative stress and lipid metabolism in rats with high fat diet induced non-alcoholic fatty liver disease. *Food Funct.* **2014**, *5*, 3216–3223. [CrossRef] [PubMed]

137. Sohn, W.; Jun, D.W.; Lee, K.N.; Lee, H.L.; Lee, O.Y.; Choi, H.S.; Yoon, B.C. Lactobacillus paracasei induces M2-Dominant Kupffer Cell Polarization in a Mouse Model of Nonalcoholic Steatohepatitis. *Dig. Dis. Sci.* **2015**, *60*, 3340–3350. [CrossRef] [PubMed]

138. Ting, W.J.; Kuo, W.W.; Hsieh, D.J.; Yeh, Y.L.; Day, C.H.; Chen, Y.H.; Chen, R.J.; Padma, V.V.; Chen, Y.H.; Huang, C.Y. Heat killed lactobacillus reuteri GMNL-263 reduces fibrosis effects on the liver and heart in high fat diet-hamsters via TGF-β suppression. *Int. J. Mol. Sci.* **2015**, *16*, 25881–25896. [CrossRef] [PubMed]

139. Cortez-Pinto, H.; Borralho, P.; Machado, J.; Lopes, M.T.; Gato, I.V.; Santos, A.M.; Guerreiro, A.S. Microbiota modulation with synbiotic decreases liver fibrosis in a high fat choline deficient diet mice model of nonalcoholic steatohepatitis (NASH). *Port. J. Gastroenterol.* **2016**. in press.

140. Loguercio, C.; de Simone, T.; Federico, A.; Terracciano, F.; Tuccillo, C.; di Chicco, M.; Carteni, M. Gut-liver axis: A new point of attack to treat chronic liver damage? *Am. J. Gastroenterol.* **2002**, *97*, 2144–2146. [CrossRef] [PubMed]

141. Loguercio, C.; Federico, A.; Tuccillo, C.; Terracciano, F.; D'Auria, M.V.; de Simone, C.; del Vecchio Blanco, C. Beneficial effects of a probiotic VSL#3 on parameters of liver dysfunction in chronic liver diseases. *J. Clin. Gastroenterol.* **2005**, *39*, 540–543. [PubMed]

142. Aller, R.; de Luis, D.A.; Izaola, O.; Conde, R.; Gonzalez Sagrado, M.; Primo, D.; de la Fuente, B.; Gonzalez, J. Effect of a probiotic on liver aminotransferases in nonalcoholic fatty liver disease patients: A double blind randomized clinical trial. *Eur. Rev. Med. Pharmacol. Sci.* **2011**, *15*, 1090–1095. [PubMed]

143. Malaguarnera, M.; Vacante, M.; Antic, T.; Giordano, M.; Chisari, G.; Acquaviva, R.; Mastrojeni, S.; Malaguarnera, G.; Mistretta, A.; Li Volti, G.; *et al.* Bifidobacterium longum with fructo-oligosaccharides in patients with non alcoholic steatohepatitis. *Dig. Dis. Sci.* **2012**, *57*, 545–553. [CrossRef] [PubMed]

144. Wong, V.W.; Won, G.L.; Chim, A.M.; Chu, W.C.; Yeung, D.K.; Li, K.C.; Chan, H.L. Treatment of nonalcoholic steatohepatitis with probiotics. A proof-of-concept study. *Ann. Hepatol.* **2013**, *12*, 256–262. [PubMed]

145. Nabavi, S.; Rafraf, M.; Somi, M.H.; Homayouni-Rad, A.; Asghari-Jafarabadi, M. Effects of probiotic yogurt consumption on metabolic factors in individuals with nonalcoholic fatty liver disease. *J. Dairy Sci.* **2014**, *97*, 7386–7393. [CrossRef] [PubMed]

146. Eslamparast, T.; Poustchi, H.; Zamani, F.; Sharafkhah, M.; Malekzadeh, R.; Hekmatdoost, A. Synbiotic supplementation in nonalcoholic fatty liver disease: A randomized, double-blind, placebo-controlled pilot study. *Am. J. Clin. Nutr.* **2014**, *99*, 535–542. [CrossRef] [PubMed]

147. Sepideh, A.; Karim, P.; Hossein, A.; Leila, R.; Hamdollah, M.; Mohammad, E.G.; Mojtaba, S.; Mohammad, S.; Ghader, G.; Seyed Moayed, A. Effects of multistrain probiotic supplementation on glycemic and inflammatory indices in patients with nonalcoholic fatty liver disease: A double-blind randomized clinical trial. *J. Am. Coll.Nutr.* **2015**, 1–6. [CrossRef] [PubMed]

148. Lirussi, F.; Mastropasqua, E.; Orando, S.; Orlando, R. Probiotics for non-alcoholic fatty liver disease and/or steatohepatitis. *Cochrane Database Syst. Rev.* **2007**, CD005165. [CrossRef]

149. Abenavoli, L.; Scarpellini, E.; Rouabhia, S.; Balsano, C.; Luzza, F. Probiotics in non-alcoholic fatty liver disease: Which and when. *Ann. Hepatol.* **2013**, *12*, 357–363. [PubMed]

150. Kelishadi, R.; Farajian, S.; Mirlohi, M. Probiotics as a novel treatment for non-alcoholic fatty liver disease; a systematic review on the current evidences. *Hepat. Mon.* **2013**, *13*, e7233. [CrossRef] [PubMed]

151. Ma, Y.Y.; Li, L.; Yu, C.H.; Shen, Z.; Chen, L.H.; Li, Y.M. Effects of probiotics on nonalcoholic fatty liver disease: A meta-analysis. *World J. Gastroenterol.* **2013**, *19*, 6911–6918. [CrossRef] [PubMed]

152. Eslamparast, T.; Eghtesad, S.; Hekmatdoost, A.; Poustchi, H. Probiotics and nonalcoholic fatty liver disease. *Middle East J. Dig. Dis.* **2013**, *5*, 129–136. [PubMed]

153. Buss, C.; Valle-Tovo, C.; Miozzo, S.; Alves de Mattos, A. Probiotics and synbiotics may improve liver aminotransferases levels in non-alcoholic fatty liver disease patients. *Ann. Hepatol.* **2014**, *13*, 482–488. [PubMed]

154. Gao, X.; Zhu, Y.; Wen, Y.; Liu, G.; Wan, C. Efficacy of probiotics in nonalcoholic fatty liver disease in adult and children: A meta-analysis of randomized controlled trials. *Hepatol. Res.* **2016**. in press. [CrossRef] [PubMed]

9

Vascular Damage in Patients with Nonalcoholic Fatty Liver Disease: Possible Role of Iron and Ferritin

Giuseppina Pisano, Rosa Lombardi and Anna Ludovica Fracanzani *

Department of Pathophysiology and Transplantation, Ca' Granda IRCCS Foundation, Policlinico Hospital, University of Milan, Centre of the Study of Metabolic and Liver Diseases, Via Francesco Sforza 35, 20122 Milan, Italy; pinaz81@hotmail.com (G.P.); rosalombardi@hotmail.it (R.L.)
* Correspondence: anna.fracanzani@unimi.it

Academic Editors: Amedeo Lonardo and Giovanni Targher

Abstract: Non Alcoholic Fatty Liver Disease (NAFLD) is the most common chronic liver disease in Western countries. Recent data indicated that NAFLD is a risk factor by itself contributing to the development of cardiovascular disease independently of classical known risk factors. Hyperferritinemia and mild increased iron stores are frequently observed in patients with NAFLD and several mechanisms have been proposed to explain the role of iron, through oxidative stress and interaction with insulin metabolism, in the development of vascular damage. Moreover, iron depletion has been shown to decrease atherogenesis in experimental models and in humans. This review presents the recent evidence on epidemiology, pathogenesis, and the possible explanation of the role of iron and ferritin in the development of cardiovascular damage in patients with NAFLD, and discusses the possible interplay between metabolic disorders associated with NAFLD and iron in the development of cardiovascular disease.

Keywords: NAFLD; ferritin; iron; cardiovascular disease; metabolic syndrome

1. Introduction

Non Alcoholic Fatty Liver Disease (NAFLD), the most common chronic liver disease in Western countries, was previously indicated as the hepatic expression of the metabolic syndrome (MetS) having shared many similar clinical manifestations [1]. More recently it has been proposed that NAFLD precedes the development of type 2 diabetes and metabolic syndrome [2], significantly increasing the risk of incident type 2 diabetes [3] even in non-overweight subjects [4]. Recent evidence links NAFLD to increases of cardiovascular risk, and further studies reveal that the first causes of death in NAFLD patients are cardiovascular disease (CVD) [5–8] and cancer [5,9–11], and not just liver diseases. NAFLD is also considered by recent studies to be a risk factor in itself to the development of CVD independently of classical known risk factors [12]. Increased ferritin and body iron stores are frequently observed in patients with NAFLD [13,14]. Iron, through oxidative stress and interaction with insulin metabolism [15], can promote the development of vascular damage. Moreover, iron depletion has been reported to decrease atherogenesis in experimental models and in humans [16,17].

2. Ferritin, Insulin Resistance, Metabolic Syndrome, and NAFLD

Growing evidence proposes a correlation between serum ferritin, insulin resistance, and NAFLD [18,19]. Several studies reported a link between high ferritin levels and MetS [20], and its single components [21], with a linear increase with the increasing number of MetS components [20]. Liver fat accumulation is considered to be one of the first pieces of evidence in the development of insulin resistance, and a strong association between NAFLD, insulin resistance, and MetS features has been demonstrated [19,22,23]. The association between ferritin and components of the MetS has been suggested to be related to an undiagnosed NAFLD. Zelber-Sagi et al. [24] demonstrated that insulin was the strongest predictor of increased serum ferritin levels and, vice versa, ferritin has been proposed as a marker of insulin resistance [25].

The evidence that increased ferritin levels precede the development of diabetes was demonstrated in prospective studies [26,27], however, it is not well defined if increased ferritin (expression of body iron accumulation) could induce metabolic alteration. In chronic liver disease hyperferritinemia may be caused by an augmented release of the protein from injured hepatocytes. Pro-inflammatory cytokines, in fact, stimulate the synthesis of ferritin, which is an acute phase reactant [28]. In patients with NAFLD (in whom ferritin and body iron are frequently increased [13,29]) inflammation, metabolic alterations, and hepatocytes necrosis may coexist with a mild iron overload, all leading to hyperferritinemia [30,31]. In addition, even a small amount of hepatic iron accumulation combined with other cofactors can increase oxidative stress responsible for liver cell necrosis, activation of hepatic stellate cells, and fibrosis [19,32], implying that iron could also play a role in the progression from "benign" fatty liver to non-alcoholic steatohepatitis (NASH). The same mechanisms determining liver damage might act in the vessel walls.

Epidemiological studies indicated that ferritin not only is a marker of insulin resistance but also is one of the strongest risk factors for the progression of carotid atherosclerosis [33,34]. Confirming this observation, the removal of iron by phlebotomy was found to improve insulin resistance, liver function tests [13,35], and atherosclerosis [36]; however, mainly due to the small sample size of the studies, the impact of phlebotomy in NAFLD is still debated [37].

3. Iron and Atherosclerosis

The role of iron in the development and progression of atherosclerosis has been reported in several papers. Iron deposition, especially in macrophages of arterial walls, is increased in atherosclerotic lesions [14,38], and has been proposed as a marker of cardiovascular risk [16]. The role that iron plays in atherosclerosis has been hypothesized to be an increase in vascular oxidative stress and acceleration of arterial thrombosis [39]; this could be caused by the induction of oxidative stress catalysis, promotion of insulin resistance [15], decreased plasma antioxidant activity, increased low-density lipoprotein (LDL) oxidation [40], and enhanced macrophage activation determining oxidized LDL uptake [41].

Iron depletion in experimental models has been shown to decrease atherogenesis [17], while, in humans, blood donation has been associated with decreased risk for myocardial infarction [26], and phlebotomy has been suggested to decrease the progression of peripheral vascular disease [42].

A worse cognitive performance in patients with metabolic alterations—as a potential consequence of vascular damage, or directly as a neurodegenerative alteration—has been described in relation to iron status in animal models, and more recently in humans as well [43]. In insulin resistant obese patients a worse cognitive performance was found related with brain iron load in the caudate, lenticular nucleus, hypothalamus, and hippocampus (by magnetic resonance imaging (RMI)) and with increased hepatic iron concentration. It is possible to hypothesize that in presence of insulin resistance, the excess of iron, being highly reactive and promoting the generation of hydroxyl radicals, may cause both metabolic distress in the liver and alterations in some target brain areas [44].

4. Iron and Carotid Plaques: Arterial Iron Promotes Plaque Instability

Through the use of electron paramagnetic resonance spectroscopy Stadler et al. [45] were able to quantify iron in ex vivo carotid lesions and in healthy human arteries and, in doing so, found that iron in the carotid lesions was higher than in healthy subjects. They also found a correlation between cholesterols and iron accumulation in the lesions.

Lapenna et al. [14] in studying ex vivo carotid endo-arterectomy specimens found a significant correlation between serum ferritin and low molecular weight iron. Yuan et al. and Li et al. [46,47] suggested that iron found in atherosclerotic vascular tissue, generated mostly by erythrophagocytosis, could interact with lipoproteins in macrophages and be responsible for increased oxidative stress and their transformation into foam cells in the presence of an atherogenic environment. Thus the increase of iron in macrophages might contribute to vulnerability of human atheroma. Moreover, Li *et al.* reported, in *ex vivo* human carotid atherosclerotic lesions [48], the positive correlation of transferrin receptor 1 (TfR1) expression and macrophage infiltration, ectopic lysosomal cathepsin L, and ferritin expression and they suggested that the expression of TfR1 and ferritin in CD68 positive macrophages was correlated with the severity of human carotid plaques.

5. Ferritin and Atherosclerosis

Ferritin is considered a marker of atherosclerosis progression [33] and a relationship has been proposed between its levels and carotid atherosclerosis [34] in epidemiological studies. Moreover, ferritin was found associated with carotid intima-media thickness (IMT), and with the presence of carotid plaques in a large cohort of NAFLD patients [49]. In this paper the authors described a stronger association of ferritin with plaques rather than with increased IMT, hypothesizing that iron, by favoring endothelial damage and thrombosis [39], can promote the development of atherosclerotic complications. In NAFLD ferritin can reflect oxidative stress, inflammation, and hepatic necrosis. This protein has been found strongly associated not only with parameters influencing iron stores, such as sex, age, alcohol, and genetic factors (*i.e.*, *HFE* mutations), but also with metabolic alterations defining the metabolic syndrome. However, a correlation was described between ferritin and vascular damage that was independent from factors associated with metabolic syndrome [50–52].

These data were recently confirmed in a Chinese population study in which serum ferritin was found significantly increased in patients with abnormal glucose metabolism and related with IMT progression [53].

6. *HFE* Gene Mutations in NAFLD and Atherosclerosis

Several studies analyzed the role of HFE mutations in patients with NAFLD and iron overload. Valenti *et al.* [29] demonstrated that carriers of the C282Y mutation have lower insulin release and develop NAFLD in the presence of less severe metabolic abnormalities. This suggests that heterozygosis for the HFE mutation (responsible for mild iron overload) may trigger the clinical NAFLD manifestation [29]. More controversial is the role of HFE mutations in the development of atherosclerotic damage. In fact, while the atherogenetic role of iron has been reported (as observed in macrophages of arterial walls in atherosclerotic lesions [40,41] and in the beneficial effect of iron depletion on vascular damage [17], a lack of association between HFE mutations with vascular damage has been reported [54]. A faster clearance of iron from arterial lesions could be caused by a decrease of Hepcidin, which could facilitate iron export from macrophages [49].

7. Hepcidin, Macrophage Iron, and Vascular Damage

Hepcidin, mainly produced in the liver, is defined as the key hormone regulating iron balance [55]. Hepcidin provides a defense mechanism against pathogens during inflammation by inhibiting iron recycling from macrophages and iron absorption from enterocytes. Also, in patients with metabolic disease, such as NAFLD, the deregulation of hepcidin expression/activity contributes to increased iron stores [56]. Subclinical inflammation and obesity can induce Hepcidin [57] and cause iron trapping in macrophages [58] in the presence of an atherogenic environment. Excessive iron in macrophages could be responsible for increased oxidative stress and transformation into foam cells. Sullivan *et al.* [16] suggested that increased hepcidin may generate iron induced atherogenesis and cardiovascular damages (Figure 1).

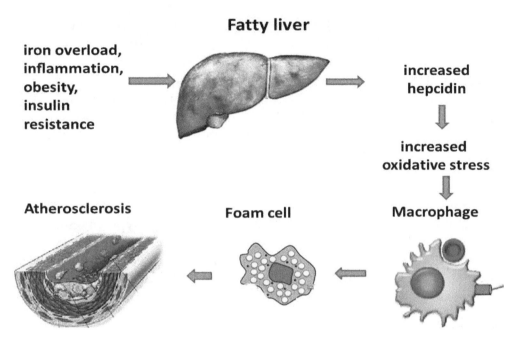

Figure 1. Simplified pathophysiological mechanisms of iron induced vascular damage through fatty liver.

Experimental Models

Findings from animal models of atherosclerosis and from studies of human atherosclerotic plaques provide evidence that elevated arterial iron levels may cause atherosclerosis. Both animal studies and clinical evidence indicate that in the presence of iron deficiency (*i.e.*, anemia) that iron can be mobilized from arterial plaques to be used in erythropoiesis with consequent iron reduction in the plaques.

Valenti *et al.* [59] reported the effect of the manipulation of intracellular iron on the release of atherogenic cytokines in human differentiating monocytes of patients with NAFLD, with Metabolic Syndrome, and with mild iron overload by treatment cells with iron salts or with hepcidin. Macrophages, but also the smooth muscle and the endothelial cells treated with iron salts, increased the release of the macrophage chemo attractant protein (MCP-1), an atherogenic chemokine that plays an important role in both the initiation and progression of atherosclerosis. Moreover, the iron salt treatment increased the IL-6 a proinflammatory cytokine involved in the acute phase response, independently of oxidative stress. IL-6 serum levels have been reported to correlate with vascular risk and with the inflammation within atherosclerotic plaques [60]. In addition it has been found that higher MCP-1 represents a negative prognostic factor in acute coronary syndromes [61]. The effect of hepcidin on MCP-1 release was similar to that of iron salts as it blocked cellular iron export. Furthermore, in patients with NAFLD and MetS, the iron-dependent induction of MCP-1 and IL-6 was found associated with the severity of vascular damage as it promoted macrophage activation by iron and may be involved in the pathogenesis of vascular damage progression. These results have also been observed in monocytes of healthy subjects in which iron treatment determined the induction of MCP-1 transcription and release, suggesting that this depicted a physiological response to increased intracellular iron availability [49].

8. Iron Depletion and Atherosclerosis

It has been reported that iron depletion decreases atherogenesis in experimental models [17]. In addition, iron reduction by frequent blood donations was found to be associated with decreased intima-media thickness [36] and decreased risk of myocardial infarction [26]. Thus, iron reduction potentially offers a benefit in atherosclerotic vascular disease acting as an anti-inflammatory process. However, the role of blood donation on cardiovascular diseases is not yet defined. The Nebraska Diet

Heart Study [62], has established a relationship between blood donation and risk of cardiovascular events. This study evaluated the cardiovascular events in 655 individuals who had donated at least one unit of blood in the preceding 10 years and in 3200 who had not. The results indicated that, compared to non-donors, the blood donors showed a significant reduction of events such as myocardial infarction, angina, or stroke. They also had fewer cardiovascular procedures and less use of nitroglycerin. Nevertheless, it is not possible to rule out that blood donors have less cardiovascular events in connection to them being in apparently good enough health to be eligible to donate blood. The beneficial effect of blood donations on cardiovascular disease has been debated in a number of epidemiological studies [13,35–37]. Interestingly, Zacharski et al. [42], in a multicenter prospective trial conducted in veteran participants with peripheral arterial disease, showed that the beneficial effect of phlebotomy was present only in younger patients. This suggests that levels of body iron stores might be operative in the early phase of atherosclerosis, while hypercoagulability and diabetes mellitus in later-stages of the diseases. Low body iron may protect against atherosclerotic CVD through different ways: (1) limiting oxidation of LDL cholesterol [63]; (2) decreasing the clinical activity of myeloperoxidase [64]; (3) increasing high density lipoprotein (HDL) and apolipoprotein A (ApoA) [65]; (4) improving nitric-oxide mediated, endothelium-dependent vasodilation [66], and, finally, improving insulin sensitivity [67].

In addition, iron depletion has been demonstrated to improve insulin resistance [13] in NAFLD, while more controversial is the beneficial effect on liver histology in NASH [68,69]. About one third of patients with NAFLD and MetS have been reported to have dysmetabolic iron overload syndrome [70], and both venesection therapy (in the absence of weight loss) and dietary treatment have been shown to improve ferritin, metabolic parameters, and liver enzymes [70,71].

An imbalance of the homoeostatic mechanisms—including the interaction of iron with hepcidin, ferritin, insulin, and with adipokines and pro-inflammatory molecules—causes parenchymal siderosis that contributes to organ damage such as pancreatic β-cell dysfunction, liver fibrosis, and atherosclerotic plaque growth and instability. Vice versa, iron depletion could exert beneficial effects, not only in NAFLD patients with mild iron overload but also in healthy frequent blood donors [72].

9. Dietary Iron, Microbiota, and CVD

Elements such as dietary macronutrients, particularly the types of fats and carbohydrates, are known factors in the etiology of type 2 diabetes, a metabolic disease closely related with NAFLD, while more controversial is the effect of dietary iron. Iron is a transitional metal, strong pro-oxidant, and catalyzer of several cellular reactions that result in the production of reactive oxygen species, thereby consequently increasing the level of oxidative stress. Graham et al. [73] reported an increase in liver cholesterol biosynthesis in mice caused by high dietary iron, showing how iron could influence cholesterol levels and cause the development of fatty liver disease. In addition, the high dietary cholesterol promotes the development of fatty liver in guinea pigs which in turn leads to the dysregulation of iron metabolism because of damaged liver [74]. Iron dextran increased oxidative stress, which was associated with the altered expression of genes related to lipid metabolism and therefore contributing to hyperlipidemia [75]. The observations, obtained in animal models, that iron can modulate lipid metabolism and therefore be associated with liver and vascular damage are very promising but not yet consolidated in humans. Also, the effect of dietary iron is not well established [76] in humans, although the intake of heme iron before and during pregnancy has been reported to correlate with the onset of diabetes, a well-known risk factor for CVD [77]. Interestingly, iron deficiency also has been reported to be associated with increased CVD risk. Iron deficiency is associated with thrombocytosis due to the lack of inhibition of thrombopoiesis with consequent increases of thrombotic complications as reported in iron-deficient children and adults [78]. In addition iron deficiency (causing anemia) increases the risk of heart failure by causing tissue ischemia with consequent increased oxidative stress, which could damage myocardial cells [79].

An updated review of cross-sectional, longitudinal, and intervention studies [79] evaluating the relation between iron and cardiovascular risk indicated that concentrations of iron within normal ranges does not have dangerous effects. In contrast, elevated amounts of non-protein-bound iron (free Fe), which has been reported to increase circulating homocysteine [80–82], seems to play a role in atherosclerosis. Free Fe catalyzes the formation of oxygen free radicals and oxidized low-density lipoprotein, which are well-established risk factors for vascular damage, thereby supporting the hypothesis that circulating homocysteine could be in part a surrogate marker for free Fe [83]. However, different iron types might act differently on the cardiovascular risk. Higher dietary intake of heme iron was found to be associated with increased cardiovascular risk; this association was not observed with non-heme and total iron intake [84]. De Oliveira Otto *et al.* [85] in a population study analyzing diet micronutrients indicated that dietary intake of non-heme iron was inversely associated with homocysteine, whereas high red meat intake (a predominant source of heme iron) was found to be associated with C-reactive protein. In addition, it is possible that the intake of nutrients containing non-heme iron (which is found in vegetables, cereals, and fruits) is more common in individuals with a healthy lifestyle (e.g., non-smokers and physically active individuals), while heme iron (abundant in red meat), which was found to be associated with insulin resistance, increased oxidative stress and CVD (Figure 2). In addition, red meat is also rich in choline and carnitine, both processed by enteric microbiota, and found to be related with atherosclerosis [86,87]. Dose-response analyses revealed a 7% increase in the risk of cardiovascular disease for each 1 mg/day increase in dietary heme iron [84].

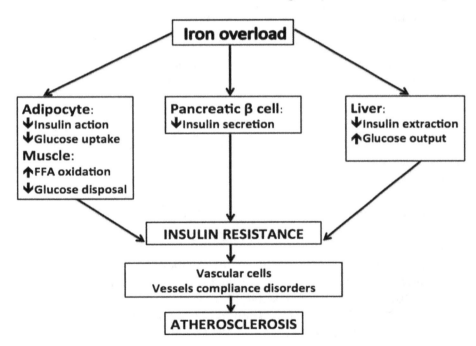

Figure 2. Effect of dietary iron overload on metabolic alterations, insulin resistance, and atherosclerosis. The downward arrows mean decrease and upward arrows mean increase. FFA: free fatty acid.

A clinically important association between bacterial infection and CVD has been reported [88]. One of the possible mechanisms in the pathogenesis of atherosclerosis could be represented by the host immunological response of extravascular tissues and/or vascular walls to bacterial agents. It is known that gut microbiota may interfere with the host metabolism by promoting multiple functions, from development of the intestinal immune system to hepatic and energy metabolism. More recently it has been reported that specific forms of gut microbiota are present in the blood of patients with diabetes and atherosclerotic plaques, thus gut microbiota could represent an environmental risk factor for CVD [89]. Gut microbiota could have a direct proatherogenic influence in atherosclerosis plaque colonization through the bloodstream after events that affect the gut barrier. Both aberrant microbiota profiles and the flux of metabolites derived from gut microbial metabolism of choline, phosphatidylcholine, and L-carnitine have been found to be associated with metabolic disease, and contribute directly to cardiovascular diseases. However, although recent data on the role of microbiota in the development of NAFLD and progression to NASH are promising, particularly in animal models, conclusive results in humans on the effect of microbiota are still missing. Oral iron intake or food rich in heme iron could alter gut microbial composition and function providing one explanation for increased vascular disease risk [90].

10. Conclusions

In patients with NAFLD, hyperferritin and mild increases in body iron store are frequently detected and associated with vascular damage. Different mechanisms have been proposed to explain the atherogenic role of iron leading to increases in vascular oxidative stress and the acceleration of arterial thrombosis. Inflammation, metabolic alterations, and hepatocytes necrosis may coexist with a mild iron overload, all leading to hyperferritinemia, which is considered to be an independent predictor of cardiovascular damage. Iron depletion, achieved by phlebotomy, has been reported to improve insulin resistance and to reduce cardiovascular risk and damage. Finally, dietary strategies, which modulate the gut microbiota and different metabolic activities, could represent efficacious tools for reducing cardiovascular risk.

Acknowledgments: The authors wish to thank Associazione Malattie Metaboliche Fegato O.N.L.U.S. for all the needed support.

Author Contributions: Giuseppina Pisano drafted the manuscript; Rosa Lombardi collected and reviewed literature; Anna Ludovica Fracanzani contributed to drafting the manuscript and provided critical revisions.

References

1.   Yki-Jarvinen, H. Non-alcoholic fatty liver disease as a cause and a consequence of metabolic syndrome. *Lancet Diabetes Endocrinol.* **2014**, *2*, 901–910. [CrossRef]

2.   Lonardo, A.; Ballestri, S.; Marchesini, G.; Angulo, P.; Loria, P. Nonalcoholic fatty liver disease: A precursor of the metabolic syndrome. *Dig. Liver Dis.* **2015**, *47*, 181–190. [CrossRef] [PubMed]

3.   Ballestri, S.; Lonardo, A.; Bonapace, S.; Byrne, C.D.; Loria, P.; Targher, G. Risk of cardiovascular, cardiac and arrhythmic complications in patients with non-alcoholic fatty liver disease. *World J. Gstroenterol.* **2014**, *20*, 1724–1745. [CrossRef] [PubMed]

4.   Fukuda, T.; Hamaguchi, M.; Kojima, T.; Hashimoto, Y.; Ohbora, A.; Kato, T.; Nakamura, N.; Fukui, M. The impact of non-alcoholic fatty liver disease on incident type 2 diabetes mellitus in non-overweight individuals. *Liver Int.* **2016**, *36*, 275–283. [CrossRef] [PubMed]

5.   Ekstedt, M.; Franzen, L.E.; Mathiesen, U.L.; Thorelius, L.; Holmqvist, M.; Bodemar, G.; Kechagias, S. Long-term follow-up of patients with NAFLD and elevated liver enzymes. *Hepatology* **2006**, *44*, 865–873. [CrossRef] [PubMed]

6.   Bhatia, L.S.; Curzen, N.P.; Calder, P.C.; Byrne, C.D. Non-alcoholic fatty liver disease: A new and important cardiovascular risk factor? *Eur. Heart J.* **2012**, *33*, 1190–1200. [CrossRef] [PubMed]

7.   Pacana, T.; Fuchs, M. The cardiovascular link to nonalcoholic fatty liver disease: A critical analysis. *Clin. Liver Dis.* **2012**, *16*, 599–613. [CrossRef] [PubMed]

8.   Lu, H.; Liu, H.; Hu, F.; Zou, L.; Luo, S.; Sun, L. Independent association between nonalcoholic fatty liver disease and cardiovascular disease: A systematic review and meta-analysis. *Int. J. Endocrinol.* **2013**, *2013*, 124958. [CrossRef] [PubMed]

9.   Ascha, M.S.; Hanouneh, I.A.; Lopez, R.; Tamimi, T.A.; Feldstein, A.F.; Zein, N.N. The incidence and risk factors of hepatocellular carcinoma in patients with nonalcoholic steatohepatitis. *Hepatology* **2010**, *51*, 1972–1978. [CrossRef] [PubMed]

10. Younossi, Z.M.; Koenig, A.B.; Abdelatif, D.; Fazel, Y.; Henry, L.; Wymer, M. Global epidemiology of non-alcoholic fatty liver disease-meta-analytic assessment of prevalence, incidence and outcomes. *Hepatology* **2015**. [CrossRef] [PubMed]

11. Reeves, H.L.; Zaki, M.Y.; Day, C.P. Hepatocellular carcinoma in obesity, type 2 diabetes, and NAFLD. *Dig. Dis. Sci.* **2016**, *61*, 1234–1245. [CrossRef] [PubMed]

12. Targher, G.; Day, C.P.; Bonora, E. Risk of cardiovascular disease in patients with nonalcoholic fatty liver disease. *N. Engl. J. Med.* **2010**, *363*, 1341–1350. [CrossRef] [PubMed]

13. Valenti, L.; Fracanzani, A.L.; Dongiovanni, P.; Bugianesi, E.; Marchesini, G.; Manzini, P.; Vanni, E.; Fargion, S. Iron depletion by phlebotomy improves insulin resistance in patients with nonalcoholic fatty liver disease and hyperferritinemia: Evidence from a case-control study. *Am. J. Gastroenterol.* **2007**, *102*, 1251–1258. [CrossRef] [PubMed]

14. Lapenna, D.; Pierdomenico, S.D.; Ciofani, G.; Ucchino, S.; Neri, M.; Giamberardino, M.A.; Cuccurullo, F. Association of body iron stores with low molecular weight iron and oxidant damage of human atherosclerotic plaques. *Free Radic. Biol. Med.* **2007**, *42*, 492–498. [CrossRef] [PubMed]

15. Dongiovanni, P.; Valenti, L.; Ludovicxp a Fracanzani, A.; Gatti, S.; Cairo, G.; Fargion, S. Iron depletion by deferoxamine up-regulates glucose uptake and insulin signaling in hepatoma cells and in rat liver. *Am. J. Pathol.* **2008**, *172*, 738–747. [CrossRef] [PubMed]

16. Sullivan, J.L. Macrophage iron, hepcidin, and atherosclerotic plaque stability. *Exp. Biol. Med.* **2007**, *232*, 1014–1020. [CrossRef] [PubMed]

17. Lee, T.S.; Shiao, M.S.; Pan, C.C.; Chau, L.Y. Iron-deficient diet reduces atherosclerotic lesions in apoe-deficient mice. *Circulation* **1999**, *99*, 1222–1229. [CrossRef] [PubMed]

18. Trombini, P.; Piperno, A. Ferritin, metabolic syndrome and NAFLD: Elective attractions and dangerous liaisons. *J. Hepatol.* **2007**, *46*, 549–552. [CrossRef] [PubMed]

19. Ballestri, S.; Nascimbeni, F.; Romagnoli, D.; Lonardo, A. The independent predictors of NASH and its individual histological features. Insulin resistance, serum uric acid, metabolic syndrome, ALT and serum total cholesterol are a clue to pathogenesis and candidate targets for treatment. *Hepatol. Res.* **2016**. [CrossRef] [PubMed]

20. Bozzini, C.; Girelli, D.; Olivieri, O.; Martinelli, N.; Bassi, A.; De Matteis, G.; Tenuti, I.; Lotto, V.; Friso, S.; Pizzolo, F.; *et al.* Prevalence of body iron excess in the metabolic syndrome. *Diabetes Care* **2005**, *28*, 2061–2063. [CrossRef] [PubMed]

21. Piperno, A.; Trombini, P.; Gelosa, M.; Mauri, V.; Pecci, V.; Vergani, A.; Salvioni, A.; Mariani, R.; Mancia, G. Increased serum ferritin is common in men with essential hypertension. *J. Hypertens.* **2002**, *20*, 1513–1518. [CrossRef] [PubMed]

22. Neuschwander-Tetri, B.A. Nonalcoholic steatohepatitis and the metabolic syndrome. *Am. J. Med. Sci.* **2005**, *330*, 326–335. [CrossRef] [PubMed]

23. Non-alcoholic Fatty Liver Disease Study Group; Lonardo, A.; Bellentani, S.; Argo, C.K.; Ballestri, S.; Byrne, C.D.; Caldwell, S.H.; Cortez-Pinto, H.; Grieco, A.; Machado, M.V.; *et al.* Epidemiological modifiers of non-alcoholic fatty liver disease: Focus on high-risk groups. *Dig. Liver Dis.* **2015**, *47*, 997–1006.

24. Zelber-Sagi, S.; Nitzan-Kaluski, D.; Halpern, Z.; Oren, R. NAFLD and hyperinsulinemia are major determinants of serum ferritin levels. *J. Hepatol.* **2007**, *46*, 700–707. [CrossRef] [PubMed]

25. Fernandez-Real, J.M.; Ricart-Engel, W.; Arroyo, E.; Balanca, R.; Casamitjana-Abella, R.; Cabrero, D.; Fernandez-Castaner, M.; Soler, J. Serum ferritin as a component of the insulin resistance syndrome. *Diabetes Care* **1998**, *21*, 62–68. [CrossRef] [PubMed]

26. Salonen, J.T.; Tuomainen, T.P.; Nyyssonen, K.; Lakka, H.M.; Punnonen, K. Relation between iron stores and non-insulin dependent diabetes in men: Case-control study. *BMJ* **1998**, *317*, 727. [CrossRef] [PubMed]

27. Jiang, R.; Manson, J.E.; Meigs, J.B.; Ma, J.; Rifai, N.; Hu, F.B. Body iron stores in relation to risk of type 2 diabetes in apparently healthy women. *JAMA* **2004**, *291*, 711–717. [CrossRef] [PubMed]

28. Harrison, P.M.; Arosio, P. The ferritins: Molecular properties, iron storage function and cellular regulation. *Biochim. Biophys. Acta* **1996**, *1275*, 161–203. [CrossRef]

29. Valenti, L.; Dongiovanni, P.; Fracanzani, A.L.; Santorelli, G.; Fatta, E.; Bertelli, C.; Taioli, E.; Fiorelli, G.; Fargion, S. Increased susceptibility to nonalcoholic fatty liver disease in heterozygotes for the mutation responsible for hereditary hemochromatosis. *Dig. Liver Dis.* **2003**, *35*, 172–178. [CrossRef]

30. Fargion, S.; Mattioli, M.; Fracanzani, A.L.; Sampietro, M.; Tavazzi, D.; Fociani, P.; Taioli, E.; Valenti, L.; Fiorelli, G. Hyperferritinemia, iron overload, and multiple metabolic alterations identify patients at risk for nonalcoholic steatohepatitis. *Am. J. Gastroenterol.* **2001**, *96*, 2448–2455. [CrossRef] [PubMed]

31. Bugianesi, E.; Manzini, P.; D'Antico, S.; Vanni, E.; Longo, F.; Leone, N.; Massarenti, P.; Piga, A.; Marchesini, G.; Rizzetto, M. Relative contribution of iron burden, hfe mutations, and insulin resistance to fibrosis in nonalcoholic fatty liver. *Hepatology* **2004**, *39*, 179–187. [CrossRef] [PubMed]

32. Rakha, E.A.; Adamson, L.; Bell, E.; Neal, K.; Ryder, S.D.; Kaye, P.V.; Aithal, G.P. Portal inflammation is associated with advanced histological changes in alcoholic and non-alcoholic fatty liver disease. *J. Clin. Pathol.* **2010**, *63*, 790–795. [CrossRef] [PubMed]

33. Kiechl, S.; Willeit, J.; Egger, G.; Poewe, W.; Oberhollenzer, F. Body iron stores and the risk of carotid atherosclerosis: Prospective results from the bruneck study. *Circulation* **1997**, *96*, 3300–3307. [CrossRef] [PubMed]

34. Wolff, B.; Volzke, H.; Ludemann, J.; Robinson, D.; Vogelgesang, D.; Staudt, A.; Kessler, C.; Dahm, J.B.; John, U.; Felix, S.B. Association between high serum ferritin levels and carotid atherosclerosis in the study of health in pomerania (SHIP). *Stroke J. Cereb. Circ.* **2004**, *35*, 453–457.

35. Aigner, E.; Theurl, I.; Theurl, M.; Lederer, D.; Haufe, H.; Dietze, O.; Strasser, M.; Datz, C.; Weiss, G. Pathways underlying iron accumulation in human nonalcoholic fatty liver disease. *Am. J. Clin. Nutr.* **2008**, *87*, 1374–1383. [PubMed]

36. Engberink, M.F.; Geleijnse, J.M.; Durga, J.; Swinkels, D.W.; de Kort, W.L.; Schouten, E.G.; Verhoef, P. Blood donation, body iron status and carotid intima-media thickness. *Atherosclerosis* **2008**, *196*, 856–862. [CrossRef] [PubMed]

37. Adams, L.A.; Crawford, D.H.; Stuart, K.; House, M.J.; St Pierre, T.G.; Webb, M.; Ching, H.L.; Kava, J.; Bynevelt, M.; MacQuillan, G.C.; *et al.* The impact of phlebotomy in nonalcoholic fatty liver disease: A prospective, randomized, controlled trial. *Hepatology* **2015**, *61*, 1555–1564. [CrossRef] [PubMed]

38. Nagy, E.; Eaton, J.W.; Jeney, V.; Soares, M.P.; Varga, Z.; Galajda, Z.; Szentmiklosi, J.; Mehes, G.; Csonka, T.; Smith, A.; *et al.* Red cells, hemoglobin, heme, iron, and atherogenesis. *Arterioscler. Thromb. Vasc. Biol.* **2010**, *30*, 1347–1353. [CrossRef] [PubMed]

39. Day, S.M.; Duquaine, D.; Mundada, L.V.; Menon, R.G.; Khan, B.V.; Rajagopalan, S.; Fay, W.P. Chronic iron administration increases vascular oxidative stress and accelerates arterial thrombosis. *Circulation* **2003**, *107*, 2601–2606. [CrossRef] [PubMed]

40. Valenti, L.; Valenti, G.; Como, G.; Burdick, L.; Santorelli, G.; Dongiovanni, P.; Rametta, R.; Bamonti, F.; Novembrino, C.; Fracanzani, A.L.; *et al.* HFE gene mutations and oxidative stress influence serum ferritin, associated with vascular damage, in hemodialysis patients. *Am. J. Nephrol.* **2007**, *27*, 101–107. [CrossRef] [PubMed]

41. Kraml, P.J.; Klein, R.L.; Huang, Y.; Nareika, A.; Lopes-Virella, M.F. Iron loading increases cholesterol accumulation and macrophage scavenger receptor I expression in THP-1 mononuclear phagocytes. *Metabolism* **2005**, *54*, 453–459. [CrossRef] [PubMed]

42. Zacharski, L.R.; Chow, B.K.; Howes, P.S.; Shamayeva, G.; Baron, J.A.; Dalman, R.L.; Malenka, D.J.; Ozaki, C.K.; Lavori, P.W. Reduction of iron stores and cardiovascular outcomes in patients with peripheral arterial disease: A randomized controlled trial. *JAMA* **2007**, *297*, 603–610. [CrossRef] [PubMed]

43. Schroder, N.; Figueiredo, L.S.; de Lima, M.N. Role of brain iron accumulation in cognitive dysfunction: Evidence from animal models and human studies. *J. Alzheimers Dis.* **2013**, *34*, 797–812. [PubMed]

44. Blasco, G.; Puig, J.; Daunis, I.E.J.; Molina, X.; Xifra, G.; Fernandez-Aranda, F.; Pedraza, S.; Ricart, W.; Portero-Otin, M.; Fernandez-Real, J.M. Brain iron overload, insulin resistance, and cognitive performance in obese subjects: A preliminary MRI case-control study. *Diabetes Care* **2014**, *37*, 3076–3083. [CrossRef] [PubMed]

45. Stadler, N.; Lindner, R.A.; Davies, M.J. Direct detection and quantification of transition metal ions in human atherosclerotic plaques: Evidence for the presence of elevated levels of iron and copper. *Arterioscler. Thromb. Vasc. Biol.* **2004**, *24*, 949–954. [CrossRef] [PubMed]

46. Yuan, X.M.; Li, W. The iron hypothesis of atherosclerosis and its clinical impact. *Ann. Med.* **2003**, *35*, 578–591. [CrossRef] [PubMed]

47. Li, W.; Ostblom, M.; Xu, L.H.; Hellsten, A.; Leanderson, P.; Liedberg, B.; Brunk, U.T.; Eaton, J.W.; Yuan, X.M. Cytocidal effects of atheromatous plaque components: The death zone revisited. *FASEB J.* **2006**, *20*, 2281–2290. [CrossRef] [PubMed]

48. Li, W.; Xu, L.H.; Forssell, C.; Sullivan, J.L.; Yuan, X.M. Overexpression of transferrin receptor and ferritin related to clinical symptoms and destabilization of human carotid plaques. *Exp. Biol. Med.* **2008**, *233*, 818–826. [CrossRef] [PubMed]

49. Valenti, L.; Swinkels, D.W.; Burdick, L.; Dongiovanni, P.; Tjalsma, H.; Motta, B.M.; Bertelli, C.; Fatta, E.; Bignamini, D.; Rametta, R.; *et al.* Serum ferritin levels are associated with vascular damage in patients with nonalcoholic fatty liver disease. *Nutr. Metab. Cardiovasc. Dis.* **2011**, *21*, 568–575. [CrossRef] [PubMed]

50. Forouhi, N.G.; Harding, A.H.; Allison, M.; Sandhu, M.S.; Welch, A.; Luben, R.; Bingham, S.; Khaw, K.T.; Wareham, N.J. Elevated serum ferritin levels predict new-onset type 2 diabetes: Results from the epic-norfolk prospective study. *Diabetologia* **2007**, *50*, 949–956. [CrossRef] [PubMed]

51. Wrede, C.E.; Buettner, R.; Bollheimer, L.C.; Scholmerich, J.; Palitzsch, K.D.; Hellerbrand, C. Association between serum ferritin and the insulin resistance syndrome in a representative population. *Eur. J. Endocrinol.* **2006**, *154*, 333–340. [CrossRef] [PubMed]

52. Kim, C.H.; Kim, H.K.; Bae, S.J.; Park, J.Y.; Lee, K.U. Association of elevated serum ferritin concentration with insulin resistance and impaired glucose metabolism in korean men and women. *Metabolism* **2011**, *60*, 414–420. [CrossRef] [PubMed]

53. Zhou, F.L.; Gao, Y.; Tian, L.; Yan, F.F.; Chen, T.; Zhong, L.; Tian, H.M. Serum ferritin is associated with carotid atherosclerotic plaques but not intima-media thickness in patients with abnormal glucose metabolism. *Clin. Chim. Acta* **2015**, *450*, 190–195. [CrossRef] [PubMed]

54. Engberink, M.F.; Povel, C.M.; Durga, J.; Swinkels, D.W.; de Kort, W.L.; Schouten, E.G.; Verhoef, P.; Geleijnse, J.M. Hemochromatosis (HFE) genotype and atherosclerosis: Increased susceptibility to iron-induced vascular damage in c282y carriers? *Atherosclerosis* **2010**, *211*, 520–525. [CrossRef] [PubMed]

55. Pietrangelo, A. Hemochromatosis: An endocrine liver disease. *Hepatology* **2007**, *46*, 1291–1301. [CrossRef] [PubMed]

56. Barisani, D.; Pelucchi, S.; Mariani, R.; Galimberti, S.; Trombini, P.; Fumagalli, D.; Meneveri, R.; Nemeth, E.; Ganz, T.; Piperno, A. Hepcidin and iron-related gene expression in subjects with dysmetabolic hepatic iron overload. *J. Hepatol.* **2008**, *49*, 123–133. [CrossRef] [PubMed]

57. Bekri, S.; Gual, P.; Anty, R.; Luciani, N.; Dahman, M.; Ramesh, B.; Iannelli, A.; Staccini-Myx, A.; Casanova, D.; Ben Amor, I.; *et al.* Increased adipose tissue expression of hepcidin in severe obesity is independent from diabetes and NASH. *Gastroenterology* **2006**, *131*, 788–796. [CrossRef] [PubMed]

58. Theurl, I.; Theurl, M.; Seifert, M.; Mair, S.; Nairz, M.; Rumpold, H.; Zoller, H.; Bellmann-Weiler, R.; Niederegger, H.; Talasz, H.; *et al.* Autocrine formation of hepcidin induces iron retention in human monocytes. *Blood* **2008**, *111*, 2392–2399. [CrossRef] [PubMed]

59. Valenti, L.; Dongiovanni, P.; Motta, B.M.; Swinkels, D.W.; Bonara, P.; Rametta, R.; Burdick, L.; Frugoni, C.; Fracanzani, A.L.; Fargion, S. Serum hepcidin and macrophage iron correlate with MCP-1 release and vascular damage in patients with metabolic syndrome alterations. *Arterioscler. Thromb. Vasc. Biol.* **2011**, *31*, 683–690. [CrossRef] [PubMed]

60. Luc, G.; Bard, J.M.; Juhan-Vague, I.; Ferrieres, J.; Evans, A.; Amouyel, P.; Arveiler, D.; Fruchart, J.C.; Ducimetiere, P.; Group, P.S. C-reactive protein, interleukin-6, and fibrinogen as predictors of coronary heart disease: The prime study. *Arterioscler. Thromb. Vasc. Biol.* **2003**, *23*, 1255–1261. [CrossRef] [PubMed]

61. Amasyali, B.; Kose, S.; Kursaklioglu, H.; Barcin, C.; Kilic, A. Monocyte chemoattractant protein-1 in acute coronary syndromes: Complex vicious interaction. *Int. J. Cardiol.* **2009**, *136*, 356–357. [CrossRef] [PubMed]

62. Meyers, D.G.; Strickland, D.; Maloley, P.A.; Seburg, J.K.; Wilson, J.E.; McManus, B.F. Possible association of a reduction in cardiovascular events with blood donation. *Heart* **1997**, *78*, 188–193. [CrossRef] [PubMed]

63. Meyers, D.G.; Jensen, K.C.; Menitove, J.E. A historical cohort study of the effect of lowering body iron through blood donation on incident cardiac events. *Transfusion* **2002**, *42*, 1135–1139. [CrossRef] [PubMed]

64. Sullivan, J.L. Stored iron and vascular reactivity. *Arterioscler. Thromb. Vasc. Biol.* **2005**, *25*, 1532–1535. [CrossRef] [PubMed]

65. Jialal, I. Evolving lipoprotein risk factors: Lipoprotein(a) and oxidized low-density lipoprotein. *Clin. Chem.* **1998**, *44*, 1827–1832. [PubMed]

66. Duffy, S.J.; Biegelsen, E.S.; Holbrook, M.; Russell, J.D.; Gokce, N.; Keaney, J.F., Jr.; Vita, J.A. Iron chelation improves endothelial function in patients with coronary artery disease. *Circulation* **2001**, *103*, 2799–2804. [CrossRef] [PubMed]

67. Fernandez-Real, J.M.; Lopez-Bermejo, A.; Ricart, W. Iron stores, blood donation, and insulin sensitivity and secretion. *Clin. Chem.* **2005**, *51*, 1201–1205. [CrossRef] [PubMed]

68. Beaton, M.D.; Chakrabarti, S.; Levstik, M.; Speechley, M.; Marotta, P.; Adams, P. Phase II clinical trial of phlebotomy for non-alcoholic fatty liver disease. *Aliment. Pharmacol. Ther.* **2013**, *37*, 720–729. [CrossRef] [PubMed]

69. Valenti, L.; Fracanzani, A.L.; Dongiovanni, P.; Rovida, S.; Rametta, R.; Fatta, E.; Pulixi, E.A.; Maggioni, M.; Fargion, S. A randomized trial of iron depletion in patients with nonalcoholic fatty liver disease and hyperferritinemia. *World J. Gstroenterol.* **2014**, *20*, 3002–3010. [CrossRef] [PubMed]

70. Dongiovanni, P.; Fracanzani, A.L.; Fargion, S.; Valenti, L. Iron in fatty liver and in the metabolic syndrome: A promising therapeutic target. *J. Hepatol.* **2011**, *55*, 920–932. [CrossRef] [PubMed]

71. Piperno, A.; Vergani, A.; Salvioni, A.; Trombini, P.; Vigano, M.; Riva, A.; Zoppo, A.; Boari, G.; Mancia, G. Effects of venesections and restricted diet in patients with the insulin-resistance hepatic iron overload syndrome. *Liver Int.* **2004**, *24*, 471–476. [CrossRef] [PubMed]

72. Fernandez-Real, J.M.; Manco, M. Effects of iron overload on chronic metabolic diseases. *Lancet Diabetes Endocrinol.* **2014**, *2*, 513–526. [CrossRef]

73. Graham, R.M.; Chua, A.C.; Carter, K.W.; Delima, R.D.; Johnstone, D.; Herbison, C.E.; Firth, M.J.; O'Leary, R.; Milward, E.A.; Olynyk, J.K.; *et al.* Hepatic iron loading in mice increases cholesterol biosynthesis. *Hepatology* **2010**, *52*, 462–471. [CrossRef] [PubMed]

74. Ye, P.; Cheah, I.K.; Halliwell, B. A high-fat and cholesterol diet causes fatty liver in guinea pigs. The role of iron and oxidative damage. *Free Radic. Res.* **2013**, *47*, 602–613. [CrossRef] [PubMed]

75. Silva, M.; da Costa Guerra, J.F.; Sampaio, A.F.; de Lima, W.G.; Silva, M.E.; Pedrosa, M.L. Iron dextran increases hepatic oxidative stress and alters expression of genes related to lipid metabolism contributing to hyperlipidaemia in murine model. *BioMed Res. Int.* **2015**, *2015*, 272617. [CrossRef] [PubMed]

76. Munoz-Bravo, C.; Gutierrez-Bedmar, M.; Gomez-Aracena, J.; Garcia-Rodriguez, A.; Navajas, J.F. Iron: Protector or risk factor for cardiovascular disease? Still controversial. *Nutrients* **2013**, *5*, 2384–2404. [CrossRef] [PubMed]

77. Qiu, C.; Zhang, C.; Gelaye, B.; Enquobahrie, D.A.; Frederick, I.O.; Williams, M.A. Gestational diabetes mellitus in relation to maternal dietary heme iron and nonheme iron intake. *Diabetes Care* **2011**, *34*, 1564–1569. [CrossRef] [PubMed]

78. Franchini, M.; Targher, G.; Montagnana, M.; Lippi, G. Iron and thrombosis. *Ann. Hematol.* **2008**, *87*, 167–173. [CrossRef] [PubMed]

79. Lapice, E.; Masulli, M.; Vaccaro, O. Iron deficiency and cardiovascular disease: An updated review of the evidence. *Curr. Atheroscler. Rep.* **2013**, *15*. [CrossRef] [PubMed]

80. Wang, X.; Qin, X.; Demirtas, H.; Li, J.; Mao, G.; Huo, Y.; Sun, N.; Liu, L.; Xu, X. Efficacy of folic acid supplementation in stroke prevention: A meta-analysis. *Lancet* **2007**, *369*, 1876–1882. [CrossRef]

81. Smulders, Y.M.; Blom, H.J. The homocysteine controversy. *J. Inherit. Metab. Dis.* **2011**, *34*, 93–99. [CrossRef] [PubMed]

82. Debreceni, B.; Debreceni, L. Why do homocysteine-lowering B vitamin and antioxidant E vitamin supplementations appear to be ineffective in the prevention of cardiovascular diseases? *Cardiovasc. Ther.* **2012**, *30*, 227–233. [CrossRef] [PubMed]

83. Baggott, J.E.; Tamura, T. Homocysteine, iron and cardiovascular disease: A hypothesis. *Nutrients* **2015**, *7*, 1108–1118. [CrossRef] [PubMed]

84. Fang, X.; An, P.; Wang, H.; Wang, X.; Shen, X.; Li, X.; Min, J.; Liu, S.; Wang, F. Dietary intake of heme iron and risk of cardiovascular disease: A dose-response meta-analysis of prospective cohort studies. *Nutr. Metab. Cardiovasc. Dis.* **2015**, *25*, 24–35. [CrossRef] [PubMed]

85. De Oliveira Otto, M.C.; Alonso, A.; Lee, D.H.; Delclos, G.L.; Jenny, N.S.; Jiang, R.; Lima, J.A.; Symanski, E.; Jacobs, D.R., Jr.; Nettleton, J.A. Dietary micronutrient intakes are associated with markers of inflammation but not with markers of subclinical atherosclerosis. *J. Nutr.* **2011**, *141*, 1508–1515. [CrossRef] [PubMed]

86.   Koeth, R.A.; Wang, Z.; Levison, B.S.; Buffa, J.A.; Org, E.; Sheehy, B.T.; Britt, E.B.; Fu, X.; Wu, Y.; Li, L.; *et al.* Intestinal microbiota metabolism of L-carnitine, a nutrient in red meat, promotes atherosclerosis. *Nat. Med.* **2013**, *19*, 576–585. [CrossRef] [PubMed]

87.   Wang, Z.; Klipfell, E.; Bennett, B.J.; Koeth, R.; Levison, B.S.; Dugar, B.; Feldstein, A.E.; Britt, E.B.; Fu, X.; Chung, Y.M.; *et al.* Gut flora metabolism of phosphatidylcholine promotes cardiovascular disease. *Nature* **2011**, *472*, 57–63. [CrossRef] [PubMed]

88.   Budzynski, J.; Wisniewska, J.; Ciecierski, M.; Kedzia, A. Association between bacterial infection and peripheral vascular disease: A review. *Int. J. Angiol.* **2016**, *25*, 3–13. [PubMed]

89.   Stock, J. Gut microbiota: An environmental risk factor for cardiovascular disease. *Atherosclerosis* **2013**, *229*, 440–442. [CrossRef] [PubMed]

90.   Goldsmith, J.R.; Sartor, R.B. The role of diet on intestinal microbiota metabolism: Downstream impacts on host immune function and health, and therapeutic implications. *J. Gastroenterol.* **2014**, *49*, 785–798. [CrossRef] [PubMed]

10

Liver Fat Measured by MR Spectroscopy: Estimate of Imprecision and Relationship with Serum Glycerol, Caeruloplasmin and Non-Esterified Fatty Acids

Michael France [1,*], See Kwok [2], Handrean Soran [3], Steve Williams [4], Jan Hoong Ho [3,*], Safwaan Adam [4], Dexter Canoy [5], Yifen Liu [6] and Paul N. Durrington [6]

[1] Department of Clinical Biochemistry, Cobbett House, Central Manchester Foundation Trust, Oxford Road, Manchester M13 9WL, UK

[2] Cardiovascular Trials Unit, The Old St Mary's Hospital, Hathersage Road, Oxford Road, Manchester M13 9WL, UK; sk7@doctors.org.uk

[3] Department of Medicine, Central Manchester Foundation Trust, Oxford Road, Manchester M13 9WL, UK; hsoran@aol.com

[4] Department of Imaging Science, University of Manchester, Oxford Road, Manchester M13 9PT, UK; steve.williams@manchester.ac.uk (S.W.); s.adam@doctors.org.uk (S.A.)

[5] Cancer Epidemiology Unit, University of Oxford, Richard Doll Building, Roosevelt Drive, Oxford OX3 7LF, UK; dexter.canoy@ceu.ox.ac.uk

[6] School of Biomedicine, 3rd floor, Core Technology Facility, 46 Grafton Street, Manchester M13 9NT, UK; yifen.liu@manchester.ac.uk (Y.L.); paul.durrington@manchester.ac.uk (P.N.D.)

* Correspondence: michael.france@cmft.nhs.uk (M.F.); jan.ho@doctors.org.uk (J.H.H.);

Academic Editors: Amedeo Lonardo and Giovanni Targher

Abstract: Magnetic resonance spectroscopy (MRS) is a non-invasive method for quantitative estimation of liver fat. Knowledge of its imprecision, which comprises biological variability and measurement error, is required to design therapeutic trials with measurement of change. The role of adipocyte lipolysis in ectopic fat accumulation remains unclear. We examined the relationship between liver fat content and indices of lipolysis, and determine whether lipolysis reflects insulin resistance or metabolic liver disease. Imprecision of measurement of liver fat was estimated from duplicate measurements by MRS at one month intervals. Patients provided fasting blood samples and we examined the correlation of liver fat with indices of insulin resistance, lipolysis and metabolic liver disease using Kendall Tau statistics. The coefficient of variation of liver fat content was 14.8%. Liver fat was positively related to serum insulin (T = 0.48, $p = 0.042$), homeostasis model assessment (HOMA)-B% (T = −0.48, $p = 0.042$), and body mass index (BMI) (T = 0.59, $p = 0.012$); and inversely related to HOMA-S% (T = −0.48, $p = 0.042$), serum glycerol (T = −0.59, $p = 0.014$), and serum caeruloplasmin (T = 0.055, $p = 0.047$). Our estimate of total variability in liver fat content (14.8%) is nearly twice that of the reported procedural variability (8.5%). We found that liver fat content was significantly inversely related to serum glycerol but not to non-esterified fatty acids (NEFA), suggesting progressive suppression of lipolysis. Reduction of caeruloplasmin with increasing liver fat may be a consequence or a cause of hepatic steatosis.

Keywords: fatty liver; NEFA; glycerol; lipolysis; insulin; magnetic resonance spectroscopy

1. Introduction

Nonalcoholic fatty liver disease (NAFLD) is associated with the histological finding of hepatic steatosis or steatohepatitis and has a number of causes [1–4]. Steatosis is defined as a liver fat content of greater than 5% [3,5], and may be detected by ultrasonography in patients investigated for abnormal serum transaminase levels. It is a common finding in patients with hypertriglyceridaemia and is frequently accompanied by insulin resistance and other features of metabolic syndrome. Although the condition is usually benign, 10% of patients do progress to nonalcoholic steatohepatitis (NASH), of whom 25% may proceed to cirrhosis [2].

Magnetic resonance spectroscopy (MRS) is a non-invasive and effective method in assessment of hepatic fat accumulation with high diagnostic accuracy and correspondence with histopathologic grade being demonstrated [6]. Imprecision in the measurement of liver fat content by MRS comprises biological variability and measurement error. It is an important consideration in the design of therapeutic trials aiming to measure change in liver fat content. We estimated imprecision from duplicate measurements at an interval of one month and compared our estimate with variability reported after immediate repetition of MRS in 10 individuals with similar characteristics. Although it has been suggested that accumulation of liver fat in metabolic syndrome is driven by increased hepatic fatty acid delivery due to adipocyte insulin resistance [7], raised levels of non-esterified fatty acids (NEFA) are not always found in hepatic steatosis [8]. We investigated the relationship between liver fat and indices of lipolysis and metabolic liver disease as these have the potential to influence biological variability.

2. Results

The distribution of differences between duplicate liver fat measurements was sufficiently normal (Shapiro–Wilk 0.7612) to calculate imprecision from the differences, with coefficient of variation 14.8%. The median body mass index (BMI) was 30.8 kg/m^2 (range 20.2–40.4) with 2 patients having a BMI <25 kg/m^2. MR image of the abdomen and a spectrum from the liver from one patient are shown in Figure 1. Both water and triglyceride signals are visible at high signal-to-noise. Median liver fat content was 44 g·kg^{-1} water (range, 10–332). Triglycerides were greater than 1.7 mmol·L^{-1} in 10 out of 11 patients. Hyperinsulinaemia was present in all patients although only one had a fasting plasma glucose in the impaired glucose tolerance range >6.1 mmol·L^{-1} and one in the diabetes range at 7.5 mmol·L^{-1}. Nine patients had supra-normal β cell function with (homeostasis model assessment (HOMA)-B% >100%) and all patients had impaired insulin sensitivity (HOMA-S% < 100%, median 43.9% and range 13.3–91.9). Table 1 shows the correlation of metabolic parameters related to insulin resistance, alcohol intake, ferritin, iron studies, α-1 antitrypsin (A1AT), and caeruloplasmin with the average of the two liver fat measurements.

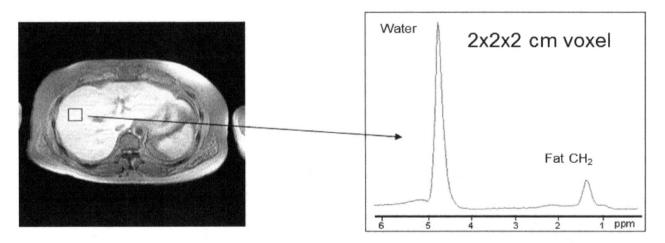

Figure 1. Transverse magnetic resonance (MR) image through the abdomen and localised MR spectrum recorded from the 2 × 2 × 2 cm voxel placed over the liver. The frequency axis of the spectrum is expressed in parts per million (ppm).

Table 1. Kendall Tau rank correlation between liver fat and metabolic parameters.

Measurement	Tau	p Value
BMI kg·m^{-2}	0.59	0.012
NEFA umol·L^{-1}	−0.22	0.3
Glycerol umol·L^{-1}	−0.59	0.014
Glucose mmol·L^{-1}	0.13	0.5
Insulin mU·L^{-1}	0.48	0.042
HOMA-S%	−0.48	0.042
HOMA-B%	0.48	0.042
Triglyceride mmol·L^{-1}	0.37	0.1
Caeruloplasmin g·L^{-1}	−0.55	0.047
Iron umol·L^{-1}	0.15	0.5
TIBC umol·L^{-1}	0.24	0.3
Iron % saturation of TIBC	0.31	0.2
Ferritin µg·L^{-1}	0.4	0.1
Alcohol units/week	−0.17	0.5
A1AT g·L^{-1}	−0.22	0.3

BMI: body mass index, NEFA: non-esterified fatty acids, HOMA-S%: homeostatic model assessment—insulin sensitivity, HOMA-B%: homeostatic model assessment—β cell function, TIBC: total iron binding capacity, A1AT: α-1 antitrypsin.

The correlations between insulin, glycerol, and caeruloplasmin and liver fat are illustrated in Figure 2. Insulin (Figure 2a) and HOMA-B% were positively related to liver fat whereas HOMA-S% was inversely related (these are identical because insulin concentration is a component of all three and the ranked pairs of observations in this small series, by chance, are the same). NEFA and glycerol (Figure 2b) were inversely related to liver fat, but this inverse correlation was only significant for glycerol. The median NEFA was 302 umol·L^{-1} with range 138–491 umol·L^{-1}, and all were in the lower half of the reference range (130–1050 umol·L^{-1}). Glycerol (reference range 27–37 umol·L^{-1}) had a wider range of 10–210 umol·L^{-1} and median 90 umol·L^{-1} reflecting suppression with high liver fat and high levels with low liver fat. Glucose, triglycerides, alcohol intake, ferritin, iron, % iron binding capacity, and A1AT were not related to liver fat but caeruloplasmin (Figure 2c) was inversely related. One patient had a caeruloplasmin level below the lower reference interval but Wilson's disease was excluded by follow-up studies. There were no differences in liver fat content between the following groups: "untreated with statins or fibrates", "statin monotherapy" or "fibrate monotherapy" ($p = 0.5$), or between groups either taking or not taking Omacor ($p = 0.2$).

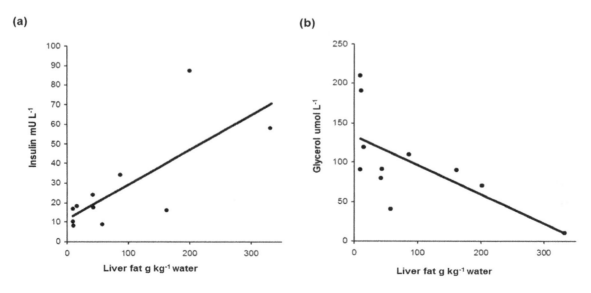

Figure 2. *Cont.*

(c)

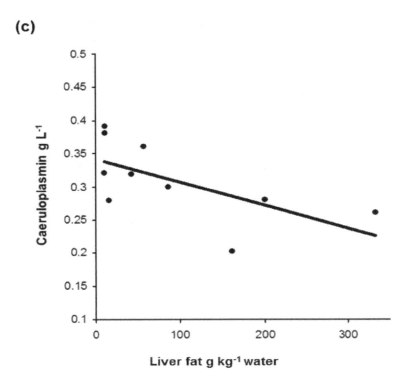

Figure 2. Relationship of insulin (**a**); glycerol (**b**); and caeruloplasmin (**c**) with liver fat content.

3. Discussion

Our data on repeat MRS at one month intervals showed a coefficient of variation of 14.8%, which is higher than the coefficient of variation of 8.5% observed between repeat MRS taken at 10 min intervals [5]. This difference likely reflects the technical challenge of repositioning the subject and reproducing conditions of the scan after one month. This would also have been contributed by alterations in hepatic adiposity in the subjects during the time period. It is important to take account of the overall imprecision of repeated measurements of liver fat in the design of therapeutic trials. Duplicate measurements improved the estimate of liver fat content in this study.

In this group of patients, we found no evidence of increased lipolysis despite increasing insulin resistance with increasing liver fat content. Higher liver fat content was significantly associated with lower serum glycerol but not NEFA. Glycerol was suppressed to quite low levels with increasing liver fat. In fact, in the subject with liver fat >30 $g \cdot kg^{-1}$ water, glycerol was almost completely suppressed. NEFA levels are in the lower half of the reference range with a downward trend as liver fat increased. It is interesting that the relationship between liver fat and glycerol is stronger than that of NEFA. Glycerol is regarded as a better reflection of adipocyte lipolysis than NEFA because, unlike NEFA, once released it cannot be taken up by the adipocyte again [9]. Our findings, therefore, do not accord with the hypothesis that increased delivery of NEFA secondary to adipocyte insulin resistance causes ectopic hepatic fat accumulation [1]. Indeed, the role of increased lipolysis in ectopic fat accumulation has been questioned in a previous study [8], with an alternative mechanism of diversion of chylomicron fatty acid to ectopic storage sites due to dysfunctional adipose tissue being proposed. It is suggested that this occurs with down regulation of NEFA trafficking and preservation of serum NEFA. Furthermore, obese subjects have been shown to have a reduction in NEFA release per unit of adipose tissue with no difference in NEFA levels compared with lean controls, and have reduced adipose tissue lipolysis [10].

The range of liver fat found in our subjects was similar to that found in the Dallas Heart Study [5]. Despite fatty liver having been reported by ultrasonography, 6 patients had a level of liver fat below the 95th centile of 5.6 $g \cdot kg^{-1}$ water cut-off established in a sub-set of the Dallas Heart Study's population without risk factors for fatty liver and normal serum transaminase levels. This may reflect the qualitative nature of hepatic ultrasound assessment of liver fat but may also reflect variability in liver fat content, particularly at near normal levels. Our subjects were not required to fast for the MRS because this has been shown not to contribute to variability [5].

The observed negative relationship of caeruloplasmin with hepatic steatosis is unexplained. Transferrin, A1AT, and caeruloplasmin are acute phase proteins, all of which increases with inflammation. Decreasing caeruloplasmin is, therefore, unlikely to reflect the inflammatory component of steatohepatitis. The decrease in caeruloplasmin could reflect reduced secretion of holoprotein due to failure to incorporate copper, an occurrence similar to that in Wilson's disease, decreased synthesis, and increased catabolism. Our results are consistent with a recent report demonstrating reduced hepatic copper related to the severity of steatosis in patients with NAFLD [11]. Furthermore, a reduction in caeruloplasmin measured as copper oxidase activity has been noted in alcoholic liver disease implying reduced incorporation of copper into caeruloplasmin [12]. The role of hepatic copper in steatosis remains undefined. One of our patients had a false positive caeruloplasmin test for Wilson's disease with a value below the lower limit of the reference range, suggesting a potential need to adjust the cut-off in the context of NAFLD.

4. Materials and Methods

4.1. Subjects

We recruited eleven patients (10 males and 1 female) attending the lipid outpatient clinic who had elevated serum alanine transaminase (ALT) levels and established hepatic steatosis demonstrated by ultrasonography. Their baseline characteristics are shown in Table 2.

Table 2. Baseline characteristics of study participants.

Population Characteristics	Median (Range)	Reference Range
Gender ($n = 11$)	10 males/1 female	-
Age	51 (32–67)	-
BMI kg·m^{-2}	29.6 (20.2–40.4)	<25% *
Alcohol (units)	3 (Male)	0–24
	5 (Female)	0–14
TC mmol·L^{-1}	5.7 (4.6–8.5)	<4.0 *
HDL mmol·L^{-1}	Female 1.26	Female > 1.2 *
	Male 1.34 (0.2–1.49)	Male > 1.0 *
TG mmol·L^{-1}	2.7 (0.6–6.0)	<1.7 *
NEFA umol·L^{-1}	302 (138–491)	130–1050
Glycerol umol·L^{-1}	90 (10–210)	27–137
Insulin mU·L^{-1}	17.2 (8.3–87.4)	3.4–6.4 **
Glucose mmol·L^{-1}	5.6 (5.0–7.5)	<6.1
HOMA-S%	43.9 (13.3–91.9)	100%
HOMA-B%	126.4 (92.6–254.5)	100%
Liver fat g·kg^{-1} water	44.0 (10.0–332.0)	<5.6 (95th centile)
ALT U·L^{-1}	56 (19–119)	5–40
Iron umol·L^{-1}	20.2 (10.2–28.1)	7–29
TIBC umol·L^{-1}	65 (50–74)	45–70
Iron % of TIBC	33 (17.6–49.4)	<50% ***
Ferritin µg·L^{-1}	187 (41.4–549.7)	15–200
Caeruloplasmin g·L^{-1}	0.31 (0.2–0.39)	0.25–0.63
A1AT g·L^{-1}	1.32 (1.07–1.95)	1.0–2.0

BMI: body mass index; TC: total cholesterol; HDL: high density cholesterol; TG: triglyceride; NEFA: non-esterified fatty acids; HOMA-S%: homeostatic model assessment—insulin sensitivity; HOMA-B%: homeostatic model assessment—β cell function; ALT: alanine transaminase; TIBC: total iron binding capacity; A1AT: α-1 antitrypsin; Reference ranges are 95th % confidence intervals unless otherwise indicated. * Clinic target levels; ** Interquartile range; *** British Society for Haematology Guideline 2000 on screening for haemochromatosis.

A diagnosis of fatty liver was made by exclusion. The presence of biliary obstruction or other structural abnormalities were excluded on ultrasonography. Autoimmune liver disease, chronic hepatitis and metabolic liver disease were excluded by the presence of normal immunoglobulin levels, absence of autoantibody markers, negative serological tests for hepatitis B and C, and measurements of serum ferritin, iron saturation, caeruloplasmin, and α-1 antitrypsin (A1AT). No patient had any clinical manifestations of Wilson's disease. Excess alcohol consumption (greater than 24 units per week for men and 14 units per week for women) was excluded on detailed history. Patients treated with hypoglycaemic agents were excluded. The study was restricted to subjects with ALT levels less than three times the upper limit of normal (120 $U \cdot L^{-1}$). All patients were following a cardioprotective diet and were also provided with advice regarding recommended levels of physical activity which comprises 150 min of moderate intensity aerobic physical activity or 75 min of high intensity aerobic physical activity per week in combination with muscle-strengthening activities for at least 2 days a week. Drug treatment was unchanged for six months prior to and during the study. Daily drug treatment was targeted at treatment of combined dyslipidaemia and consisted of no treatment ($N = 3$), statin monotherapy (Simvastatin 10 mg o.d., Simvastatin 40 mg o.d. and Atorvastatin 80 mg o.d.) ($N = 3$), statin in combination with Omacor (Atorvastatin 80 mg o.d. with Omacor 2 g per day) ($N = 1$), fibrate monotherapy (Fenofibrate 160 mg o.d. and 200 mg o.d.) ($N = 2$), fibrate in combination with Omacor (Fenofibrate 267 mg o.d. with Omacor 2 g per day) ($N = 1$), and Omacor monotherapy (4 g per day) ($N = 1$). None of the patients were on thyroxine, β blockers, thiazolidinediones or thiazide diuretics. All patients provided blood samples in clinic following a minimum of 12 h fasting and had their height and weight measured, which was used to calculate their body mass index (BMI) as weight (kg) $\times$ height (m^{-2}).

4.2. Laboratory Methods

Serum total cholesterol, high density lipoprotein cholesterol (HDL), triglycerides, iron, total iron binding capacity (TIBC), % iron saturation of TIBC, and fluoride oxalate plasma glucose were measured routinely using the standard laboratory protocols of the Department of Clinical Biochemistry at the Central Manchester University Hospital NHS Foundation Trust (CMFT) using a Roche Modular P Analyzer. Serum caeruloplasmin was measured by a nephelometric assay on the Beckman Array Analyser using a Beckman calibrator. Serum ferritin was measured using the standard laboratory protocol of the Department of Clinical Haematology at CMFT on a Beckman Access Analyser with reagents supplied by Beckman Coulter. Serum glycerol was measured using Sigma Aldrich GPO PAP reagents and serum NEFA were measured using Wako NEFA C ACS-ACOD reagents (Wako Chemicals GmbH, Neuss, Germany) on a Roche Cobas Mira analyzer (Roche, Basel, Switzerland). Serum insulin was measured by an "in house" method using a polyclonal anti-porcine insulin, raised in guinea-pig obtained from Diagnostics Scotland, Carluke, Scotland, UK and using ^{125}I labeled Insulin (DSL-1620, 185kBq, DSL Ltd.) obtained through Oxford Bio-Innovation Ltd., Bicester, UK. HOMA-S% and HOMA-B% were calculated using the Oxford University Calculator HOMA2 2004 [13].

4.3. Estimation of Liver Fat

Two MRS of the liver were performed, at one month intervals, in each patient using a Philips 1.5 Tesla *Achieva* MR scanner (Amsterdam, The Netherlands). After subjects were positioned to allow access to an area free of blood vessels, fully relaxed (repetition time, TR = 6 s) and localised ^{1}H MR spectra were obtained from a 2 × 2 × 2 cm volume using PRESS localization without water suppression (echo time, TE = 23 ms, 32 averages). T_2 relaxation times (the time constant for decay of transverse components of magnetisation (M_{xy})) for water and fat were estimated from a series of 5 spectra recorded in each session (8 averages, TR = 1600) at TE values of 23, 50, 100, 150, and 200 ms. Analysis of the spectra was performed using the AMARES routine in the jMRUI deconvolution software (MRUI consortium) [14], which provided a ratio of intracellular triglyceride to water. The ratio was corrected for T_2 relaxation time differences between water and fat [15,16]. In order to provide consistency between serial scans, the second scan performed after a one month interval was obtained in a similar position with the aid of the first scan. The MRS procedure was well tolerated with only one patient experiencing claustrophobia.

4.4. Statistical Methods

The standard deviation of MRS estimates of liver fat was calculated from the differences between the two scans as $\sqrt{[\sum (\text{differences}^2)/22]}$. The normality of the distribution of differences was assessed using the Shapiro–Wilk W test. All other data are expressed as median (range) because of their non-parametric distribution. Correlation between variables was calculated as the Kendall Tau rank statistic with a 2 tailed probability of <0.05 being regarded as significant. The Kruskal Wallace one way analysis of variance test was used to assess the differences in liver fat content between 3 groups defined by drug treatment as: "no statin or fibrate treatment", "statin monotherapy", and "fibrate monotherapy", which were mutually exclusive, and between 2 groups defined as "Omacor treated" or "not Omacor treated".

The study was designed to estimate the variability of sequential measures of liver fat to inform power calculation for future studies. The estimate was considered sufficiently robust after 11 patients, after review by our statistician.

5. Main Messages

Variability of repeat scans performed one month apart is nearly twice that observed with immediate repetition, and should be taken into account in the design of interventional trials with liver fat content as the endpoint. Glycerol is inversely related to liver fat content suggesting down regulation of fatty acid trafficking consistent with the new paradigm for the pathogenesis of fatty liver. Caeruloplasmin is inversely related to liver fat content, which is as yet unexplained.

Acknowledgments: Support from the Manchester Wellcome Trust Clinical Research Facility and the National Institute of Health Research (NIHR) Biomedical Research Centre is acknowledged.

Author Contributions: Michael France, See Kwok and Paul N. Durrington were involved in the design of the study. Michael France, See Kwok, Handrean Soran, Yifen Liu, Safwaan Adam and Jan Hoong Ho wrote the first draft and all authors were involved in production of the final manuscript. Dexter Canoy advised on and critically appraised the statistical analysis. Steve Williams designed the magnetic resonance protocol and supervised the liver scans.

References

1.   Kopec, K.L.; Burns, D. Nonalcoholic fatty liver disease: A review of the spectrum of disease, diagnosis, and therapy. *Nutr. Clin. Pract.* **2011**, *26*, 565–576. [CrossRef] [PubMed]
2.   Cheung, O.; Sanyal, A.J. Recent advances in nonalcoholic fatty liver disease. *Curr. Opin. Gastroenterol.* **2010**, *26*, 202–208. [CrossRef] [PubMed]
3.   Tessari, P.; Coracina, A.; Cosma, A.; Tiengo, A. Hepatic lipid metabolism and non-alcoholic fatty liver disease. *Nutr. Metab. Cardiovasc. Dis.* **2009**, *19*, 291–302. [CrossRef] [PubMed]
4.   Mehta, S.R. Advances in the treatment of nonalcoholic fatty liver disease. *Ther. Adv. Endocrinol. Metab.* **2010**, *1*, 101–115. [CrossRef] [PubMed]
5.   Szczepaniak, L.S.; Nurenberg, P.; Leonard, D.; Browning, J.D.; Reingold, J.S.; Grundy, S.; Hobbs, H.H.; Dobbins, R.L. Magnetic resonance spectroscopy to measure hepatic triglyceride content: Prevalence of hepatic steatosis in the general population. *Am. J. Physiol. Endocrinol. Metab.* **2005**, *288*, E462–E468. [CrossRef] [PubMed]
6.   Georgoff, P.; Thomasson, D.; Louie, A.; Fleischman, E.; Dutcher, L.; Mani, H.; Kottilil, S.; Morse, C.; Dodd, L.; Kleiner, D.; et al. Hydrogen-1 MR spectroscopy for measurement and diagnosis of hepatic steatosis. *AJR Am. J. Roentgenol.* **2012**, *199*, 2–7. [CrossRef] [PubMed]

7. Baldeweg, S.E.; Golay, A.; Natali, A.; Balkau, B.; del Prato, S.; Coppack, S.W. Insulin resistance, lipid and fatty acid concentrations in 867 healthy Europeans. European Group for the Study of Insulin Resistance (EGIR). *Eur. J. Clin. Investig.* **2000**, *30*, 45–52. [CrossRef]

8. McQuaid, S.E.; Hodson, L.; Neville, M.J.; Dennis, A.L.; Cheeseman, J.; Humphreys, S.M.; Ruge, T.; Gilbert, M.; Fielding, B.A.; Frayn, K.N.; et al. Downregulation of adipose tissue fatty acid trafficking in obesity: A driver for ectopic fat deposition? *Diabetes* **2011**, *60*, 47–55. [CrossRef] [PubMed]

9. Galton, D.J.; Wallis, S. The regulation of adipose cell metabolism. *Proc. Nutr. Soc.* **1982**, *41*, 167–173. [CrossRef] [PubMed]

10. Kolditz, C.I.; Langin, D. Adipose tissue lipolysis. *Curr. Opin. Clin. Nutr. Metab. Care* **2010**, *13*, 377–381. [CrossRef] [PubMed]

11. Aigner, E.; Strasser, M.; Haufe, H.; Sonnweber, T.; Hohla, F.; Stadlmayr, A.; Solioz, M.; Tilg, H.; Patsch, W.; Weiss, G.; et al.   A role for low hepatic copper concentrations in nonalcoholic Fatty liver disease. *Am. J. Gastroenterol.* **2010**, *105*, 1978–1985. [CrossRef] [PubMed]

12. Uhlikova, E.; Kupcova, V.; Szantova, M.; Turecky, L. Plasma copper and ceruloplasmin in patients with alcoholic liver steatosis. *Bratisl. Lek. List.* **2008**, *109*, 431–433.

13. Levy, J.C.; Matthews, D.R.; Hermans, M.P. Correct homeostasis model assessment (HOMA) evaluation uses the computer program. *Diabetes Care* **1998**, *21*, 2191–2192. [CrossRef] [PubMed]

14. Vanhamme, L.; van den Boogaart, A.; van Huffel, S. Improved method for accurate and efficient quantification of MRS data with use of prior knowledge. *J. Magn. Reson.* **1997**, *129*, 35–43. [CrossRef] [PubMed]

15. Stefan, D.; di Cesare, F.; Andrasescu, A.; Popa, E.; Lazariev, A.; Vescovo, E.; Strbak, O.; Williams, S.; Starcuk, Z.; Cabanas, M.; et al. Quantitation of magnetic resonance spectroscopy signals: The jMRUI software package. *Meas. Sci. Technol.* **2010**, *20*, 104035–104044. [CrossRef]

16. Thomas, E.L.; Saeed, N.; Hajnal, J.V.; Brynes, A.; Goldstone, A.P.; Frost, G.; Bell, J.D. Magnetic resonance imaging of total body fat. *J. Appl. Physiol.* **1998**, *85*, 1778–1785. [PubMed]

11

Bidirectional Relationships and Disconnects between NAFLD and Features of the Metabolic Syndrome

Patrick Wainwright [1] and Christopher D. Byrne [2,3,*]

[1] Clinical Biochemistry, University Hospital Southampton, Tremona Road, Southampton SO16 6YD, UK; patrick.wainwright@uhs.nhs.uk

[2] Nutrition and Metabolism, Faculty of Medicine, University of Southampton, Tremona Road, Southampton SO16 6YD, UK

[3] Southampton National Institute for Health Research Biomedical Research Centre, University Hospital Southampton, Tremona Road, Southampton SO16 6YD, UK

* Correspondence: C.D.Byrne@soton.ac.uk

Academic Editors: Amedeo Lonardo and Giovanni Targher

Abstract: Non-alcoholic fatty liver disease (NAFLD) represents a wide spectrum of liver disease from simple steatosis, to steatohepatitis, (both with and without liver fibrosis), cirrhosis and end-stage liver failure. NAFLD also increases the risk of hepatocellular carcinoma (HCC) and both HCC and end stage liver disease may markedly increase risk of liver-related mortality. NAFLD is increasing in prevalence and is presently the second most frequent indication for liver transplantation. As NAFLD is frequently associated with insulin resistance, central obesity, dyslipidaemia, hypertension and hyperglycaemia, NAFLD is often considered the hepatic manifestation of the metabolic syndrome. There is growing evidence that this relationship between NAFLD and metabolic syndrome is bidirectional, in that NAFLD can predispose to metabolic syndrome features, which can in turn exacerbate NAFLD or increase the risk of its development in those without a pre-existing diagnosis. Although the relationship between NAFLD and metabolic syndrome is frequently bidirectional, recently there has been much interest in genotype/phenotype relationships where there is a disconnect between the liver disease and metabolic syndrome features. Such potential examples of genotypes that are associated with a dissociation between liver disease and metabolic syndrome are patatin-like phospholipase domain-containing protein-3 (PNPLA3) (I148M) and transmembrane 6 superfamily member 2 protein (TM6SF2) (E167K) genotypes. This review will explore the bidirectional relationship between metabolic syndrome and NAFLD, and will also discuss recent insights from studies of PNPLA3 and TM6SF2 genotypes that may give insight into how and why metabolic syndrome features and liver disease are linked in NAFLD.

Keywords: NAFLD; metabolic syndrome; insulin resistance; PNPLA3

1. Introduction

Non-alcoholic fatty liver disease (NAFLD) is a considerable public health concern, and is the commonest cause for chronic liver disease in the developed world [1,2]. Worldwide prevalence of NAFLD is estimated to be in the region of 20% in the general population [3]. NAFLD represents a disease spectrum ranging from hepatic steatosis, to non-alcoholic steatohepatitis, to cirrhosis, end-stage liver failure and hepatocellular carcinoma. The accepted definition of NAFLD is a hepatic triglyceride content of greater than 5.5%, as determined from analysis of the Dallas Heart Study cohort [4]. The metabolic syndrome is a collection of underlying risk factors for cardiovascular disease with an estimated prevalence in the USA of 34% [5].

The relationship between NAFLD, obesity, insulin resistance and type 2 diabetes is a complex one. NAFLD has traditionally been considered to be the hepatic manifestation of the metabolic syndrome, due to the close association between NAFLD and the various component features of the metabolic syndrome such as abdominal obesity, hypertension, elevated fasting plasma glucose, raised serum triglycerides and low high-density lipoprotein cholesterol (HDL-C) concentrations. Many epidemiological studies have demonstrated an association between NAFLD and the metabolic syndrome [6–8].

There is now a growing body of evidence supporting the idea that there is a bidirectional relationship between NAFLD and features of the metabolic syndrome, with insulin resistance being the central pathophysiological process common to both conditions. As such there currently exists and "chicken and egg" debate in the literature regarding the temporal relationship between NAFLD and the metabolic syndrome, with no clear consensus about which is considered to generally occur first. A recent study has demonstrated a reciprocal causality between NAFLD and metabolic syndrome in a Chinese population, with metabolic syndrome being found to have a greater effect on incident NAFLD in terms of causality than NAFLD does on incident metabolic syndrome [9].

In addition to this there are recognised situations whereby there is an apparent disconnect between NAFLD and insulin resistance/metabolic syndrome features, and these generally arise as a result of particular genetic polymorphisms such as in the patatin-like phospholipase domain-containing protein-3 (PNPLA3) gene.

This review will attempt to review the available evidence regarding the bidirectional relationship between NAFLD and components of the metabolic syndrome, as well as to explore the potential disconnects that may exist between the two due to genetic variability and inherited metabolic disease.

2. Association between NAFLD and Components of the Metabolic Syndrome

There have been various diagnostic criteria available for the diagnosis of metabolic syndrome, and these have changed subtly over recent years. The most commonly used criteria are those published by the International Diabetes Federation in 2009. It should be noted that these most recent criteria advocate using population- and country- specific definitions for abdominal obesity [10]. Table 1 outlines the various diagnostic criteria available.

NAFLD can occur in individuals who are not obese [11,12], however this is more unusual and generally NAFLD is closely related to increased central adiposity. NAFLD is commonly associated with all of the component features of the metabolic syndrome, and nearly two thirds of people with obesity and type 2 diabetes demonstrate hepatic steatosis [13,14]. One study identified hepatic steatosis via ultrasonography in 50% of patients with hyperlipidaemia [15]. NAFLD is also associated with arterial hypertension and cross-sectional studies have demonstrated that approximately 50% of people with essential hypertension also have NAFLD [16,17]. Importantly, in those people with NAFLD the presence of multiple features of the metabolic syndrome is associated with more severe liver disease and a higher likelihood of progression to NASH and cirrhosis [18,19].

Table 1. Diagnostic criteria available for metabolic syndrome.

Criteria	WHO (1999)	NCEP (2001)	IDF (2005)	IDF (2009)
Required	Insulin resistance	Nil	Waist circumference ≥94 cm in men, ≥80 cm in women	Nil
Number of features	≥2 of:	≥3 of:	≥2 of:	≥3 of:
Obesity	Waist/hip ratio of >0.9 in men, >0.85 in women or BMI ≥ 30	Waist circumference ≥ 102 cm in men, ≥88 cm in women		Waist circumference—population specific definitions
Triglycerides	≥150 mg/dL (1.7 mmol/L)	≥150 mg/dL (1.7 mmol/L)	≥150 mg/dL (1.7 mmol/L)	≥150 mg/dL (1.7 mmol/L)
HDL-cholesterol	<40 mg/dL (1 mmol/L) in men, <50 mg/dL (1.3 mmol/L) in women	<40 mg/dL (1 mmol/L) in men, <50 mg/dL (1.3 mmol/L) in women	<40 mg/dL (1 mmol/L) in men, <50 mg/dL (1.3 mmol/L) in women	<40 mg/dL (1 mmol/L) in men, <50 mg/dL (1.3 mmol/L) in women
Hypertension	≥140/90 mmHg	≥135/85 mmHg	≥135/85 mmHg	≥135/85 mmHg
Glucose		110 mg/dL (6.1 mmol/L)	100 mg/dL (5.6 mmol/L)	100 mg/dL (5.6 mmol/L)
Microalbuminuria	Albumin/creatinine ratio > 30 mg/g; albumin excretion rate > 20 mcg/min			

WHO, World Health Organisation; NCEP, National Cholesterol Education Program; IDF, international diabetes federation.

3. NAFLD as a Risk Factor for and Precursor to the Metabolic Syndrome

There is evidence to suggest that NAFLD, rather than being simply the hepatic manifestation of the metabolic syndrome, may in fact be a necessary first step in its development.

When the link between NAFLD and insulin resistance was initially described by Day et al, it was proposed as part of a "two hit hypothesis" [20]. Here, the "first hit" was increased triglyceride accumulation as a result of insulin resistance and increased delivery of free fatty acids to the liver, followed by a "second hit" of hepatic oxidative stress resulting in increased lipid peroxidation. This was said to then lead inexorably to hepatocyte injury, inflammation and fibrosis, with the potential for progressive liver damage. It has subsequently been suggested that pathogenesis of NAFLD may in fact reflect "multiple parallel hits" which all contribute to an environment of hepatic inflammation with the involvement of cytokines and adipokines from extrahepatic tissues such as the gut and adipose tissue [21].

From a basic science perspective, there is reason to believe that hepatic lipid accumulation could be a cause and a perpetuating factor for the development of insulin resistance. There is currently much interest in fully elucidating the role that protein kinase C-ε (PKC-ε) may play in this relationship. An elegant study conducted by Samuel et al investigated PKC-ε and how it may link NAFLD and insulin resistance [22].

They observed that rats that were fed a 3 day high-fat diet developed marked hepatic steatosis and hepatic insulin resistance as determined by hyperinsulinaemic-euglycaemic clamp studies. Here, PKC-ε was activated but other forms of PKC were not. Crucially, the authors then went on to attenuate the expression of PKC-ε using an anti-sense oligonucelotide directed at PKC-ε and they noted that this protected the rats from steatosis-induced hepatic insulin resistance and also reversed defects that they had observed in insulin receptor signalling function. It should be noted that both hepatic diacylglycerol and triacylglycerol content were not affected by this intervention suggesting that the hepatic lipid accumulation is a prerequisite for insulin resistance. This relationship has also been investigated in humans, in a study of 37 obese non-diabetic individuals awaiting bariatric surgery [23]. Here it was observed that hepatic diacylglycerol content from liver biopsy specimens was the strongest predictor of insulin resistance and accounted for 64% of the variability in insulin sensitivity. Hepatic diacylglycerol content was strongly correlated with activation of PKC-ε. Given this evidence, a model has emerged whereby increases in liver diacylglycerol content result in activation of PKC-ε, translocation of PKC-ε in the cell membrane, inhibition of hepatic insulin signalling and the resulting generation and maintenance of hepatocyte insulin resistance.

More recently there has been interest in the hepatokine, fetuin B. This compound has been shown to be increased in obese rodents [24]. It has also been shown that overnutrition in experimental mice results in hepatic steatosis, and this alters the hepatocyte protein secretion profile leading to increased secretion of fetuin B [25]. The authors of this study went on to further study the effects of fetuin B *in vivo* and observed that injecting recombinant fetuin B intraperitoneally into mice significantly impaired glucose tolerance when compared with controls. In addition to this, silencing fetuin B gene expression using short hairpin RNA was found to increase glucose tolerance. As such, fetuin B provides an example of how hepatic steatosis can be linked to the development of insulin resistance and thus the metabolic syndrome. Other hepatokines such as FGF21 and selenoprotein P are thought to be play a role in the pathophysiology of insulin resistance with action on the liver and other tissues, however it is less clear how they fit into the relationship between hepatic steatosis and the metabolic syndrome.

It is known that most people with NAFLD also have insulin resistance, however most do not exhibit all of the features of the metabolic syndrome [26]. This could indicate that hepatic steatosis is required as a prerequisite for the development of further metabolic disease such as altered glucose and lipid metabolism. There is now a significant body of clinical evidence for NAFLD preceding, and being a strong risk factor for, development of the metabolic syndrome and its various components. A large prospective cohort study looked at 17,920 individuals from a Han Chinese population and followed them up over a 6 years period [27]. These individuals did not have metabolic syndrome at baseline, and the authors identified NAFLD as an independent risk factor for its development with an adjusted hazard ratio of 1.55 (95% confidence intervals 1.39–1.72). This observation of NAFLD as an independent risk factor for the development of the metabolic syndrome has also been made in a variety of other populations such as North American [28], western Australian [29], Korean [30], Japanese [31] and south Indian [32].

A large prospective cohort study of over 22,000 Korean men demonstrated that NAFLD is an independent risk factor for incident arterial hypertension, and that risk increases with severity of NAFLD [33]. This study replicated the findings of an earlier, smaller prospective study which demonstrated that NAFLD was an independent risk factor for the development of prehypertension [34]. Another prospective cohort study examined 1521 people and stratified them on the basis of their fatty liver index score (a surrogate marker of hepatic steatosis) [35]. It was observed that NAFLD, as diagnosed using fatty liver index score, was an independent risk factor for incident arterial hypertension. Finally, a retrospective cohort study of 11,448 individuals without hypertension revealed that the development of incident fatty liver disease over a five years period was associated with increased risk of incident hypertension [36].

A retrospective study of a Korean occupational cohort of 13,218 individuals observed that development of new fatty liver was associated with incident diabetes [37]. There are many prospective studies in the literature that demonstrate that NAFLD, and the surrogate markers with which it is associated, is a key risk factor and precursor for the development of type 2 diabetes [29,38–46]. Table 2 summarises the characteristics of these key studies.

Of particular interest is a longitudinal cohort study in which the authors followed up 358 individuals (109 with NAFLD, 249 without NAFLD) over an 11 years period [29]. After excluding those who had type 2 diabetes at baseline, they observed that those with NAFLD were significantly more likely to develop diabetes during the follow up period than those without. Similarly, they observed the same regarding who would go on to develop the metabolic syndrome. Also, a retrospective study of a Korean occupational cohort of 12,853 individuals demonstrated that the clustering of insulin resistance, overweight/obesity and hepatic steatosis markedly increased risk of incident type 2 diabetes [47]. The fully adjusted odds ratio for those with all 3 factors and risk of incident diabetes at 5 years follow-up was 14.13 (95% confidence intervals 8.99–22.21).

In addition to this, a meta-analysis has been performed recently which concluded that the presence of NAFLD doubles an individual's risk of developing type 2 diabetes in later life [48]. It would seem that there may be subsets of patients with NAFLD that have different levels of risk of type 2 diabetes, with one small study suggesting that the presence of biopsy-proven NASH is a greater risk factor than steatosis alone [41]. This is consistent with the accepted notion that individuals with nonalcoholic steatohepatitis (NASH) will tend to have a greater burden of metabolic disease.

Table 2. Characteristics of prospective studies linking hepatic steatosis to the development of type 2 diabetes.

Study	Country/Population	Sample Size	NAFLD Diagnostic Method/Surrogate Marker Used	Duration of Follow-Up	Key Findings	Limitations of Study
Vozarova 2002 [38]	Pima Indians aged 18–50	173 women, 278 men	ALT, AST and GGT concentrations	6.9 years average	High baseline ALT associated with increased risk of incident DM	Only surrogate markers used, no control for alcohol/hep C
Lee 2003 [39]	Korean men aged 25–55	4088 men	GGT concentration	4 years	Strong relationship between baseline GGT and risk of incident DM	Only studied men, only used surrogate marker
Hanley 2005 [40]	USA non-Hispanic whites and African American adults	910 women, 715 men	ALT, AST and ALP concentrations	5.2 years average	ALT and ALP in upper quartile at baseline significantly increased risk of metabolic syndrome	Only surrogate markers used for NAFLD diagnosis
Ekstedt 2006 [41]	Swedish NAFLD patients	87 men, 42 women	Biopsy-proven NAFLD	13.7 years average	Marked increase in proportion of patients with DM over period of study	No control group, no baseline glycaemic data to compare
Monami 2008 [42]	Florence aged 40–75	3124 total	ALT, AST and GGT concentrations	40 months average	Baseline GGT near upper limit of normal predicts incident DM	Study population participated in screening programme for diabetes, may not be representative
Goessling 2008 [43]	New England adults, all white	1575 women, 1237 men	ALT and AST concentrations	20 years	Increased ALT associated with higher risk of DM and metabolic syndrome, increased AST associated with incident DM risk	Homogenous study population, only surrogate markers used
Adams 2009 [29]	Western Australian adults	115 women, 243 men	NAFLD diagnosed with ALT after exclusion of other causes	11 years	NAFLD associated with higher risk of incident diabetes	Not an independent predictor if adjusted for WC, hypertension or insulin resistance
Ryu 2010 [44]	Korean men aged 30–65	9148 men	GGT concentrations	4.1 years average	Increase in GGT during study period predicted incident metabolic syndrome	Did not use accepted criteria for diagnosis of metabolic syndrome
Balkau 2010 [45]	Western France, aged 30–65	1950 women, 1861 men	NAFLD diagnosed using fatty liver index (FLI) score	9 years	Higher FLI score at baseline predicted incident DM	Used FLI rather than formal diagnostic methods
Sung 2011 [46]	Korean adults	7236 men, 3855 women	NAFLD diagnosed with ultrasound scan	5 years	Presence of fatty liver on ultrasound strongly predicted incident DM	Ultrasound relatively insensitive for diagnosis

ALT, alanine aminotransferase; AST, aspartate aminotransferase; GGT, gamma-glutamyl transferase; DM, diabetes mellitus; ALP, alkaline Phosphatase; NAFLD, non-alcoholic fatty liver disease; WC, waist circumference.

4. Metabolic Syndrome as an Initiating or Aggravating Factor for Liver Disease

In addition to the evidence from the literature that NAFLD may predispose individuals to developing or worsening insulin resistance and the metabolic syndrome, there is also growing evidence that insulin resistance may contribute to progressive liver damage.

Of particular interest is the role played by plasminogen activator inhibitor 1 [49]. PAI-1 is a member of the serine protease inhibitor family, and acts as a key mediator in the fibrinolytic system. In tissues with a significant degree of fibrosis, concentrations of PAI-1 are elevated leading to an inhibition of tissue proteolytic activities, a decreased rate of collagen degradation and increased tissue fibrogenesis [49]. Increased PAI-1 levels are associated with obesity, insulin resistance, type 2 diabetes and dyslipidaemia [50,51]. Specifically it has been shown that PAI-1 concentrations measured in subcutaneous adipose tissue biopsy samples from individuals with nascent metabolic syndrome are significantly higher than those in control samples [52]. It has also been observed in a human hepatocyte cell line that tumour necrosis factor α (TNF-α) is able to induce the expression of PAI-1, leading to increased hepatic fibrosis and atherosclerosis in insulin-resistant individuals [53]. There is also a wealth of evidence in the literature regarding the role of PAI-1 in initiating and perpetuating hepatic fibrosis [49]. As such this provides evidence of a causative role for insulin resistance and obesity in the generation of ongoing hepatic fibrosis.

In addition to this, there is evidence that other inflammatory cytokines originating from white adipose tissue as a result of obesity and insulin resistance may play a significant role in hepatic fibrosis and inflammation. It has been known for some time that white adipose tissue is not metabolically inert but is a complex organ that can become active in the obese, insulin-resistant state leading to the production of various pro-inflammatory cytokines [54,55]. These cytokines include interleukin-1β (IL-1β), interleukin-6 (IL-6), interleukin-8 (IL-8), interleukin-18 (IL-18), complement component 3 (C3), TNF-α, PAI-1, adiponectin, leptin, resistin, apelin, vaspin and visfatin. There is evidence that these inflammatory mediators could play a role in the progression of liver disease from "simple" steatosis to NASH [56,57], and also that they may stimulate the differentiation of stellate cells in the liver into myofibroblast-like cells resulting in a more fibrogenic environment [58]. IL-1β, IL-6 and TNF-α are traditionally considered to be pro-inflammatory cytokines, and are all thought to play a role in the pathogenesis of NASH and its associated fibrosis [59,60]. More recently it has been suggested that the balance of pro- and anti-inflammatory mediators can lead to alterations in the gut microbiota and that this may have a significant impact on the progression of hepatic steatosis to NASH [61]. It has also been suggested that apoptosis of hepatocytes could be an important factor in liver damage and specifically progression to NASH [62,63]. Recent findings indicate that patients with a higher degree of insulin resistance exhibit greater evidence for apoptosis of hepatocytes in liver biopsy specimens of morbidly obese individuals, and it has been speculated that this may be mediated by inflammatory cytokines [64]. These studies all provide evidence for a causative link between insulin resistance and hepatic damage mediated in part by inflamed, endocrinologically-active adipose tissue.

There is also clinical evidence that insulin resistance and the metabolic syndrome can cause a worsening of liver disease. A retrospective study of 103 individuals with NAFLD examined histological findings from paired liver biopsy specimens with an average interval of 3 years [65]. The authors observed marked variability in the progression of histological features of NAFLD between the 2 time points, but noted that those individuals with diabetes were at higher risk than non-diabetic people for progression of fibrosis. It is also established in the literature that metabolic syndrome and type 2 diabetes are strongly associated with severe liver disease such as cirrhosis and hepatocellular carcinoma [66–69]. It appears from the literature that individuals with type 2 diabetes and NAFLD combined are at markedly greater risk of more severe liver disease than those with NAFLD alone, and their liver-related mortality is greater.

There are a variety of cross-sectional studies available that demonstrate that metabolic syndrome and its components are associated with an increased risk of NAFLD in a variety of populations including North American [70], Mexican [71], Taiwanese [72] and Japanese [26]. However, given the cross-sectional nature of these studies they do not provide real evidence of a causative link. Of interest is a recent longitudinal prospective cohort study of 15,791 Han Chinese individuals followed up over a 6 years period [73]. They observed 3913 new cases of NAFLD in this population, and risk of incident NAFLD was markedly higher in those with metabolic syndrome. After adjusting for possible confounding factors such as age, diet, sex, smoking status and level of physical activity, the hazard ratio for incident NAFLD was found to be 1.94 (95% confidence intervals 1.78–2.13). The authors also observed that hazard ratios for incident NAFLD increased the more components of the metabolic syndrome were present at baseline, reaching 3.51 (95% confidence intervals 3.15–3.91) when 3 components were present as compared with individuals who exhibited no metabolic syndrome components. Figure 1 summarises the bidirectional relationship between hepatic steatosis and the metabolic syndrome with regards to the various aspects described above.

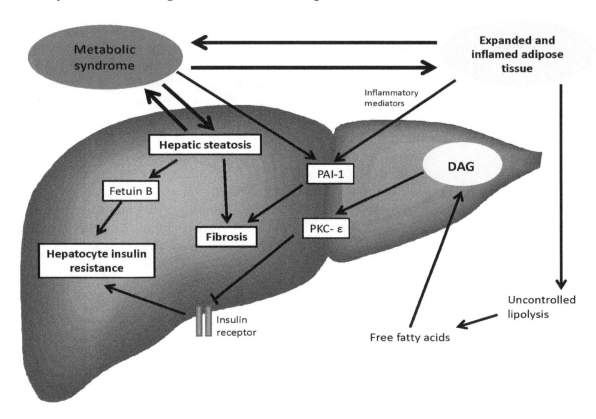

Figure 1. Schematic demonstrating the bidirectional interactions between hepatic steatosis and metabolic syndrome and aspects of how these are mediated. DAG: diacylglycerols; PKC-ε: protein kinase C-ε; PAI-1: plasminogen activator inhibitor-1.

5. Evidence for a Disconnection between Hepatic Steatosis and Metabolic Syndrome

Despite the clear bidirectional causal links between NAFLD and the metabolic syndrome, there are certain situations where this appears to not be the case. In such scenarios there is a clinical disconnect between NAFLD and insulin resistance. Several groups have demonstrated that it is possible experimentally to induce either insulin resistance or hepatic steatosis individually without the presence of the other. The first evidence that hepatic steatosis could occur independently of insulin resistance was published in 2007 [74]. Here mice were raised which over-expressed acyl-CoA:diacylglycerol acyltransferase 2 (DGAT 2), an enzyme which acts to catalyze the final step of hepatic triglyceride biosynthesis. These mice were observed to develop marked hepatic steatosis in the absence of any abnormalities in plasma glucose and insulin levels, glucose and insulin tolerance, or infusion rates during hyperinsulinaemic euglycaemic clamp experiments. A subsequent study investigated variability in the DGAT2 gene to see if this relationship could also be found in humans. The authors investigated 187 individuals from south Germany, and observed 2 single nucleotide polymorphisms (SNPs) in DGAT2 that were associated with smaller decreases in liver fat following an exercise programme than wild type genotype [75]. There were no observed changes in insulin sensitivity among the different genotypes and thus the authors concluded that DGAT2 may play a role in mediating a disconnection between insulin resistance and hepatic steatosis. Additionally, it has been observed that inhibiting secretion of very low density lipoprotein (VLDL) from the liver by a genetic modification or diet-induced choline deficiency in a mouse model results in accumulation of hepatic triglyceride without causing insulin resistance [76,77].

More recently, there has been much interest focused on the patatin-like phospholipase domain-containing protein-3 (PNPLA3) gene, which encodes for a protein called adiponutrin. The exact role of this adiponutrin is currently unclear, however it is recognised as being a membrane-associated protein expressed in hepatic and adipose tissue that possesses lipogenic and lipolytic activities. There is evidence to suggest that it is located in lipid droplets and may play a role in triglyceride hydrolysis [78]. PNPLA3 gene expression is upregulated following the post-prandial insulin spike, and downregulated following fasting. It was reported in 2008 that a particular allele in PNPLA3 (I148M or rs738409) was strongly associated with increased hepatic steatosis and hepatic inflammation, with individuals homozygous for I148M exhibiting twice the level of hepatic fat content than non-carriers [79]. Interestingly, it was also observed that I148M carrier frequency was highest in Hispanic populations who are thought to have highest susceptibility to NAFLD, and regression analysis demonstrated that the presence or absence of this PNPLA3 variant along with another (453I) accounted for 72% of the observed ethnic differences in levels of hepatic steatosis from the Dallas Heart Study. It was subsequently reported that the I148M variant has a marked effect on enzyme activity and results in a disruption to normal hydrolysis of triglycerides leading to impaired secretion of very low density lipoproteins (VLDL) [80,81]. Interestingly, it has subsequently been demonstrated that the association between the I148M variant and NAFLD in independent of insulin sensitivity as measured by hyperinsulinaemic euglycaemic clamp, as well as central obesity [82,83]. Therefore the PNPLA3 I148M variant provides an example of how hepatic steatosis can occur in humans independently of insulin resistance and the metabolic syndrome.

A similar scenario has been identified more recently with the transmembrane 6 superfamily member 2 (TM6SF2) gene. TM6SF2 is expressed largely in the liver and intestine and is thought to play a key role in the regulation of hepatic fat metabolism and the secretion of triglyceride-rich lipoproteins. As with PNPLA3, it is thought to be located in lipid droplets and siRNA inhibition is associated with increased hepatocellular triglyceride concentration and lipid droplet lipid content [84]. Variation in this gene has been shown to be associated with susceptibility to NAFLD independently of variation in PNPLA3, with the variant being identified as E167K or rs58542926 [85]. The allele frequency of this variant was shown to be 7.2% in European populations. A subsequent study of 361 individuals, including 226 patients with biopsy-proven NAFLD, has shown that this variant has a modest effect on NAFLD susceptibility and is associated with a slightly higher risk of developing NASH [86]. A further study of 1074 individuals demonstrated an association between this variant and advanced fibrosis and cirrhosis that occurred independently of potential confounding factors such as age, BMI, presence of type 2 diabetes and PNPLA3 genotype status [87]. However, it should be noted that 2 studies looking at this variant in Japanese [88] and Chinese [89] populations of individuals with biopsy-proven NAFLD failed to show an association between it and fibrosis stage or general histological severity. The Japanese study had relatively small numbers with 211 individuals and just 2 who were homozygous for E167K, and it should be noted that both of these studies focused on a single ethnic group that may not be directly applicable to other populations. A meta-analysis of 10 published studies looked at the relationship between the E167K variant and the presence of NAFLD in a total of 5537 study participants [90]. This revealed a carrier frequency of up to 7%, and demonstrated a moderate effect on the risk of developing NAFLD with an odds ratio of 2.13 (95% confidence interval 1.36–3.30). Crucially, it has been shown in a recent Finnish study that this variant is associated with preserved insulin sensitivity and a lack of hypertriglyceridaemia suggesting that this represents a distinct subtype of NAFLD similar to that associated with the PNPLA3 I148M variant [91]. Figure 2 demonstrates the relationship between the 2 described genetic variants and the lipid droplet within the hepatocyte.

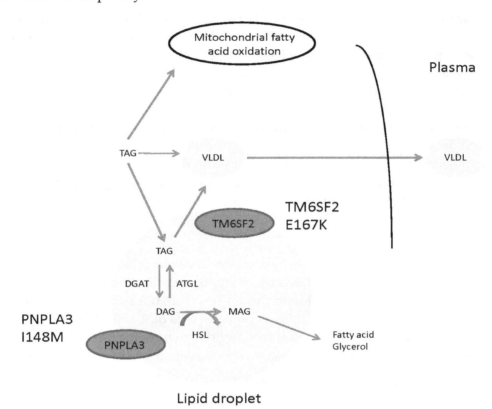

Figure 2. Interaction between PNPLA3 and TM6SF2 variants and lipid metabolism in the hepatic lipid droplet. TAG; triacylglycerol; DAG; diacylglycerol; MAG; monoacylglycerol; VLDL; very low density lipoprotein; DGAT; diglyceride acyltransferase; ATGL; adipose triglyceride lipase; HSL; hormone sensitive lipase.

Further evidence for a dissociation between hepatic steatosis and insulin resistance may be found in the case of familial hypobetalipoproteinaemia (FHBL). Patients with FHBL have very low or absent levels of apolipoprotein B and this leads to an impairment of very low density lipoprotein export from the liver and consequently intra-hepatic accumulation of triglyceride. Amaro *et al.* [92] investigated a small number of overweight or obese patients with FHBL and observed that these individuals had greater insulin sensitivity than BMI- and hepatic triglyceride content-matched subjects with NAFLD alone. The authors speculate that this would support the assertion that hepatic steatosis is a marker rather than a cause of the metabolic syndrome, however this was a very small study and it is not clear how applicable these findings are to the wider population of people with NAFLD. It has also been observed that lysosomal acid lipase deficiency (LAL-D), a rare autosomal recessive inherited condition, can lead to hepatic steatosis in the absence of metabolic syndrome [93].

There is also evidence that adipose triacylglycerol lipase (ATGL) may play a role in a potential dissociation between insulin resistance and hepatic steatosis [94]. ATGL acts to initiate hydrolysis of stored lipid by selectively cleaving triacylglycerols and not diacylglycerols or monoacylglycerols. Knock-out studies have demonstrated that ATGL-deficient mice experience a marked hepatic steatosis [95] and similarly overexpression of the ATGL gene leads to a reduction in liver fat in mice [96]. One study investigated the effects of ATGL gene manipulation on insulin sensitivity in mice, and here the authors observed that while ATGL knock-out mice do develop marked hepatic steatosis this does not result in any changes to their hepatocyte insulin sensitivity [97]. Hepatic ATGL overproduction in the same mice resulted in reduced hepatic steatosis, and interestingly the authors did observe a mild increase in insulin sensitivity although this was not sufficiently large to result in improvements in fasting glucose concentrations or insulinaemia.

Further insights into a possible disconnection between hepatic steatosis and insulin resistance can be gained by looking at disorders of fatty acid oxidation. In health, fasting stimulates gluconeogenesis in the liver fuelled by oxidation of fatty acids. If fatty acid oxidation is impaired this can lead to fasting hypoglycaemia and accumulation of lipids resulting in hepatic steatosis [98]. In such situations individuals will exhibit enhanced glucose tolerance, therefore exhibiting the disconnection. This occurs in numerous inborn errors of fatty acid oxidation such as medium chain acyl-CoA dehydrogenase deficiency (MCADD) and carnitine palmitoyl transferase II (CPT-2) deficiency [99]. Additionally, peroxisome proliferator-activated receptor alpha (PPARα) stimulates the expression of many genes involved in fatty acid oxidation. Experimental mice who have undergone PPARα knock-out develop marked hepatic steatosis after being exposed to a high fat diet, and after fasting demonstrate hypoglycaemia and increased insulin sensitivity [100].

6. Conclusions

It is clear from the literature that there is a complicated causal relationship between NAFLD and the metabolic syndrome. NAFLD is considered by many to represent the hepatic manifestation of the metabolic syndrome however rigidly sticking to this dogma does not appreciate the complexity of the relationship. Clearly the two clinical entities share many aspects of their pathophysiology, and insulin resistance is at the centre of both. There is sufficient evidence now for not only reciprocal causality between these disease states, but also each acting as a perpetuating or exacerbating factor for the other.

There are, however, many aspects of the interactions between NAFLD and the metabolic syndrome that are yet to be fully elucidated, and this is clearly demonstrated by the situations where there is an apparent disconnect or dissociation between them. Arguably, the hepatic steatosis that occurs in these situations due to genetic variation and inborn errors of metabolic can be considered a separate clinical entity to that which is associated with insulin resistance and the metabolic syndrome. However, focusing on the mechanisms that underlie these observations of dissociation could prove valuable for identifying new therapeutic targets in metabolic disease.

Acknowledgments: Christopher D. Byrne is supported in part by the Southampton National Institute for Health Research Biomedical Research Centre.

Author Contributions: Patrick Wainwright and Christopher D. Byrne conceived and designed the review; Patrick Wainwright completed the first draft; Christopher D. Byrne critically reviewed the draft and revised it with changes to the text and figures; Patrick Wainwright and Christopher D. Byrne completed the final draft and prepared it for submission.

Abbreviations

The following abbreviations are used in this manuscript:

NAFLD	Non-alcoholic fatty liver disease
PNPLA3	Patatin-like phospholipase domain-containing protein-3
TM6SF2	Transmembrane 6 superfamily member 2 protein
HDL-C	High density lipoprotein cholesterol
NASH	Non-alcoholic steatohepatitis
PKC-ε	Protein kinase C-ε
FLI	Fatty liver index
PAI-1	Plasminogen activator inhibitor-1
TNF-α	Tumour necrosis factor-α

IL	Interleukin
DAG	Diacylglycerols
DGAT	Diacylglycerol acyltransferase
SNP	Single nucleotide polymorphism
VLDL	Very low density lipoprotein
TAG	Triacylglycerol
MAG	Monoacylglycerol
ATGL	Adipose triglyceride lipase
HSL	Hormone sensitive lipase
FHBL	Familial hypobetalipoproteinaemia
BMI	Body mass index

References

1. Anstee, Q.M.; McPherson, S.; Day, C.P. How big a problem is nonalcoholic fatty liver disease? *BMJ* **2011**, *343*, d3897. [CrossRef] [PubMed]
2. Targher, G.; Byrne, C.D. Clinical review. Nonalcoholic fatty liver disease: A novel cardiometabolic risk factor for type 2 diabetes and its complications. *J. Clin. Endocrinol. Metab.* **2013**, *98*, 483–495. [CrossRef] [PubMed]
3. Chalasani, N.; Younossi, Z.; Lavine, J.E.; Diehl, A.M.; Brunt, E.M.; Cusi, K.; Charlton, M.; Sanyal, A.J. The diagnosis and management of non-alcoholic fatty liver disease: Practice guideline by the American Association for the Study of Liver Diseases, American College of Gastroenterology, and the American Gastroenterological Association. *Hepatology* **2012**, *55*, 2005–2023. [CrossRef] [PubMed]
4. Browning, J.D.; Szczepaniak, L.S.; Dobbins, R.; Nuremberg, P.; Horton, J.D.; Cohen, J.C.; Grundy, S.M.; Hobbs, H.H. Prevalence of hepatic steatosis in an urban population in the United States: Impact of ethnicity. *Hepatology* **2004**, *40*, 1387–1395. [CrossRef] [PubMed]
5. Aguilar, M.; Bhuket, T.; Torres, S.; Liu, B.; Wong, R.J. Prevalence of the metabolic syndrome in the United States 2003–2012. *JAMA* **2015**, *313*, 1973–1974. [CrossRef] [PubMed]
6. Cortez-Pinto, H.; Camilo, M.E.; Baptista, A.; de Oliveira, A.G.; de Moura, M.C. Non-alcoholic fatty liver: Another feature of the metabolic syndrome? *Clin. Nutr.* **1999**, *18*, 353–358. [CrossRef]
7. Bedogni, G.; Miglioli, L.; Masutti, F.; Tiribelli, C.; Marchesini, G.; Bellentani, S. Prevalence of and risk factors for nonalcoholic fatty liver disease: The Dionysos nutrition and liver study. *Hepatology* **2005**, *42*, 44–52. [CrossRef] [PubMed]
8. Souza, M.R.; Diniz Mde, F.; Medeiros-Filho, J.E.; Araujo, M.S. Metabolic syndrome and risk factors for non-alcoholic fatty liver disease. *Arq. Gastroenterol.* **2012**, *49*, 89–96. [CrossRef] [PubMed]
9. Zhang, Y.; Zhang, T.; Zhang, C.; Tang, F.; Zhong, N.; Li, H.; Song, X.; Lin, H.; Liu, Y.; Xue, F. Identification of reciprocal causality between non-alcoholic fatty liver disease and metabolic syndrome by a simplified Bayesian network in a Chinese population. *BMJ Open* **2015**, *5*, e008204. [CrossRef] [PubMed]
10. Alberti, K.G.; Eckel, R.H.; Grundy, S.M.; Zimmet, P.Z.; Cleeman, J.I.; Donato, K.A.; Fruchart, J.C.; James, W.P.; Loria, C.M.; Smith, S.C.; *et al.* Harmonizing the metabolic syndrome. *Circulation* **2009**, *120*, 1640–1645. [CrossRef] [PubMed]
11. Kim, H.J.; Kim, H.J.; Lee, K.E.; Kim, S.K.; Ahn, C.W.; Lim, S.K.; Kim, K.R.; Lee, H.C.; Huh, K.B.; *et al.* Metabolic significance of nonalcoholic fatty liver disease in nonobese, nondiabetic adults. *Arch. Intern. Med.* **2004**, *164*, 2169–2175. [CrossRef] [PubMed]
12. Sinn, D.H.; Gwak, G.Y.; Park, H.N.; Kim, J.E.; Min, Y.W.; Kim, K.M.; Kim, Y.J.; Choi, M.S.; Lee, J.H.; Koh, K.C.; *et al.* Ultrasonographically detected non-alcoholic fatty liver disease is an independent predictor for identifying patients with insulin resistance in non-obese, non-diabetic middle-aged Asian adults. *Am. J. Gastroenterol.* **2012**, *107*, 561–567. [CrossRef] [PubMed]
13. Targher, G.; Bertolini, L.; Padovani, R.; Rodella, S.; Tessari, R.; Zenari, L.; Day, C.; Arcaro, G. Prevalence of nonalcoholic fatty liver disease and its association with cardiovascular disease among type 2 diabetic patients. *Diabetes Care* **2007**, *30*, 1212–1218. [CrossRef] [PubMed]
14. Leite, N.C.; Salles, G.F.; Araujo Antonio, L.E.; Villela-Noqueira, C.A.; Cardosa, C.R. Prevalence and associated factors of non-alcoholic fatty liver disease in patients with type-2 diabetes mellitus. *Liver Int.* **2009**, *29*, 113e9. [CrossRef] [PubMed]

15. Assy, N.; Kaita, K.; Mymin, D.; Levy, C.; Rosser, B.; Minuk, G. Fatty infiltration of liver in hyperlipidemic patients. *Dig. Dis. Sci.* **2000**, *45*, 1929–1934. [CrossRef] [PubMed]

16. Lopez-Suarez, A.; Guerrero, J.M.; Elvira-Gonzalez, J.; Beltran-Robles, M.; Canas-Hormigo, F.; Bascunana-Quirell, A. Nonalcoholic fatty liver disease is associated with blood pressure in hypertensive and nonhypertensive individuals from the general population with normal levels of alanine aminotransferase. *Eur. J. Gastroenterol. Hepatol.* **2011**, *23*, 1011–1017. [CrossRef] [PubMed]

17. Lau, K.; Lorbeer, R.; Haring, R.; Schmidt, C.O.; Wallaschofski, H.; Nauck, M.; John, U.; Baumeister, S.E.; Volzke, H. The association between fatty liver disease and blood pressure in a population-based prospective longitudinal study. *J. Hypertens.* **2010**, *28*, 1829–1835. [CrossRef] [PubMed]

18. Marchesini, G.; Bugianesi, E.; Forlani, G.; Cerelli, F.; Lenzi, M.; Manini, R.; Natale, S.; Vanni, E.; Villanova, N.; Melchionda, N. Nonalcoholic fatty liver, steatohepatitis, and the metabolic syndrome. *Hepatology* **2003**, *37*. [CrossRef] [PubMed]

19. Ryan, M.C.; Wilson, A.M.; Slavin, J.; Best, J.D.; Jenkins, A.J.; Desmond, P.V. Associations between liver histology and severity of the metabolic syndrome in subjects with nonalcoholic fatty liver disease. *Diabetes Care* **2005**, *28*, 1222–1224. [CrossRef] [PubMed]

20. Day, C.P.; James, O.F. Steatohepatitis: A tale of two "hits"? *Gastroenterology* **1998**, *114*, 842–845. [CrossRef]

21. Tilg, H.; Moschen, A.R. Evolution of inflammation in nonalcoholic fatty liver disease: The multiple parallel hits hypothesis. *Hepatology* **2010**, *52*, 1836–1846. [CrossRef] [PubMed]

22. Samuel, V.T.; Liu, Z.-X.; Wang, A.; Beddow, S.A.; Geisler, J.G.; Kahn, M.; Zhang, X.; Monia, B.P.; Bhanot, S.; Shulman, G.I. Inhibition of protein kinase Cε prevents hepatic insulin resistance in nonalcoholic fatty liver disease. *J. Clin. Investig.* **2007**, *117*, 739–745. [CrossRef] [PubMed]

23. Kumashiro, N.; Erion, D.M.; Zhang, D.; Kahn, M.; Beddow, S.A.; Chu, X.; Still, C.D.; Gerhard, G.S.; Han, X.; Dziura, J.; et al. Cellular mechanism of insulin resistance in nonalcoholic fatty liver disease. *PNAS* **2011**, *108*, 16381–16385. [CrossRef] [PubMed]

24. Choi, J.W.; Wang, X.; Joo, J.I.; Kim, D.H.; Oh, T.S.; Choi, D.K.; Yun, J.W. Plasma proteome analysis in diet-induced obesity-prone and obesity resistant rats. *Proteomics* **2010**, *10*, 4386–4400. [CrossRef] [PubMed]

25. Meex, R.C.; Hoy, A.J.; Morris, A.; Brown, R.D.; Lo, J.C.; Burke, M.; Goode, R.J.; Kingwell, B.A.; Kraakman, M.J.; Febbraio, M.A.; et al. Fetuin B is a secreted hepatocyte factor linking steatosis to impaired glucose metabolism. *Cell Metab.* **2015**, *22*, 1078–1089. [CrossRef] [PubMed]

26. Hamaguchi, M.; Takeda, N.; Kojima, T.; Ohbora, A.; Kato, T.; Sarhui, H.; Fukui, M.; Nagata, C.; Takeda, J. Identification of individuals with non-alcoholic fatty liver disease by the diagnostic criteria for the metabolic syndrome. *World J. Gastroenterol.* **2012**, *18*, 1508–1516. [CrossRef] [PubMed]

27. Zhang, T.; Zhang, Y.; Zhang, C.; Tang, F.; Li, H.; Zhang, Q.; Lin, H.; Wu, S.; Liu, Y.; Xue, F. Prediction of metabolic syndrome by non-alcoholic fatty liver disease in northern urban Han Chinese population: A prospective cohort study. *PLoS ONE* **2014**, *9*, e96651.

28. Smits, M.M.; Ioannou, G.N.; Boyko, E.J.; Utzschneider, K.M. Non-alcoholic fatty liver disease as an independent manifestation of the metabolic syndrome: Results of a US national survey in three ethnic groups. *J. Gastroenterol. Hepatol.* **2013**, *28*, 664–670. [CrossRef] [PubMed]

29. Adams, L.A.; Waters, O.R.; Knuiman, M.W.; Elliott, R.R.; Olynyk, J.K. NAFLD as a risk factor for the development of diabetes and the metabolic syndrome: An eleven-year follow-up study. *Am. J. Gastroenterol.* **2009**, *104*, 861–867. [CrossRef] [PubMed]

30. Ryoo, J.H.; Choi, J.M.; Moon, S.Y.; Suh, Y.J.; Shin, J.Y.; Shin, H.C.; Park, S.K. The clinical availability of non alcoholic fatty liver disease as an early predictor of the metabolic syndrome in Korean men: 5-year's prospective cohort study. *Atherosclerosis* **2013**, *227*, 398–403. [CrossRef] [PubMed]

31. Hamaguchi, M.; Kojima, T.; Itoh, Y.; Harano, Y.; Fujii, K.; Nakajima, T.; Kato, T.; Takeda, N.; Okuda, J.; Ida, K.; et al. The severity of ultrasonographic findings in nonalcoholic fatty liver disease reflects the metabolic syndrome and visceral fat accumulation. *Am. J. Gastroenterol.* **2007**, *102*, 2708–2715. [CrossRef] [PubMed]

32. Mohan, V.; Farooq, S.; Deepa, M.; Ravikumar, R.; Pitchumoni, C.S. Prevalence of non-alcoholic fatty liver disease in urban south Indians in relation to different grades of glucose intolerance and metabolic syndrome. *Diabetes Res. Clin. Pract.* **2009**, *84*, 84–91. [CrossRef] [PubMed]

33. Rhoo, J.H.; Suh, Y.J.; Shin, H.C.; Cho, Y.K.; Choi, J.M.; Park, S.K. Clinical association between non-alcoholic fatty liver disease and the development of hypertension. *J. Gastroenterol. Hepatol.* **2014**, *29*, 1926–1931.

34. Rhoo, J.H.; Ham, W.T.; Choi, J.M.; Kang, M.A.; An, S.H.; Lee, J.K.; Shin, H.C.; Park, S.K. Clinical significance of non-alcoholic fatty liver disease as a risk factor for prehypertension. *J. Korean Med. Sci.* **2014**, *29*, 973–979.

35. Huh, J.H.; Ahn, S.V.; Koh, S.B.; Choi, E.; Kim, J.Y.; Sung, K.C.; Kim, E.J.; Park, J.B. A prospective study of fatty liver index and incident hypertension: The KoGES-ARIRANG study. *PLoS ONE* **2015**, *10*, e0143560.

36. Sung, K.C.; Wild, S.H.; Byrne, C.D. Development of new fatty liver, or resolution of existing fatty liver, over five years of follow-up, and risk of incident hypertension. *J. Hepatol.* **2014**, *60*, 1040–1045. [CrossRef] [PubMed]

37. Sung, K.C.; Wild, S.H.; Byrne, C.D. Resolution of fatty liver and risk of incident diabetes. *J. Clin. Endocrinol. Metab.* **2013**, *93*, 3637–3643. [CrossRef] [PubMed]

38. Vozarova, B.; Stefan, N.; Lindsay, R.S.; Saremi, A.; Pratley, R.E.; Bogardus, C.; Tataranni, P.A. High alanine Aminotransferase is associated with decreased hepatic insulin sensitivity and predicts the development of type 2 diabetes. *Diabetes* **2002**, *51*, 1889–1895. [CrossRef] [PubMed]

39. Lee, D.H.; Ha, M.H.; Kim, J.H.; Christiani, D.C.; Gross, M.D.; Steffes, M.; Blomhoff, R.; Jacobs, D.R. Gamma glutamyltransferase and diabetes—A 4 years follow-up study. *Diabetologia* **2003**, *46*, 359–364. [PubMed]

40. Hanley, A.J.; Williams, K.; Festa, A.; Wagenknecht, L.E.; D'Agostino, R.B.; Haffner, S.M. Liver markers and development of the metabolic syndrome: The insulin resistance atherosclerosis study. *Diabetes* **2005**, *54*, 3140–3147. [CrossRef] [PubMed]

41. Ekstedt, M.; Franzén, L.E.; Mathiesen, U.L.; Thorelius, L.; Holmqvist, M.; Bodemar, G.; Kechagias, S. Long-term follow-up of patients with NAFLD and elevated liver enzymes. *Hepatology* **2006**, *44*, 865–873. [CrossRef] [PubMed]

42. Monami, M.; Bardini, G.; Lamanna, C.; Pala, L.; Cresci, B.; Francesconi, P.; Buiatti, E.; Rotella, C.M.; Mannucci, E. Liver enzymes and risk of diabetes and cardiovascular disease: Results of the Firenze Bagno a Ripoli (FIBAR) study. *Metabolism* **2008**, *57*, 387–392. [CrossRef] [PubMed]

43. Goessling, W.; Massaro, J.M.; Vasan, R.S.; D'Agostino, R.B.; Ellison, R.C.; Fox, C.S. Aminotransferase levels and 20-year risk of metabolic syndrome, diabetes, and cardiovascular disease. *Gastroenterology* **2008**, *135*, 1935–1944. [CrossRef] [PubMed]

44. Ryu, S.; Chang, Y.; Woo, H.Y.; Yoo, S.H.; Choi, N.K.; Lee, W.Y.; Kim, I.; Song, J. Longitudinal increase in gamma-glutamyltransferase within the reference interval predicts metabolic syndrome in middle-aged Korean men. *Metabolism* **2010**, *59*, 683–689. [PubMed]

45. Balkau, B.; Lange, C.; Vol, S.; Fumeron, F.; Bonnet, F. Group Study D.E.S.I.R. Nine-year incident diabetes is predicted by fatty liver indices: The French D.E.S.I.R. study. *BMC Gastroenterol.* **2010**, *10*, 56–66. [CrossRef] [PubMed]

46. Sung, K.C.; Kim, S.H. Interrelationship between fatty liver and insulin resistance in the development of type 2 diabetes. *J. Clin. Endocrinol. Metab.* **2011**, *96*, 1093–1097. [CrossRef] [PubMed]

47. Sung, K.C.; Jeong, W.S.; Wild, S.H.; Byrne, C.D. Combined influence of insulin resistance, overweight/obesity, and fatty liver as risk factors for type 2 diabetes. *Diabetes Care* **2012**, *35*, 717–722. [CrossRef] [PubMed]

48. Musso, G.; Gambino, R.; Cassader, M.; Pagano, G. Meta analysis: Natural history of non-alcoholic fatty liver disease (NAFLD) and diagnostic accuracy of non-invasive tests for liver disease severity. *Ann. Med.* **2011**, *43*, 617–649. [CrossRef] [PubMed]

49. Ghosh, A.K.; Vaughan, D.E. PAI-1 in tissue fibrosis. *J. Cell. Physiol.* **2012**, *227*, 493–507. [CrossRef] [PubMed]

50. Cesari, M.; Pahor, M.; Incalzi, R.A. Plasminogen activator inhibitor-1 (PAI-1): A key factor linking fibrinolysis and age-related subclinical and clinical conditions. *Cardiovasc. Ther.* **2010**, *28*, e72–e91. [CrossRef] [PubMed]

51. Oishi, K. Plasminogen activator inhibitor-1 and the circadian clock in metabolic disorders. *Clin. Exp. Hypertens.* **2009**, *31*, 208–219. [CrossRef] [PubMed]

52. Bremer, A.A.; Jialal, I. Adipose tissue dysfunction in nascent metabolic syndrome. *J. Obes.* **2013**, *2013*, 393192. [CrossRef] [PubMed]

53. Takeshita, Y.; Takamura, T.; Hamaguchi, E.; Shimizu, A.; Ota, T.; Sakurai, M.; Kaneko, S. Tumor necrosis factor-alpha-induced production of plasminogen activator inhibitor 1 and its regulation by pioglitazone and cerivastatin in a nonmalignant human hepatocyte cell line. *Metabolism* **2006**, *55*, 1464–1472. [CrossRef] [PubMed]

54. Baranova, A.; Gowder, S.J.; Schlauch, K.; Elariny, H.; Collantes, R.; Afendy, A.; Ong, J.P.; Goodman, Z.; Chandhoke, V.; Younossi, Z.M. Gene expression of leptin, resistin, and adiponectin in the white adipose tissue of obese patients with non-alcoholic fatty liver disease and insulin resistance. *Obes. Surg.* **2006**, *16*, 1118–1125. [CrossRef] [PubMed]

55. Baranova, A.; Schlauch, K.; Elariny, H.; Jarrar, M.; Bennett, C.; Nugent, C.; Gowder, S.J.; Younoszai, Z.; Collantes, R.; Chandhoke, V.; *et al.* Gene expression patterns in the hepatic tissue and in the visceral adipose tissue of patients with non-alcoholic fatty liver disease. *Obes. Surg.* **2007**, *17*, 1111–1118. [CrossRef] [PubMed]

56. Hubscher, S.G. Histological assessment of non-alcoholic fatty liver disease. *J. Clin. Gastroenterol.* **2006**, *40*, S5–S10. [CrossRef] [PubMed]

57. Weltman, M.D.; Farrell, G.C.; Liddle, C. Increased hepatocyte CYP2E1 expression in a rat nutritional model of hepatic steatosis with inflammation. *Gastroenterology* **1996**, *111*, 1645–1653. [CrossRef]

58. Geerts, A. History, heterogeneity, developmental biology, and functions of quiescent hepatic stellate cells. *Semin. Liver Dis.* **2001**, *21*, 3113–3135. [CrossRef] [PubMed]

59. Fain, J.N. Release of interleukins and other inflammatory cytokines by human adipose tissue is enhanced in obesity and primarily due to the nonfat cells. *Vitam. Horm.* **2006**, *74*, 443–477. [PubMed]

60. You, T.; Nicklas, B.J. Chronic inflammation: Role of adipose tissue and modulation by weight loss. *Curr. Diabetes Rev.* **2006**, *2*, 29–37. [CrossRef] [PubMed]

61. Henao-Mejia, J.; Elinav, E.; Cheng-Cheng, J.; Hao, L.; Mehal, W.Z.; Strowig, T.; Thaiss, C.A.; Kau, A.L.; Eisenbarth, S.C.; Jurczak, M.J.; *et al.* Inflammasome-mediated dysbiosis regulates progression of NAFLD and obesity. *Nature* **2012**, *482*, 179–185. [CrossRef] [PubMed]

62. Feldstein, A.E.; Canbay, A.; Angulo, P.; Taniai, M.; Burgart, L.J.; Lindor, K.D.; Gores, G.J. Hepatocyte apoptosis and fas expression are prominent features of human non alcoholic steatohepatitis. *Gastroenterology* **2003**, *125*, 437–443. [CrossRef]

63. Bantel, H.; Ruck, P.; Gregor, M.; Shulze-Oshtoff, K. Detection of elevated caspase activation and early apoptosis in lever disease. *Eur. J. Cell Biol.* **2001**, *80*, 230–239. [CrossRef] [PubMed]

64. Civera, M.; Urios, A.; Garcia-Torres, M.L.; Ortega, J.; Martinez-Valls, J.; Cassinello, N.; Del Olmo, J.A.; Ferrandez, A.; Rodrigo, J.M.; Montoliu, C. Relationship between insulin resistance, inflammation and liver cell apoptosis in patients with severe obesity. *Diabetes Metab. Res. Rev.* **2010**, *26*, 187–192. [CrossRef] [PubMed]

65. Adams, L.A.; Sanderson, S.; Lindor, K.D.; Angulo, P. The histological course of non-alcoholic fatty liver disease: A longitudinal study of 103 patients with sequential liver biopsies. *J. Hepatol.* **2005**, *42*, 132–138. [CrossRef] [PubMed]

66. El-Serag, H.B.; Tran, T.; Everhart, J.E. Diabetes increases the risk of chronic liver disease and hepatocellular carcinoma. *Gastroenterology* **2004**, *126*, 460–468. [CrossRef] [PubMed]

67. Hamaguchi, M.; Kojima, T.; Takeda, N.; Nakagawa, T.; Taniguchi, H.; Fujii, K.; Omatsu, T.; Nakajima, T.; Sarui, H.; Shimazaki, M.; *et al.* The metabolic syndrome as a predictor of nonalcoholic fatty liver disease. *Ann. Intern. Med.* **2005**, *143*, 722–728. [CrossRef] [PubMed]

68. Porepa, L.; Ray, J.G.; Sanchez-Romeu, P.; Booth, G.L. Newly diagnosed diabetes mellitus as a risk factor for serious liver disease. *CMAJ* **2010**, *182*, E526–E531. [CrossRef] [PubMed]

69. Emerging Risk Factors, Collaboration; Seshasai, S.R.; Kaptoge, S.; Thompson, A.; Di Angelantonio, E.; Gao, P.; Sarwar, N.; Whincup, P.H.; Mukamal, K.J.; Gillum, R.F.; *et al.* Diabetes mellitus, fasting glucose, and risk of cause-specific death. *N. Engl. J. Med.* **2011**, *364*, 829–841.

70. Graham, R.C.; Burke, A.; Stettler, N. Ethnic and sex differences in the association between metabolic syndrome and suspected nonalcoholic fatty liver disease in a nationally representative sample of US adolescents. *J. Pediatr. Gastroenterol. Nutr.* **2009**, *49*, 442–449. [CrossRef] [PubMed]

71. Castro-Martinez, M.G.; Banderas-Lares, D.Z.; Ramirez-Martinez, J.C.; Escobedode, I.P.J. Prevalence of nonalcoholic fatty liver disease in subjects with metabolic syndrome. *Cir. Cir.* **2012**, *80*, 128–133. [PubMed]

72. Tsai, C.H.; Li, T.C.; Lin, C.C. Metabolic syndrome as a risk factor for non-alcoholic fatty liver disease. *South Med. J.* **2008**, *101*, 900–905. [CrossRef] [PubMed]

73. Zhang, T.; Zhang, C.; Zhang, Y.; Tang, F.; Li, H.; Zhang, Q.; Lin, H.; Wu, S.; Liu, Y.; Xue, F. Metabolic syndrome and its components as predictors of non-alcoholic fatty liver disease in a northern urban Han Chinese population: A prospective cohort study. *Atherosclerosis* **2015**, *240*, 144–148. [CrossRef] [PubMed]

74. Monetti, M.; Levin, M.C.; Watt, M.J.; Sajan, M.P.; Marmor, S.; Hubbard, B.K.; Stevens, R.D.; Bain, J.R.; Newgard, C.B.; Farese, R.V.; *et al.* Dissociation of hepatic steatosis and insulin resistance in mice overexpressing DGAT in the liver. *Cell Metab.* **2007**, *6*, 69–78. [CrossRef] [PubMed]

75. Kantartzis, K.; Machicao, F.; Machann, J.; Schick, F.; Fritsche, A.; Haring, H.U.; Stefan, N. The *DGAT2* gene is a candidate for the dissociation between fatty liver and insulin resistance in humans. *Clin. Sci.* **2009**, *116*, 531–537. [CrossRef] [PubMed]

76. Niebergall, L.J.; Jacobs, R.L.; Chaba, T.; Vance, D.E. Phosphatidylcholine protects against steatosis in mice but not non-alcoholic steatohepatitis. *Biochim. Biophys. Acta* **2011**, *1811*, 1177–1185. [CrossRef] [PubMed]

77. Jacobs, R.L.; Zhao, Y.; Koonen, D.P.; Sletten, T.; Su, B.; Lingrell, S.; Cao, G.; Peake, D.A.; Kuo, M.S.; Proctor, S.D.; *et al.* Impaired *de novo* choline synthesis explains why phosphatidylethanolamine N-methyltransferase-deficient mice are protected from diet-induced obesity. *J. Biol. Chem.* **2010**, *285*, 22403–22413. [CrossRef] [PubMed]

78. Chamoun, Z.; Vacca, F.; Parton, R.G.; Gruenberg, J. PNPLA3/adiponutrin functions in lipid droplet formation. *Biol. Cell* **2013**, *105*, 219–233. [CrossRef] [PubMed]

79. Romeo, S.; Kozlitina, J.; Xing, C.; Pertsemlidis, A.; Cox, D.; Pennacchio, L.A.; Boerwinkle, E.; Cohen, J.C.; Hobbs, H.H. Genetic variation in *PNPLA3* confers susceptibility to nonalcoholic fatty liver disease. *Nat. Genet.* **2008**, *40*, 1461–1465. [CrossRef] [PubMed]

80. Romeo, S.; Sentinelli, F.; Dash, S.; Yeo, G.S.; Savage, D.B.; Leonetti, F.; Capoccia, D.; Incani, M.; Maglio, C.; Iacovino, M.; *et al.* Morbid obesity exposes the association between PNPLA3 I148M (rs738409) and indices of hepatic injury in individuals of European descent. *Int. J. Obes.* **2010**, *34*, 190–194. [CrossRef] [PubMed]

81. Romeo, S.; Sentinelli, F.; Cambuli, V.M.; Incani, M.; Congiu, T.; Matta, V.; Pilia, S.; Huang-Doran, I.; Cossu, E.; Loche, S.; *et al.* The 148M allele of the PNPLA3 gene is associated with indices of liver damage early in life. *J. Hepatol.* **2010**, *53*, 335–338. [CrossRef] [PubMed]

82. Shen, J.; Wong, G.L.; Chan, H.L.; Chan, H.Y.; Yeung, D.K.; Chan, R.S.; Chim, A.M.; Chan, A.W.; Choi, P.C.; Woo, J.; *et al.* PNPLA3 gene polymorphism accounts for fatty liver in community subjects without metabolic syndrome. *Aliment. Pharmacol. Ther.* **2014**, *39*, 532–539. [CrossRef] [PubMed]

83. Kantartzis, K.; Peter, A.; Machicao, F.; Machann, J.; Wagner, S.; Konigsrainer, I.; Konigsrainer, A.; Schick, F.; Fritsche, A.; Haring, H.U.; *et al.* Dissociation between fatty liver and insulin resistance in humans carrying a variant of the patatin-like phospholipase 3 gene. *Diabetes* **2009**, *58*, 2616–2623. [CrossRef] [PubMed]

84. Mahdessian, H.; Taxiarchis, A.; Popov, S.; Silveira, A.; Franco-Cereceda, A.; Hamsten, A.; Eriksson, P.; van't Hooft, F. TM6SF2 is a regulator of liver fat metabolism influencing triglyceride secretion and hepatic lipid droplet content. *PNAS* **2014**, *111*, 8913–8918. [CrossRef] [PubMed]

85. Kozlitina, J.; Smagris, E.; Stender, S.; Nordestgaard, B.G.; Zhou, H.H.; Tybjærg-Hansen, A.; Vogt, T.F.; Hobbs, H.H.; Choen, J.C. Exome-wide association study identifies a TM6SF2 variant that confers susceptibility to nonalcoholic fatty liver disease. *Nat. Genet.* **2014**, *46*, 352–356. [CrossRef] [PubMed]

86. Sookoian, S.; Castano, G.O.; Scian, R.; Mallardi, P.; Fernandez Gianotti, T.; Burqueno, A.L.; San Martino, J.; Pirola, C.J. Genetic variation in transmembrane 6 superfamily member 2 and the risk of nonalcoholic fatty liver disease and histological disease severity. *Hepatology* **2015**, *61*, 515–525. [CrossRef] [PubMed]

87. Liu, Y.L.; Reeves, H.L.; Burt, A.D.; Tiniakos, D.; McPherson, S.; Leathart, L.B.; Allison, M.E.; Alexander, G.J.; Piquet, A.C.; Anty, R. TM6SF2 rs58542926 influences hepatic fibrosis progression in patients with non-alcoholic fatty liver disease. *Nat. Commun.* **2014**, *5*, 4309. [CrossRef] [PubMed]

88. Akuta, N.; Kawamura, Y.; Arase, Y.; Suzuki, F.; Sezaki, S.; Hosaka, T.; Kobayashi, M.; Kobayashi, M.; Saitoh, S.; Suzuki, Y. Relationships between genetic variations of PNPLA3, TM6SF2 and histological features of nonalcoholic fatty liver disease in Japan. *Gut Liver* **2015**. [CrossRef] [PubMed]

89. Wong, V.W.; Wong, G.L.; Tse, C.H.; Chan, H.L. Prevalence of the TM6SF2 variant and non-alcoholic fatty liver disease in Chinese. *J. Hepatol.* **2014**, *61*, 708–709. [CrossRef] [PubMed]

90. Pirola, C.J.; Sookoian, S. The dual and opposite role of the TM6SF2-rs58542926 variant in protecting against cardiovascular disease and conferring risk for nonalcoholic fatty liver: A meta-analysis. *Hepatology* **2015**, *62*, 1742–1756. [CrossRef] [PubMed]

91. Zhou, Y.; Llaurado, G.; Oresic, M.; Hyotylainen, T.; Orho-Melander, M.; Yki-Jarvinen, H. Circulating triacylglycerol signatures and insulin sensitivity in NAFLD associated with the E167K variant in TM6SF2. *J. Hepatol.* **2015**, *62*, 657–663. [CrossRef] [PubMed]

92.   Amaro, A.; Fabbrini, E.; Kars, M.; Yue, P.; Schechtman, K.; Schonfeld, G.; Klein, S. Dissociation between intrahepatic triglyceride content and insulin resistance in familial hypobetalipoproteinemia. *Gastroenterology* **2010**, *139*, 149–153. [CrossRef] [PubMed]

93.   Reiner, Z.; Guardamagna, O.; Nair, D.; Soran, H.; Hovingh, K.; Bertolini, S.; Jones, S.; Coric, M.; Calandra, S.; Hamilton, J. Lysosomal acid lipase deficiency–an under-recognized cause of dyslipidaemias and liver dysfunction. *Atherosclerosis* **2014**, *235*, 21–30. [CrossRef] [PubMed]

94.   Stefan, N.; Staiger, H.; Haring, H.U. Dissociation between fatty liver and insulin resistance: The role of adipose triacylglycerol lipase. *Diabetologia* **2011**, *54*, 7–9. [CrossRef] [PubMed]

95.   Haemmerle, G.; Lass, A.; Zimmermann, R.; Gorkiewicz, G.; Meyer, C.; Rozman, J.; Heldmaier, G.; Maier, R.; Theussl, C.; Eder, S. Defective lipolysis and altered energy metabolism in mice lacking adipose triglyceride lipase. *Science* **2006**, *312*, 734–737. [CrossRef] [PubMed]

96.   Reid, B.N.; Ables, G.P.; Otlivanchik, O.A.; Schoiswohl, G.; Zechner, R.; Blaner, W.S.; Goldberg, I.J.; Schwabe, R.F.; Chua, S.C.; Huang, L.S. Hepatic overexpression of hormone-sensitive lipase and adipose triglyceride lipase promotes fatty acid oxidation, stimulates direct release of free fatty acids, and ameliorates steatosis. *J. Biol. Chem.* **2008**, *283*, 13087–13099. [CrossRef] [PubMed]

97.   Turpin, S.N.; Hoy, A.J.; Brown, A.D.; Rudaz, C.G.; Honeyman, J.; Matzaris, M.; Watt, M.J. Adipose triacylglycerol lipase is a major regulator of hepatic lipid metabolism but not insulin sensitivity in mice. *Diabetologia* **2011**, *54*, 146–156. [CrossRef] [PubMed]

98.   Bennett, M.J. Pathophysiology of fatty acid oxidation disorders. *J. Inherit. Metab. Dis.* **2010**, *33*, 533–537. [CrossRef] [PubMed]

99.   Sun, Z.; Lazar, M.A. Dissociating fatty liver and diabetes. *Trends Endocrinol. Metab.* **2013**, *24*, 4–12. [CrossRef] [PubMed]

100.   Kersten, S.; Seydoux, J.; Peters, J.M.; Gonzalez, F.J.; Desvergne, B.; Wahli, W. Peroxisome proliferator-activated receptor alpha mediates the adaptive response to fasting. *J. Clin. Invest.* **1999**, *103*, 1489–1498. [CrossRef] [PubMed]

12

NAFLD and Chronic Kidney Disease

Morgan Marcuccilli [1],* **and Michel Chonchol** [2],*

1   Division of Renal Diseases and Hypertension, University of Colorado Hospital, Aurora, CO 80045, USA
2   Division of Renal Diseases and Hypertension, University of Colorado Denver,
    13199 East Montview Boulevard, Suite 495, Aurora, CO 80045, USA
*   Correspondence: morgan.marcuccilli@ucdenver.edu (M.M.); michel.chonchol@ucdenver.edu (M.C.)

Academic Editors: Amedeo Lonardo and Giovanni Targher

Abstract: Non-alcoholic fatty liver disease (NAFLD) is the most common cause of chronic liver disease in developed countries and it is now considered a risk factor for cardiovascular disease. Evidence linking NAFLD to the development and progression of chronic kidney disease (CKD) is emerging as a popular area of scientific interest. The rise in simultaneous liver-kidney transplantation as well as the significant cost associated with the presence of chronic kidney disease in the NAFLD population make this entity a worthwhile target for screening and therapeutic intervention. While several cross-sectional and case control studies have been published to substantiate these theories, very little data exists on the underlying cause of NAFLD and CKD. In this review, we will discuss the most recent publications on the diagnosis of NAFLD as well new evidence regarding the pathophysiology of NAFLD and CKD as an inflammatory disorder. These mechanisms include the role of obesity, the renin-angiotensin system, and dysregulation of fructose metabolism and lipogenesis in the development of both disorders. Further investigation of these pathways may lead to novel therapies that aim to target the NAFLD and CKD. However, more prospective studies that include information on both renal and liver histology will be necessary in order to understand the relationship between these diseases.

Keywords: non-alcoholic fatty liver disease; chronic kidney disease; non-alcoholic steatohepatitis; inflammation; review

1. Introduction

Non-alcoholic fatty liver disease (NAFLD) is the most common cause of chronic liver disease worldwide [1]. It is defined as the accumulation of fat (>5%) in liver cells in the absence of excessive alcohol intake or other causes of liver disease including autoimmune, drug-induced, or viral hepatitis [2]. The histologic spectrum of NAFLD ranges from simple steatosis to non-alcoholic steatohepatitis (NASH), liver fibrosis, and cirrhosis [2]. This disease reportedly affects up to 30% of the general population in Western countries, especially in patients with metabolic syndrome, obesity, and type II diabetes [3]. Given the high prevalence of this disease, it has recently been associated with hepatocellular carcinoma (HCC) [3]. In addition, NASH as the primary indication for liver transplantation has increased from 1.2% to 9.7% in the last decade [3]. NAFLD is considered to be an independent risk factor for cardiovascular disease and there is accumulating evidence to support a causative role in the development of chronic kidney disease (CKD) [3].

In addition to NAFLD, CKD represents a significant health burden in the Western adult population, and it affects over 25% of individuals older than 65 years [4]. CKD is defined as decreased estimated glomerular filtration (eGFR) and/or the presence of significant proteinuria (>500 mg) [5]. In the United States, over 400,000 people currently receive some form of renal replacement therapy, and this number is expected to reach 2.2 million by 2030 [6]. However, less than half of CKD patients develop end stage renal disease due to the high risk of mortality associated with cardiovascular events [7]. Furthermore, the incidence of simultaneous liver-kidney transplantation continues to increase exponentially over the last five years [3]. An analysis of the United Network Organ Sharing (UNOS) database during the years 2002–2011, revealed that 35% of patients transplanted for NAFLD-related cirrhosis progressed to stage 3b-4 CKD within two years after liver transplantation in comparison to 10% of patients transplanted for other etiologies [8]. Despite these findings, CKD often goes unrecognized and in the Third National Health and Nutrition Survey (NHANES III), among all individuals with moderately decreased GFR (<60 mL/min; Stage 3), the awareness is approximately 8% [9].

The similarity in traditional risk factors for CKD including hypertension, obesity, dyslipidemia, and insulin resistance make it difficult to determine a causational relationship with NAFLD adjusting for "hepatorenal" and "cardiorenal" features [5]. While a multitude of cross-sectional and longitudinal studies exist, there is still very little prospective data linking NAFLD to CKD. In addition, underlying mechanisms related to inflammation, oxidative stress, and fibrogenesis are currently being investigated in the development of kidney injury in the presence of fatty liver disease [5]. In this review, we will examine new data on the diagnosis of NAFLD, current evidence linking NAFLD to CKD, and new studies revealing the underlying pathophysiology and potential treatments of these globally burdensome diseases.

2. Diagnosis and Screening

2.1. Imaging

Liver biopsy remains the gold standard of diagnosis for NAFLD or NASH. Histologic classifications range from simple steatosis to advanced periportal or perisinusoidal fibrosis [10]. However, a considerable proportion of patients are not diagnosed with NAFLD by biopsy, and this method is unreliable secondary to subjectivity of histologic interpretation as well as sample bias related to patchiness of its distribution in the liver [10]. Ultrasonography remains the recommended first-line imaging modality for diagnosing hepatic lipid accumulation in clinical practice. This method of screening is limited if >30% of hepatocytes are steatoic given its reliance of echogenicity or contrast [5]. A recent meta-analysis has shown that the overall sensitivity and specificity of ultrasonography for the detection of moderate to severe fatty liver compared to histology were 84.8% and 93.6% [11].

Other methods of diagnosis include magnetic resonance imaging (MRI), which can assess decreased liver signal intensity, and proton magnetic resonance spectroscopy, which is used for measuring the area under the lipid spectrum relative to water spectrum [12]. These diagnostic techniques are excellent for assessing the quantitative severity of liver fat accumulation, however, they cannot discriminate simple steatosis from lipid accumulation associated with inflammation and fibrosis (i.e., NASH) [12]. According to systematic review, simple steatosis and NASH are considered different disease states each with its own pathogenesis and cardiovascular risk. In addition, it may be possible that NASH can occur in the absence of simple steatosis and the pathogenesis leading to the progression to fibrosis/cirrhosis is still not entirely clear [13]. Nevertheless, NASH is often progressive, with development of advanced fibrosis in 30%–40% of patients, cirrhosis in 15%–20%, and liver failure in 2%–4% [5].

Another modality for the assessment of NAFLD that has recently gained popularity is the use of transient elastography (TE; Fibroscan®, Echosens, Paris, France), which measures liver stiffness using an ultrasound probe [14]. A new physical parameter based on the properties of ultrasonic signals acquired by this machine has been recently developed to assess liver steatosis known as the controlled attenuation parameter (CAP) score. [14]. A recent study measured the CAP score on 62 patients with CKD stage III and IV in order to quantify liver steatosis and concluded that 53 patients had NAFLD with a positive correlation between severity of liver steatosis and serum creatinine ($p < 0.01$). Limitations included the cross-sectional format of this investigation, which does not allow conclusions to be causal, as well as the absence of a control group of non-steatotic patients, or confirmation of findings by liver biopsy in comparison to CAP score [14]. This study determined that that the severity of liver steatosis is negatively correlated with kidney function, and it documents the value of ultra-sonographic elastography as an effective non-invasive screening method for the diagnosis of NAFLD [14].

2.2. Liver Enzymes and Biomarkers

In addition to imaging, many investigators have explored the use of serum tests in NAFLD ideally for diagnosis, monitoring progression, response to therapeutic intervention, and determining the prognosis of the disease. Mildly elevated serum aminotransferase levels are the primary abnormality seen in patients with NAFLD, however, liver enzymes (LFTs) may be normal in up to 78% of patients with NAFLD [15]. A recent study published by Mikolasevic and associates examined the use of liver enzymes *versus* CAP score in the detection of NAFLD in patients with CKD and coronary artery disease (CAD). This was a cross-sectional study of 202 patients with CKD, end-stage renal disease (ESRD), renal transplant recipients (RTRs) and patients with proven CAD matched against individuals without elevated LFTs and normal kidney function [15]. According to the CAP findings, 76.9% of CKD patients, 82% ESRD patients, 74% RTRs, and 69.1% CAD patients had CAP > 238 decibels to milliwatt (dB.m) and thus by definition NAFLD. However, the results demonstrated that LFTs correlated with liver stiffness acquired with TE only in CAD patients, and therefore is not a reliable marker of the detection of NAFLD in patients with renal disease [15].

While several other biomarkers have been implicated in the diagnosis and screening of NAFLD, there is still a lack of reproducibility in their clinical application. Tumor necrosis factor (TNF-α), which plays an important role in insulin resistance through inhibition of the tyrosine kinase activity of the insulin receptor, has recently gained attention for its potential value [16]. One study reported that patients with NASH had significantly higher serum TNF-α than those with simple steatosis, while another recent study further stated that patients with NASH had higher levels of TNF-α messenger ribonucleic acid (mRNA) than healthy controls with a sensitivity 66.7% and a specificity 74.1% [16]. Still, there are no known studies reporting the relationship of TNF-α as a marker of both NAFLD and CKD. Other potential biomarkers include interleukin-6 (IL-6), adiponectin, and pentraxin-3 (PTX3) are also under investigation [16].

The development of panels has also shown promise in non-invasive testing for NAFLD. There are scoring systems available for the prediction of the presence NASH as well as for prognosis of advanced fibrosis (see Table 1) [17–25]. Diagnostic panels are thought to be more applicable for patients with a BMI > 35 and the presence of hypertension as well as age >50 years [26]. FIB-4 score is a prognostic panel composed of age, alanine aminotransferase (ALT), aspart aminotransferase (AST), and platelet count [27]. A recent study published in *Hepatology Intl.* compared these scoring systems in an effort to identify the presence of CKD in patients with NAFLD. A total of 755 patients diagnosed with NAFLD by ultrasound were assessed for glomerular filtration rate, AST to ALT ratio, AST to platelet ratio, FIB-4 score, NAFLD fibrosis score, and BARD score [27]. The results revealed that a cut-off value of 1.100 for FIB-4 score gave a sensitivity of 68.85% and a specificity of 71.07% for predicting CKD, and only the FIB-4 score, older age, higher uric acid level, and elevated diastolic blood pressure were independent predictors of CKD in comparison to the other scoring panels [27]. While this study was cross-sectional and limited by ultrasound diagnosis of NAFLD, the investigators concluded that a high noninvasive fibrosis score is associated with an increased risk of prevalent CKD, and that FIB-4 is the better predictor than other fibrosis scores in excluding the presence of CKD in patients with NAFLD [27]. Ideally, a combination of non-invasive imaging and serum biomarkers will be verified for practical application in the clinical detection of both NAFLD and CKD.

Table 1. Non-alcoholic fatty liver disease (NAFLD) prognostic panels for fibrosis.

Reference	Test	Components	PPV%	NPV%
Rosenberg [17]	Original European Liver Fibrosis Panel	age, HA, TIMP1, PIIINP for score $\leqslant 1$	80	98
Ratziu [18]	BAAT score	BMI $\geqslant 28$ kg/m^2 age $\geqslant 50$ years, ALT $\geqslant 2 \times$ ULN triglycerides $\geqslant 1.7$ mmol/L	33	100
Ratziu [19]	Fibrotest	$\alpha 2$ macroglobulin, haptoglobin, GGT, Total bilirubin, apolipoprotein A1	54	90
Angulo [20]	NAFLD Fibrosis Score	age, hyperglycemia, BMI, platelet count, albumin, AAR	56	93
Harrison [21]	BARD	BMI $\geqslant 28$ kg/m^2, AAR $\geqslant 0.8$, diabetes	43	96
Cales [22]	Fibrometer NAFLD	glucose, AST, ferritin, ALT, body weight, age	87.9	92.1
Shah [23]	FIB4 index	age, ALT, AST, platelet count	43	90
Sumida [24]	NAFIC score	serum ferritin ($\geqslant 200$ ng/mL for female, $\geqslant 300$ ng/mL for male), fasting insulin $\geqslant 10$	32	96
Younossi [25]	NAFLD Diagnostic Panel	diabetes, gender, BMI, triglycerides, apoptotic and necrotic CK18 fragments	57.7	85

This table demonstrates various prognostic panels for predicting the severity of fibrosis in NAFLD with respect to their positive predictive value (PPV) and negative predictive value (NPV) as determined by each study and its components. Abbreviations: BAAT=body mass index, aspart aminotransferase, age, triglycerides, HA = hyaluronic acid, TIMP1 = tissue inhibitor of matrix metalloproteinase, PIIINP = N-terminal propeptide of type III procollagen, BMI = body mass index, ALT = alanine aminotransferase, ULN = upper limit of normal , BARD = body mass index, aspart aminotransferase, alanine aminotransferase, diabetes, GGT = gamma-glutamyl transpeptidase, AAR = aspart aminotransferase alanine aminotransferase ratio, AST = aspart transaminase, CK18 = creatinine kinase 18.

3. Epidemiologic Evidence Linking Chronic Kidney Disease (CKD) to Non-Alcoholic Fatty Liver Disease (NAFLD)

As stated above, the similarity in risk factors for NAFLD and CKD including obesity, diabetes, and hypertension make it difficult to delineate a direct association between the diagnosis of fatty liver disease and the development and progression of renal disease. A recent meta-analysis of thirty-three studies for a total of over two-thousand participants found that NAFLD was associated with an increased prevalence odd ratio (OR) 2.12, 95% confidence interval (CI), 1.69–2.66 as well as incidence hazard ratio (HR) 1.79, 95% CI 1.65–1.95 of CKD [28]. In Table 2, there several large cross-sectional as well as case control studies of patients with NAFLD showing the prevalence of CKD between 4%–40% (see Table 2) [29–50]. In addition, there appears to be a correlation between the severity of NAFLD and the progression of CKD [51]. However, nearly half of these studies use ultrasound for the diagnosis of NAFLD or NASH as opposed to biopsy [29–50]. Other limitations include the use of Modification of Diet in Renal Disease (MDRD) and the Chronic Kidney Disease Epidemiology Collaboration (CKD-EPI) algorithms to calculate eGFR, neither of which are reliable in the presence of obesity or cirrhosis [5]. There is also substantial variability in the patient groups studied in regards ethnicity, age, risk factors, and selection bias using hospital based cohorts that often represent a population with advanced disease [29–50]. Fortunately, the majority of the studies found a correlation between NAFLD and CKD with adjustment for these factors, as well as co-morbidities such as insulin resistance and metabolic syndrome [29–50].

While the prevalence of CKD in NAFLD appears to be substantial, studies that examine the incidence of CKD in NAFLD are not as robust [5]. The Valpolicella Heart Diabetes Study of 1760 patients with type 2 diabetes with preserved kidney function followed over a six-year period found an increased incidence of CKD in patients with NAFLD (HR 1.49; CI 95%, 1.1–2.2) independent of sex, age, blood pressure, duration of diabetes and smoking [31]. Additionally, a retrospective study on a cohort of 8329 non-diabetic, non-hypertensive men with normal kidney function revealed that NAFLD was associated with an increased incidence of CKD (HR 1.60; CI 95%, 1.3–2.0) over a three year period after adjustment for age, cholesterol, and other factors [31]. However, both of these studies also used ultrasound for the diagnosis of NAFLD [31,32]. Finally, none of these studies have used renal biopsy to examine the pathology of their CKD. In the future, randomized studies with larger cohorts of patients and longer follow-up and histologically confirmed fatty liver disease are needed to verify a causal relationship between NAFLD and CKD.

Table 2. Principal retrospective studies of the association between nonalcoholic fatty liver disease and the prevalence of chronic kidney disease (CKD).

Study	Characteristics	CKD Diagnosis and Prevalence	Liver Disease Diagnosis and Prevalence	Risk Factors Adjusted in Analysis
Targher, 2008 [29]	Outpatient; $n = 103$; HTN 63%	eGFR < 60 mL/min/1.73 m² (CKD-EPI) and/or overt proteinuria; 15%	Ultrasound; 48%	Age, sex, BMI, waist circumference, HTN, alcohol consumption, diabetes duration, HbA1c, LDL cholesterol, Tg
Campos, 2008 [30]	Hospital; $n = 197$; HTN 56%, DM 26%	eGFR < 60 mL/min/1.73 m² (CKD-EPI); 10%	Liver biopsy: NAFLD 63%, NASH 32%	Age, gender, BMI, waist circumference, HTN
Chang, 2008 [31]	Population; $n = 8329$; DM 0%, HTN 0%, metabolic syndrome 6%	eGFR < 60 mL/min/1.73 m² (MDRD) or morning proteinuria >1+; 4%	Ultrasound; 73%	Age, eGFR, dyslipidemia, BMI, CRP, sys BP
Targher, 2008 [32]	Population; $n = 1760$; DM 100%, HTN 65%, metabolic syndrome 55%	eGFR < 60 mL/min/1.73 m² (MDRD) or ACR = 300 mg/g; 31%	Ultrasound; 30%	Age, gender, BMI, waist circumference, BP, LDL-C, Tg, smoking, DM duration, medications
Targher, 2010 [33]	Outpatient; $n = 202$ adults; HTN 35%, DM 0%	eGFR < 60 mL/min/1.73 m² and/or ACR ≥ 30 mg/g; 37.8%	Ultrasound	Age, sex, BMI, systolic BP, alcohol consumption, diabetes duration, HbA1c, Tg, medication use
Targher, 2010 [34]	Hospital; $n = 160$; DM 6%, HTN 60%, metabolic syndrome 29%	eGFR < 60 mL/min/1.73 m² (CKD-EPI) or ACR = 30 mg/g; 14%	Biopsy: NASH 100%	Age, sex, BMI, waist circumference, smoking, systolic BP; insulin resistance
Yilmaz, 2010 [35]	Hospital; $n = 87$; DM 0%, HTN 30%, metabolic syndrome 27%	eGFR < 60 mL/min/1.73 m² (CKD-EPI) or ACE 30–300 mg/d; 16%	Biopsy; NAFLD 100%, NASH 67%	Age, gender, BMI, waist circumference, BP, lipids, smoking, insulin resistance, metabolic syndrome
Soderberg, 2010 [36]	Hospital; $n = 125$; DM 24%, HTN 37%, metabolic syndrome 31%	eGFR < 60 mL/min/1.73 m² (CKD-EPI); 27%	Biopsy; NAFLD 67%, NASH 33%	Age, BMI, HTN, smoking, DM, metabolic syndrome
Wong 2010 [37]	Hospital; $n = 51$; DM 50%, HTN 37%, metabolic syndrome 65%	eGFR < 60 mL/min/1.73 m² (CKD-EPI) or ACR > 30 mg/g; 8%	Biopsy; NAFLD 100%, NASH 33%	Age, BMI, DM, HTN, waist circumference, metabolic syndrome, smoking
Lau 2010 [38]	Population; $n = 2858$; DM 8.9%, HTN 47%, metabolic syndrome 24%	eGFR < 60 mL/min/1.73 m² (CKD-EPI) or ACR > 30 mg/g; 8%	Ultrasound; 30%	Age, BMI, metabolic syndrome, HTN, dyslipidemia, smoking
Yasui 2011 [39]	Hospital; $n = 169$; DM 31%, HTN 34%, metabolic syndrome 30%	eGFR < 60 mL/min/1.73 m² (CKD-EPI) or am proteinuria 1+; 14%	Biopsy; NAFLD 100%, NASH 53%	BMI, HTN, waist circumference, dyslipidemia, smoking, DM
Machado 2012 [40]	Hospital; $n = 148$; HTN 67%	eGFR < 60 mL/min/1.73 m²; 8%	Biopsy; NAFLD 100%	Age, sex, HTN, DM, dyslipidemia
Targher 2012 [41]	Hospital; $n = 343$; DM 100%, HTN 43%, metabolic syndrome 46%	eGFR < 60 mL/min/1.73 m² (MDRD) or ACR > 30 mg/g; 40%	Ultrasound 53%	Age, gender, BMI, family history, systolic BP, dyslipidemia, smoking DM, medications, microalbuminuria
Sirota 2012 [42]	Population; $n = 11469$; HTN 24%	eGFR < 60 mL/min/1.73 m² and/or ACR > 30 mg/g; 42%	Ultrasound	Age, sex, race, HTN, diabetes, waist circumference, dyslipidemia, insulin resistance
Armstrong 2012 [43]	Population; $n = 146$; DM 0%, HTN 36%	eGFR < 60 mL/min/1.73 m² (CKD-EPI); 25%	Ultrasound; 50%	BMI, HTN

Table 2. *Cont.*

Study	Characteristics	CKD Diagnosis and Prevalence	Liver Disease Diagnosis and Prevalence	Risk Factors Adjusted in Analysis
Musso 2012 [44]	Hospital; n = 80; DM 0%, HTN 52%, metabolic syndrome 31%	eGFR < 60 mL/min/1.73 m^2 (CKD-EPI) or ACR > 30 mg/d; 20%	Biopsy; NAFLD 50%, NASH 20%	Age, gender, BMI, waist circumference, HTN, smoking, metabolic syndrome
Francque 2012 [45]	Hospital; n = 230; DM 0%, HTN 50%, metabolic syndrome 47%	eGFR < 60 mL/min/1.73 m^2 (CKD-EPI) or proteinuria > 300 mg/d; 9%	Biopsy; NAFLD 100%, NASH 52%	Age, BMI, HTN, waist circumference, smoking, metabolic syndrome
Casoinic 2012 [46]	Hospital; n = 145; DM 100%; HTN 55%; metabolic syndrome 80%	eGFR < 60 mL/min/1.73 m^2 (CKD-EPI) or ACE 30–300 mg/g; 10%	Ultrasound; 51%	Age, gender, CRP
Xia 2012 [47]	Population; n = 1141; DM 0%, HTN 38%, metabolic syndrome 32%	eGFR < 60 mL/min/1.73 m^2 (mDRD) or ACR > 30 mg/g; 12%	Ultrasound; 41%	Age, BMI, smoking, HTN, metabolic syndrome, uric acid
Kim 2013 [48]	Hospital; n = 96; DM 100%, HTN 66%, metabolic syndrome 56%	eGFR < 60 mL/min/1.73 m^2 (MDRD) or proteinuria > 1+ am; 25%	Biopsy; NAFLD 100%, NASH 56%	Age, BMI, HTN, waist circumference, smoking, metabolic syndrome, dyslipidemia
Angulo 2013 [49]	Hospital; n = 191; DM 17%, HTN 32%, metabolic syndrome 25%	eGFR < 60 mL/min/1.73 m^2 (CKD-EPI) or am proteinuria >1+; 18%	Biopsy	Age, BMI, DM, HTN, smoking, dyslipidemia, metabolic syndrome
El Azeem 2013 [50]	Population; n = 747; DM 57%, HTN 32%, metabolic syndrome 67%	eGFR < 60 mL/min/1.73 m^2 (MDRD) or ACE > 30 mg/g; 29%	Ultrasound 35%	Age, BMI, HTN, dyslipidemia, smoking, metabolic syndrome

This table represents the major retrospective studies linking the prevalence of CKD in NAFLD. The data is organized chronologically and include the cohort, definition of CKD and NAFLD with prevalence as well as adjustment variables. Studies using liver enzymes for the diagnosis of NAFLD or survey data were not included in this review. Abbreviations: HTN = hypertension, DM = diabetes mellitus, eGFR = estimated glomerular filtration rate, CKD-EPI = chronic kidney disease epidemiology collaboration, MDRD = modification of diet in renal disease, BMI=body mass index, HbA1C = hemoglobin A1C %, LDL = low density lipoprotein, Tg = triglyceride, BP = blood pressure, CRP = c-reactive protein.

4. Mechanisms Linking NAFLD to CKD

According to the Center for Disease Control (CDC), more than one-third of U.S. adults are obese [52]. This epidemic affects over 78 million people with co-morbidities of insulin resistance, diabetes, and atherosclerosis leading to an estimated annual medical cost of 147 billion dollars [52]. The liver is the key regulator of glucose and lipid metabolism as well as the main source of inflammatory elements thought to be involved in the development of cardiovascular and kidney disease [5]. It is known that obesity is an independent risk factor for CKD and it is associated with the development of proteinuria and pathologic findings of podocyte hypertrophy and focal segmental glomerular sclerosis even in the absence of diabetes and hypertension [53]. In addition, studies have shown that obesity as well as metabolic syndrome is a strong predictor of the development of NAFLD [54]. While the complex "crosstalk" among adipose tissue, the liver, and kidneys make it difficult to delineate the specific processes underlying NAFLD as a cause of CKD, it is not surprising that these diseases may be linked. Mounting evidence on liver-kidney interactions including; altered renin-angiotensin system (RAS) activation, impaired antioxidant defense, and damaged lipogenesis is currently emerging as a major area of research (Figure 1) [51]. Understanding these mechanisms may lead to modifiable risk factors and therapeutic targets for the prevention and treatment of NAFLD and CKD.

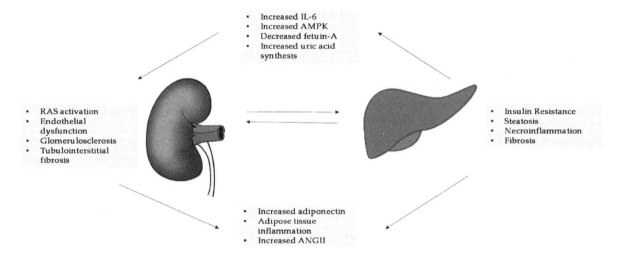

Figure 1. This figure demonstrates the various mechanisms associated with non-alcoholic fatty liver disease (NAFLD) and chronic kidney disease (CKD). The liver-kidney crosstalk in NAFLD includes altered renin-angiotensin system (RAS) and activated protein kinase (AMPK) activation, impaired antioxidant defense, and excessive dietary fructose intake, which affects renal injury through altered lipogenesis and inflammatory response. In turn, 8 the kidney reacts promoting further RAS activation, increased angiotensin II (ANGII) and uric acid production in a vicious cycle leading to fibrosis [20].

4.1. AMPK, Fetuin-A, and Adiponectin

The role of the energy sensor 5′-AMP activated protein kinase (AMPK) and its regulation of fetuin-A and adiponectin in liver and kidney fat cells is currently an area of investigation in animal models as well as human subjects [53]. Fetuin-A is a serum protein mediated through AMPK as an important promoter of insulin resistance found in both podocytes and hepatocytes [53]. Observations in fetuin-A null mice include resistance to weight gain when challenged with a high fat diet and increased insulin levels [55]. Similarly in humans, higher fetuin-A levels are associated with obesity and found in patients with NAFLD and CKD [55]. Adversely, adiponectin, which is regulated by fetuin A, is present in low levels with similar characteristics of elevated body mass index and hypertriglyceridemia [56]. Interestingly, therapeutic maneuvers including caloric restriction, exercise, and insulin sensitizing medications are associated with declines in levels of serum fetuin-A, increases in adiponectin levels, and stimulation of AMPK [53]. Although direct causation cannot be implied, it appears that increased caloric intake and adiposity initiates an inflammatory cascade through AMPK, fetuin-A, and adiponectin between fat cells in the liver and kidney leading to end-organ damage [53].

4.2. Renin-Angiotensin System (RAS) in NAFLD and CKD

The renin-angiotensin system (RAS) is also believed to play a key role in the pathogenesis of NAFLD and CKD. Adipocytes express all components of RAS and contribute up to 30% of circulating renin, angiotensin converting enzyme (ACE), and angiotensin II (AngII) [51]. The kidney and liver also express RAS constituents, and experimental studies support a role for both systemic and local activation of AngII in NAFLD and CKD. In the liver, AngII promotes insulin resistance, *de novo* lipogenesis, and pro-inflammatory cytokine production such as interleukin-6 (IL-6) and tumor growth factor-β (TGF-β) [51]. These processes are thought to trigger fibrogenesis contributing to the entire spectrum of histological changes seen with NASH [51]. In the kidney, RAS activation plays a key role in determining renal ectopic lipid deposition which is known to cause oxidative stress and inflammation through hemodynamic effects of glomerular efferent arteriole vasoconstriction leading to glomerulosclerosis [57]. In addition, a process known as the ACE2-Ang (1–7)-Mas receptor axes whose activity is known to oppose that of AngII has been shown in animal models to inhibit liver fibrosis [58]. The role of the RAS system in the liver and kidneys makes it a prime target for blockade in an attempt to attenuate fibrosis in NAFLD and CKD.

4.3. Fructose Metabolism in NAFLD and CKD

Based on the NHANESIII study, over 10% of Americans' daily calories are from fructose and consumption in high fructose corn syrup (HFCS) has increased 8% over the last decade especially amongst adolescents [59]. Several observational studies have implicated HFCS in the incidence and severity of NAFLD and CKD [51]. Fructose acts independently of calorie excess by initiating fructose phosphorylation to fructose-1-phosphate by fructokinase in the liver, ultimately leading to the accumulation of uric acid [51]. Research investigations support that uric acid promotes the development and progression of NAFLD and CKD via hepatocyte ATP depletion, which causes enhanced hepatic and renal lipogenesis, mitochondrial ROS generation, endothelial dysfunction and pro-inflammatory cytokine secretion similar to overexpression of RAS [51]. Mouse models unable to metabolize fructose are protected from obesity, metabolic syndrome, and a reduction in fructose intake or uric acid production improved experimental NAFLD and CKD [60]. Also in a recent study of 341 adult NAFLD patients, investigators evaluated whether increased fructose consumption correlates with the development of NAFLD and found that after controlling for age, gender, BMI, and total calorie intake, increased daily fructose consumption was associated with lower steatosis grade and higher fibrosis stage in comparison to groups ($p < 0.05$) [61]. Finally, a meta-analysis examined four studies that assess the association between consumption of artificially sweetened soda verses regular soda and CKD and concluded the pooled risk reduction of CKD in patients consuming artificially sweetened soda was 1.33 (95% CI 0.82–2.15) [62]. Limitations in this study include its retrospective nature, which cannot imply causation as well as variability in types of soda consumed [62]. Future prospective studies on human subjects and limitations of fructose as well as reductions in uric acid levels in patients with NAFLD and CKD are necessary to confirm these hypotheses.

4.4. Impaired Oxidative Stress

As stated above increased oxidative stress is believed to play a key role in the pathogenesis of NAFLD and CKD. Nuclear erythroid related factor-2 (Nrf2), which is expressed ubiquitously in human tissues with its highest expression in the liver and kidney, upregulates the transcription of numerous antioxidant and detoxification enzymes by binding to their antioxidant response elements [63]. Experimental data support a key protective role for Nrf2 against NAFLD and CKD using wild-type and Nrf2-null mice fed a high fat diet. Their specimens were analyzed for pathology as well as for fatty acid content and revealed the wild-type mice had increased hepatic fat deposition without fibrosis while the Nrf2-null mice had significantly more hepatic steatosis and substantial inflammation [63]. Based on these results, several natural and artificial Nrf2 activators are being evaluated in the treatment of diabetic CKD patients in the "Bardoxolone ethyl and kidney function in CKD with type 2 diabetes (BEAM)" study and previously in the "Bardoxolone methyl evaluation in patients with chronic kidney disease and type 2 diabetes: the occurrence of renal events (BEACON)" trial [64,65]. Mechanisms linked to fibroblastic growth factor 21, gut microflora, and other proteins such as sirtuin-1 are also showing promise in the development of CKD in NAFLD [51].

5. Therapeutic Interventions in NAFLD and CKD

Based on the newer mechanisms discussed as well as aims at reducing insulin resistance, several therapeutic interventions for the treatment of NAFLD are currently under investigation. The mainstay of management of for NASH is lifestyle intervention, which includes diet and exercise with a 5%–10% weight reduction associated with improvement in hepatic steatosis [5]. While there are very few studies examining the use of medications and behavioral modification in both NAFLD and CKD, the shared cardiometabolic risk factors and underlying pathophysiology may make these therapies applicable to both diseases.

RAS blockade using angiotensin converting enzyme inhibitors (ACE-) and angiotensin receptor blockers (ARBs) has been studied in NAFLD and CKD. Limited data from 223 patients in three randomized controlled trials in NAFLD suggests that ARBs attenuate steatosis, insulin resistance, and inflammatory markers independent of reduction in blood pressure [51]. In addition, telmisartan which is an ARB with peroxisome proliferator activated receptor [PPAR]-γ-regulating activity was compared to the use of valsartan in the Fatty Liver Protection by Telmisartan (FANTASY Trial) and found to cause reduction in necroinflammation, NAFLD activity score, fibrosis stage in NASH, as well as microalbuminuria [66]. Not surprisingly, the use of these medications in CKD has been extensively evaluated and based on the Collaborative Study Group Trial and several others, the use of ACE- and ARBs in patients with CKD with proteinuria is now a level one recommendation by Kidney Disease Outcomes Quality Initiative (KDOQI) [67]. A recent cross-sectional study of 191 patients with CKD III, IV, ESRD, and renal transplant recipients (n = 68) treated with ACE- or ARBs for >1 year and examined liver stiffness with the use of TE and a CAP score to evaluate whether CKD patients receiving these medications have a lower frequency of NAFLD [68]. Investigators determined that CKD-NAFLD patients taking ACE-I or ARBs had lower degree of liver stiffness in comparison to the patients not on medications (p = 0.0005) [68]. However, there was no statistical significance in degree of fibrosis or grade of steatosis in the two groups based on CAP score [68].

Evidence from recent clinical trials suggests that insulin-sensitizing agents including thiazolidinediones (TZDs) such as pioglitazone are beneficial in the treatment of NAFLD. As stated above, pioglitazone is associated with a decline in levels of serum fetuin-A and concomitant increase in adiponectin levels resulting in decreased insulin resistance [53]. A recent meta-analysis using only liver biopsy studies, found that TZDs as well as pentoxyifylline, which has shown *in vitro* to inhibit proinflammatory cytokines as well as reduce fibrogenesis, are superior to placebo for improving steatosis and lobular inflammation [69]. This review also examined studies on obeticholic acid (OCA), a semi-synthetic bile acid analogue and vitamin E, both which have been used in the treatment of NAFLD and revealed improvement in ballooning degeneration and fibrosis in comparison to placebo [69]. While many of these studies have a small cohort of patients and the histological endpoints were not standardized, the American Association for the Study of Liver Disease (AASLD) published guidelines recommending the use of vitamin E and pioglitazone in non-diabetic adults with biopsy-proven NASH [69].

Pharmacologic treatments related to disordered cholesterol metabolism and insulin resistance including statins, fibrates, metformin, and glucagon-like peptide (GLP-1) analogues have shown potential benefit in adult patients with NAFLD and NASH [5]. However, the effects of these treatments are improvement in liver enzymes, decreased plasma glucose and weight loss without changes in histologic staging of the disease. There are three major post-hoc analysis reviewing the use of statins including the "Greek Atorvastatin and Coronary-Heart-Disease Evaluation" (GREACE), and "Incremental Decrease in End Points Through Aggressive Lipid Lowering" (IDEAL) trials that showed a significant reduction in cardiovascular disease events in patients with NAFLD/NASH [70,71]. Also, the GREACE study, revealed normal liver enzymes with the use of atorvastatin *versus* usual care in a three year follow-up period [51]. Therefore, it appears that the use of statins may also be safe in this patient population. Finally, lifestyle interventions including exercise, weight loss, and gastric bypass surgery will decrease hepatic fat content and inflammation, however, require significant effort and often financial burden on individual patients [5]. However, these may be worthwhile efforts in patients with early steatosis in order to prevent progression of to NAFLD with CKD. Novel therapies including translational approaches based on the mechanisms discussed, as well as more traditional methods need to be evaluated in large randomized controlled trials for their potential value in the treatment of both NAFLD and CKD.

6. Conclusions

Based on the data presented as well as several other ongoing trials, there is substantial evidence linking NAFLD to the development of CKD. It is clear that the mechanisms underlying these diseases are complexly inter-woven requiring additional investigation with animal and human models. Furthermore, prospective studies on NAFLD and CKD must include information on hepatic and renal histology. Preventative measures including lifestyle modification aiming toward weight loss and physical activity may be of benefit in both diseases. Furthermore, physician awareness for screening of CKD in NAFLD may lead to earlier detection and treatment of this disease leading to better outcomes in patients with liver steatosis as well as more advanced fibrosis requiring organ transplantation.

Abbreviations

DM	diabetes mellitus
HTN	hypertension
Tg	triglycerides
A1C%	hemoglobin A1C
eGFR	estimated glomerular filtration rate
MDRD	Modification of Diet in Renal Disease
CKD-EPI	Chronic Kidney Disease Epidemiology Collaboration
CRP	C-reactive protein
LFTs	liver function tests
HR	hazard ration
CI	confidence interval

References

1. Vernon, G.; Baranova, A.; Younossi, Z.M. Systematic review: The epidemiology and natural history of non-alcoholic fatty liver disease and non-alcoholic steatohepatitis in adults. *Aliment. Pharmacol. Ther.* **2011**, *34*, 274–285. [CrossRef] [PubMed]
2. Chalasani, N.; Younossi, Z.; Lavine, J.E.; Diehl, A.M.; Brunt, E.M.; Cusi, K.; Charlton, M.; Sanyal, A.J. The diagnosis and management of non-alcoholic fatty liver disease: Practice guideline by the American Association for the Study of Liver Diseases, American College of Gastroenterology, and the American Gastroenterological Association. *Hepatology* **2012**, *55*, 2005–2023.
3. Loomba, R.; Sanyal, A.J. The global NAFLD epidemic. *Nat. Rev. Gastroenterol. Hepatol.* **2013**, *10*, 686–690. [CrossRef] [PubMed]

4. McCullough, K.; Sharma, P.; Ali, T.; Khan, I.; Smith, W.C.; MacLeod, A.; Black, C. Measuring the population burden of chronic kidney disease: A systematic literature review of the estimated prevalence of impaired kidney function. *Nephrol. Dial. Transplant.* **2012**, *27*, 1812–1821. [CrossRef] [PubMed]

5. Targher, G.; Chonchol, M.B.; Byrne, C.D. CKD and non-alcoholic fatty liver disease. *AJKD* **2014**, *64*, 638–652. [CrossRef] [PubMed]

6. Black, C.; Sharma, P.; Scotland, G.; McCullough, K.; McGurn, D.; Robertson, L.; Fluck, N.; MacLeod, A.; McNamee, P.; Prescott, G.; *et al.* Early referral strategies for management of people with markers of renal disease: A systematic review of the evidence of clinical effectiveness, cost-effectiveness and economic analysis. *Health Technol. Assess.* **2010**, *14*, 1–184. [CrossRef] [PubMed]

7. Athyros, V.; Tziomalos, K.; Katsiki, N.; Doumas, M.; Karagiannis, A.; Mikhailidis, D.P. Cardiovascular risk across the histological spectrum and the clinical manifestations of non-alcoholic fatty liver disease; an update. *World J. Gastroenterol.* **2015**, *21*, 6820–6834. [PubMed]

8. Singal, A.K.; Salameh, H.; Kuo, Y.F.; Wiesner, R.H. Evolving frequency and outcomes of simultaneous liver kidney transplants based on liver disease etiology. *Transplantation* **2014**, *98*, 216–221. [CrossRef] [PubMed]

9. Coresh, J.; Byrd-Holt, D.; Astor, B.C.; Briggs, J.P.; Eggers, P.W.; Lacher, D.A.; Hostetter, T.H. Chronic kidney disease awareness, prevalence, and trends among US adults, 1999 to 2000. *J. Am. Soc. Nephrol.* **2005**, *16*, 180–188. [CrossRef] [PubMed]

10. Kim, D.; Kim, W.R.; Kim, H.J.; Therneau, T.M. Association between noninvasive fibrosis markers and mortality among adults with nonalcoholic fatty liver disease in the United States. *Hepatology* **2013**, *57*, 1357–1365. [CrossRef] [PubMed]

11. Hernaez, R.; Lazo, M.; Bonekamp, S.; Kamel, I.; Brancati, F.L.; Guallar, E.; Clark, J.M. Diagnostic accuracy and reliability of ultrasonography for the detection of fatty liver: A meta-analysis. *Hepatology* **2011**, *54*, 1082–1090. [CrossRef] [PubMed]

12. Anstee, Q.M.; Targher, G.; Day, C.P. Progression of NAFLD to diabetes mellitus, cardiovascular disease or cirrhosis. *Nat. Rev. Gastroenterol. Hepatol.* **2013**, *10*, 330–344. [CrossRef] [PubMed]

13. Dowman, J.K.; Tomlinson, J.W.; Newsome, P.N. Systematic review; the diagnosis and staging of non-alcoholic fatty liver disease and non-alcoholic steatohepatitis. *Aliment. Pharmacol. Ther.* **2011**, *33*, 525–540. [CrossRef] [PubMed]

14. Mikolasevic, I.; Racki, S.; Bubic, I.; Jelic, I.; Stimac, D.; Orlic, L. Chronic kidney disease and nonalcoholic fatty liver disease proven by transient elastography. *Kidney Blood Press Res.* **2013**, *37*, 305–310. [CrossRef] [PubMed]

15. Mikolasevic, I.; Orlic, L.; Zaputovic, L.; Racki, S.; Cubranic, Z.; Anic, K.; Devcic, B.; Stimac, D. Usefulness of liver test and controlled attenuation parameter in detection of nonalcoholic fatty liver disease in patients with chronic renal failure and coronary heart disease. *Wien. Klin. Wochenschr.* **2015**, *127*, 451–458. [CrossRef] [PubMed]

16. Satapathy, S.K.; Garg, S.; Chauhan, R.; Sakhuja, P.; Malhotra, V.; Sharma, B.C.; Sarin, S.K. Beneficial effects of tumor necrosis factor-α inhibition by pentoxyfilline on clinical, biochemical, and metabolic parameters of patients with nonalcoholic steatohepatitis. *Am. J. Gastroenterol.* **2004**, *99*, 1946–1952. [CrossRef] [PubMed]

17. Rosenberg, W.M.; Voelker, M.; Thiel, R.; Becka, M.; Burt, A.; Schuppan, D.; Hubscher, S.; Roskams, T.; Pinzani, M.; Arthur, M.J. European Liver Fibrosis Group: Serum markers detect the presence of liver fibrosis: A cohort study. *Gastroenterology* **2004**, *127*, 1704–1713. [CrossRef] [PubMed]

18. Ratziu, V.; Gira, P.; Charlotte, F.; Bruckert, E.; Thibault, V.; Theodorou, I.; Khalil, L.; Turpin, G.; Opolon, P.; Poynard, T. Liver fibrosis in overweight patient. *Gastroenterology* **2000**, *118*, 1117–1123. [CrossRef]

19. Ratziu, V.; Massard, J.; Charlotte, F.; Messous, D.; Imbert-Bismut, F.; Bonyhay, L.; Tahiri, M.; Munteanu, M.; Thabut, D.; Cadranel, J.F.; *et al.* Diagnostic value of biochemical markers (FibroTest-FibroSURE) for the prediction of liver fibrosis in patients with non-alcoholic fatty liver disease. *BMC Gastroenterol.* **2006**, *6*, 6. [CrossRef] [PubMed]

20. Angulo, P.; Keach, J.C.; Batts, K.P.; Lindor, K.D. Independent predictor of liver fibrosis in patients with nonalcoholic steatohepatitis. *Hepatology* **1999**, *30*, 1356–1362. [CrossRef] [PubMed]

21. Harrison, S.A.; Oliver, D.; Arnod, H.L.; Gogia, S.; Neuschwander-Tetri, B.A. Development and validation of a simple NAFLD clinical scoring system for identifying patients without advanced disease. *Gut* **2008**, *57*, 1441–1447. [CrossRef] [PubMed]

22. Cales, P.; Laine, F.; Boursier, J.; Deugnier, Y.; Moal, V.; Oberti, F.; Hunault, G.; Rousselet, M.C.; Hubert, I.; Laafi, J.; *et al.* Comparison of blood tests for liver fibrosis specific or not to NAFLD. *J. Hepatol.* **2009**, *50*, 165–173. [CrossRef] [PubMed]

23. Shah, A.; Lydecker, A.; Murray, K.; Tetri, B.N.; Contos, M.J.; Sanyal, A.J. Nash Clinical Research Network. Comparison of noninvasive markers of fibrosis in patients with nonalcoholic fatty liver disease. *Clin. Gastroenterol. Hepatol.* **2009**, *7*, 1104–1112. [CrossRef] [PubMed]

24. Sumida, Y.; Yoneda, M.; Hyogo, H.; Yamaguchi, K.; Ono, M.; Fujii, H.; Eguchi, Y.; Suzuki, Y.; Imai, S.; Kanemasa, K.; *et al.* Japan Study Group of Nonalcoholic Fatty Liver Disease (JSG-NAFLD): A simple clinical scoring system using ferritin, fasting insulin, and type IV collagen 7S for predicting steatohepatitis in nonalcoholic fatty liver disease. *J. Gastroenterol.* **2011**, *46*, 257–268. [CrossRef] [PubMed]

25. Younossi, Z.; Page, S.; Rafiq, N.; Birerdinc, A.; Stepanova, M.; Hossain, N.; Afendy, A.; Younoszai, Z.; Goodman, Z.; Baranova, A. A biomarker panel for non-alcoholic steatohepatitis (NASH) and NASH-related fibrosis. *Obes. Surg.* **2011**, *21*, 431–439. [CrossRef] [PubMed]

26. Pearce, S.G.; Thosani, N.C.; Pan, J. Noninvasive biomarkers for the diagnosis of steatohepatitis and advanced fibrosis in NAFLD. *Biomark. Res.* **2013**, *1*, 7. [CrossRef] [PubMed]

27. Xu, H.W.; Hsu, Y.C.; Chang, C.H.; Wei, K.L.; Lin, C.L. High FIB-4 index as an independent risk factor of prevalent chronic kidney disease in patients with nonalcoholic fatty liver disease. *Hepatol. Int.* **2016**, *10*, 340–346. [CrossRef] [PubMed]

28. Musso, G.; Gambino, R.; Tabibian, J.H.; Ekstedt, M.; Kechagias, S.; Hamaguchi, M.; Hultcrantz, R.; Hagström, H.; Yoon, S.K.; Charatcharoenwitthaya, P.; *et al.* Association of non-alcoholic fatty liver disease with chronic kidney disease: A systematic review and meta-analysis. *PLoS Med.* **2014**, *11*, e1001680. [CrossRef] [PubMed]

29. Targher, G.; Bertolini, L.; Rodella, S.; Zoppini, G.; Lippi, G.; Day, C.; Muggeo, M. Non-alcoholic fatty liver disease is independently associated with an increased prevalence of chronic kidney disease and proliferative/laser-treated retinopathy in type 2 diabetic patients. *Diabetologia* **2008**, *51*, 444–450. [CrossRef] [PubMed]

30. Campos, G.M.; Bambha, K.; Vittinghoff, E.; Rabl, C.; Posselt, A.M.; Ciovica, R.; Tiwari, U.; Ferrel, L.; Pabst, M.; Bass, N.M.; *et al.* A clinical scoring system for predicting nonalcoholic steatohepatitis in morbidly obese patients. *Hepatology* **2008**, *47*, 1916–1923. [CrossRef] [PubMed]

31. Chang, Y.; Ryu, S.; Sung, E.; Woo, H.Y.; Oh, E.; Cha, K.; Jung, E.; Kim, W.S. Nonalcoholic fatty liver disease predicts chronic kidney disease in nonhypertensive and nondiabetic Korean men. *Metabolism* **2008**, *57*, 569–576. [CrossRef] [PubMed]

32. Targher, G.; Chonchol, M.; Bertolini, L.; Rodella, S.; Zenari, L.; Ciovica, R.; Tiwari, U.; Ferrel, L.; Pabst, M.; Bass, N.M.; *et al.* Increased risk of CKD among type 2 diabetics with nonalcoholic fatty liver disease. *J. Am. Soc. Nephrol.* **2008**, *19*, 1564–1570. [CrossRef] [PubMed]

33. Targher, G.; Bertolini, L.; Chonchol, M.; Rodella, S.; Zoppini, G.; Lippi, G. Nonalcoholic fatty liver disease is independently associated with an increased prevalence of chronic kidney disease and retinopathy in type 1 diabetic patients. *Diabetologia* **2010**, *53*, 1341–1348. [CrossRef] [PubMed]

34. Targher, G.; Bertolini, L.; Rodella, S.; Lippi, G.; Zoppini, G.; Chonchol, M. Relationship between kidney function and liver histology in subjects with nonalcoholic steatohepatitis. *Clin. J. Am. Soc. Nephrol.* **2010**, *5*, 2166–2171. [CrossRef] [PubMed]

35. Yilmaz, Y.; Alahdab, Y.O.; Yonal, O.; Kurt, R.; Kedrah, A.E.; Celikel, C.A.; Ozdogan, O.; Duman, D.; Imeryuz, N.; Avsar, E.; *et al.* Microalbuminuria in nondiabetic patients with nonalcoholic fatty liver disease: Association with liver fibrosis. *Metabolism* **2010**, *59*, 1327–1330. [CrossRef] [PubMed]

36. Söderberg, C.; Stål, P.; Askling, J.; Glaumann, H.; Lindberg, G.; Marmur, J.; Hultcrantz, R. Decreased survival of subjects with elevated liver function tests during a 28-year follow-up. *Hepatology* **2010**, *51*, 595–602. [CrossRef] [PubMed]

37. Wong, V.W.; Wong, G.L.; Choi, P.C.; Chan, A.W.; Li, M.K.; Chan, H.Y.; Chim, A.M.; Yu, J.; Sung, J.J.; Chan, H.L. Disease progression of non-alcoholic fatty liver disease: A prospective study with paired liver biopsies at 3 years. *Gut* **2010**, *59*, 969–974. [CrossRef] [PubMed]

38. Lau, K.; Lorbeer, R.; Haring, R.; Schmidt, C.O.; Wallaschofski, H.; Nauck, M.; John, U.; Baumeister, S.E.; Völzke, H. The association between fatty liver disease and blood pressure in a population-based prospective longitudinal study. *J. Hypertens.* **2010**, *28*, 1829–1835. [CrossRef] [PubMed]

39. Yasui, K.; Sumida, Y.; Mori, Y.; Mitsuyoshi, H.; Minami, M.; Itoh, Y.; Kanemasa, K.; Matsubara, H.; Okanoue, T.; Yoshikawa, T. Nonalcoholic steatohepatitis and increased risk of chronic kidney disease. *Metabolism* **2011**, *60*, 735–739. [CrossRef] [PubMed]

40. Machado, M.V.; Gonçalves, S.; Carepa, F.; Coutinho, J.; Costa, A.; Cortez-Pinto, H. Impaired renal function in morbid obese patients with nonalcoholic fatty liver disease. *Liver Int.* **2012**, *32*, 241–248. [CrossRef] [PubMed]

41. Targher, G.; Pichiri, I.; Zoppini, G.; Trombetta, M.; Bonora, E. Increased prevalence of chronic kidney disease in patients with Type 1 diabetes and non-alcoholic fatty liver. *Diabet. Med.* **2012**, *29*, 220–226. [CrossRef] [PubMed]

42. Sirota, J.C.; McFann, K.; Targher, G.; Chonchol, M.; Jalal, D.I. Association between nonalcoholic liver disease and chronic kidney disease: An ultrasound analysis from NHANES 1988–1994. *Am. J. Nephrol.* **2012**, *36*, 466–471. [CrossRef] [PubMed]

43. Armstrong, M.J.; Houlihan, D.D.; Bentham, L.; Shaw, J.C.; Cramb, R.; Olliff, S.; Gill, P.S.; Neuberger, J.M.; Lilford, R.J.; Newsome, P.N. Presence and severity of non-alcoholic fatty liver disease in a large prospective primary care cohort. *J. Hepatol.* **2012**, *56*, 234–240. [CrossRef] [PubMed]

44. Musso, G.; Cassader, M.; de Michieli, F.; Rosina, F.; Orlandi, F.; Gambino, R. Nonalcoholic steatohepatitis *versus* steatosis: Adipose tissue insulin resistance and dysfunctional response to fat ingestion predict liver injury and altered glucose and lipoprotein. *Metab. Hepatol.* **2012**, *56*, 933–942. [CrossRef] [PubMed]

45. Francque, S.M.; Verrijken, A.; Mertens, I.; Hubens, G.; van Marck, E.; Pelckmans, P.; Michielsen, P.; van Gaal, L. Noninvasive assessment of nonalcoholic fatty liver disease in obese or overweight patients. *Clin. Gastroenterol. Hepatol.* **2012**, *10*, 1162–1168. [CrossRef] [PubMed]

46. Casoinic, F.; Sâmpelean, D.; Bădău, C.; Prună, L. Nonalcoholic fatty liver disease–A risk factor for microalbuminuria in type 2 diabetic patients. *Rom. J. Int. Med.* **2009**, *47*, 55–59.

47. Xia, M.F.; Lin, H.D.; Li, X.M.; Yan, H.M.; Bian, H.; Chang, X.X.; He, W.Y.; Jeekel, J.; Hofman, A.; Gao, X. Renal function-dependent association of serum uric acid with metabolic syndrome and hepatic fat content in a middle-aged and elderly Chinese population. *Clin. Exp. Pharmacol. Physiol.* **2012**, *39*, 930–937. [CrossRef] [PubMed]

48. Kim, Y.S.; Jung, E.S.; Hur, W.; Bae, S.H.; Choi, J.Y.; Chang, X.X.; He, W.Y.; Jeekel, J.; Hofman, A.; Gao, X. Noninvasive predictors of nonalcoholic steatohepatitis in Korean patients with histologically proven nonalcoholic fatty liver disease. *Clin. Mol. Hepatol.* **2013**, *19*, 120–130. [CrossRef] [PubMed]

49. Angulo, P.; Bugianesi, E.; Bjornsson, E.S.; Charatcharoenwitthaya, P.; Mills, P.R.; Barrera, F.; Haflidadottir, S.; Day, C.P.; George, J. Simple noninvasive systems predict long-term outcomes of patients with nonalcoholic fatty liver disease. *Gastroenterology* **2013**, *145*, 782–789. [CrossRef] [PubMed]

50. El Azeem, H.A.; Khalek, E.A.; El-Akabawy, H.; Naeim, H.; Khalik, H.A.; Alfifi, A.A. Association between nonalcoholic fatty liver disease and the incidence of cardiovascular and renal events. *J. Saudi. Heart Assoc.* **2013**, *25*, 239–246. [CrossRef] [PubMed]

51. Musso, G.; Cassader, M.; Cohney, S.; Pinach, S.; Saba, F.; Gambino, R. Emerging liver–kidney interactions in nonalcoholic fatty liver disease. *Trends Mol. Med.* **2015**, *21*, 645–662. [CrossRef] [PubMed]

52. Ogden, C.L.; Carroll, M.D.; Kit, B.K.; Flegal, K.M. Prevalence of childhood and adult obesity in the United States, 2011–2012. *JAMA* **2014**, *311*, 806–814. [CrossRef] [PubMed]

53. Ix, J.H.; Sharma, K. Mechanisms linking obesity, chronic kidney disease, and fatty liver disease: The roles of fetuin-A, adiponectin, and AMPK. *J. Am. Soc. Nephrol.* **2010**, *21*, 406–412. [CrossRef] [PubMed]

54. Hamaguchi, M.; Kojima, T.; Takeda, N.; Nakagawa, T.; Taniguchi, H.; Fujii, K.; Omatsu, T.; Nakajima, T.; Sarui, H.; Shimazaki, M.; *et al.* The metabolic syndrome as a predictor of nonalcoholic fatty liver disease. *Ann. Intern. Med.* **2005**, *143*, 722–728. [CrossRef] [PubMed]

55. Mathews, S.T.; Rakhade, S.; Zhou, X.; Parker, G.C.; Coscina, D.V.; Grunberger, G. Fetuin-null mice are protected against obesity and insulin resistance associated with aging. *Biochem. Biophys. Res. Commun.* **2006**, *350*, 437–443. [CrossRef] [PubMed]

56. Ix, J.H.; Chertow, G.M.; Shlipak, M.G.; Brandenburg, V.M.; Ketteler, M.; Whooley, M.A. Fetuin-A and kidney function in persons with coronary artery disease—Data from the Heart and Soul Study. *Nephrol. Dial. Transplant.* **2006**, *21*, 2144–2151. [CrossRef] [PubMed]

57. De Vries, A.P.; Ruggenenti, P.; Ruan, X.Z.; Praga, M.; Cruzado, J.M.; Bajema, I.M.; D'Agati, V.D.; Lamb, H.J.; Pongrac Barlovic, D.; Hojs, R.; *et al.* Fatty kidney: Emerging role of ectopic lipid in obesity-related renal disease. *Lancet Diabetes Endocrinol.* **2014**, *2*, 417–426. [CrossRef]

58. Osterreicher, C.H.; Taura, K.; de Minicis, S.; Seki, E.; Penz-Osterreicher, M.; Kodama, Y.; Kluwe, J.; Schuster, M.; Oudit, G.Y.; Penninger, J.M.; *et al.* Angiotensin-converting-enzyme 2 inhibits liver fibrosis in mice. *Hepatology* **2009**, *50*, 929–938. [CrossRef] [PubMed]

59. Vos, M.; Kimmons, J.; Gillespie, C.; Welsh, J.; Blanck, H. Dietary fructose consumption among US children and adults: The Third National Health and Nutrition Examination Survey. *Medscape J. Med.* **2008**, *10*, 160. [PubMed]

60. Osterreicher, C.H.; Taura, K.; de Minicis, S.; Seki, E.; Penz-Osterreicher, M.; Kodama, Y.; Kluwe, J.; Schuster, M.; Oudit, G.Y.; Penninger, J.M.; *et al.* Betaine supplementation protects against high-fructose-induced renal injury in rats. *J. Nutr. Biochem.* **2014**, *25*, 353–362.

61. Abdelmalek, M.F.; Suzuki, A.; Guy, C.; Unalp-Arida, A.; Colvin, R.; Johnson, R.J.; Diehl, A.M. Nonalcoholic Steatohepatitis Clinical Research Network. Increased fructose consumption is associated with fibrosis severity in patients with nonalcoholic fatty liver disease. *Hepatology* **2010**, *51*, 1961–1971. [CrossRef] [PubMed]

62. Cheungpasitporn, W.; Thongprayoon, C.; O'Corragain, O.A.; Edmonds, P.J.; Kittanamongkolchai, W.; Erickson, S.B. Associations of sugar and artificially sweetened soda and chronic kidney disease: A systematic review and meta-analysis. *Nephrology* **2014**, *19*, 791–797. [CrossRef] [PubMed]

63. Wang, C.; Cui, Y.; Li, C.; Zhang, Y.; Xu, S.; Li, X.; Li, H.; Zhang, X. Nrf2 deletion causes "benign" simple steatosis to develop into nonalcoholic steatohepatitis in mice fed a high-fat diet. *Lipids Health Dis.* **2013**, *12*, 165–171. [CrossRef] [PubMed]

64. Pergola, P.E.; Raskin, P.; Toto, R.D.; Meyer, C.J.; Huff, W.; Grossman, E.B.; Krauth, M.A.B.; Ruiz, S.; Audhya, P.; Christ-Schmidt, H.; *et al.* Bardoxolone methyl and kidney function in CKD with type 2 diabetes. *N. Engl. J. Med.* **2011**, *365*, 327–336. [CrossRef] [PubMed]

65. De Zeeuw, D.; Akizawa, T.; Agarwal, R.; Audhya, P.; Bakris, G.L.; Chin, M.; Krauth, M.; Lambers Heerspink, H.J.; Meyer, C.J.; McMurray, J.J.; *et al.* Rationale and trial design of bardoxolone methyl evaluation in patients with chronic kidney disease and type 2 diabetes: The occurrence of renal events (BEACON). *Am. J. Nephrol.* **2013**, *37*, 212–222. [CrossRef] [PubMed]

66. Hirata, T.; Tomita, K.; Kawai, T.; Yokoyama, H.; Shimada, A.; Kikuchi, M.; Hirose, H.; Ebinuma, H.; Irie, J.; Ojiro, K.; *et al.* Effect of telmisartan or losartan for treatment of nonalcoholic fatty liver disease: Fatty Liver Protection Trial by Telmisartan or Losartan Study (FANTASY). *Int. J. Endocrinol.* **2013**, *2013*, 587140. [CrossRef] [PubMed]

67. Bain, R.; Rohde, R.; Hunsicker, L.G.; McGill, J.; Kobrin, S.; Lewis, E.J. A controlled clinical trial of angiotensin-converting enzyme inhibition in type I diabetic nephropathy: Study design and patient characteristics. The Collaborative Study Group. *J. Am. Soc. Nephrol.* **1992**, *3*, S97–S103. [PubMed]

68. Orlic, L.; Mikolasevic, I.; Lukenda, V.; Anic, K.; Jelic, I.; Racki, S. Nonalcoholic fatty liver disease and the renin-angiotensin system blockers in the patients with chronic kidney disease. *Wien. Klin. Wochenschr.* **2015**, *127*, 355–362. [CrossRef] [PubMed]

69. Singh, S.; Khera, R.; Allen, A.M.; Murad, H.; Loomba, R. Comparative effectiveness of pharmacologic interventions for non-alcoholic steatohepatitis: A systemic review and network meta-analysis. *Hepatology* **2015**, *62*, 1417–1432. [CrossRef] [PubMed]

70. Athyros, V.G.; Tziomalos, K.; Gossios, T.D.; Griva, T.; Anagnostis, P.; Kargiotis, K.; Pagourelias, E.D.; Theocharidou, E.; Karagiannis, A.; Mikhailidis, D.P. Safety and efficacy of long-term statin treatment for cardiovascular events in patients with coronary heart disease and abnormal liver tests in the Greek Atorvastatin and Coronary Heart Disease Evaluation (GREACE) Study: A post-hoc analysis. *Lancet* **2010**, *376*, 1916–1922. [CrossRef]

71. Tikkanen, M.J.; Fayyad, R.; Faergeman, O.; Olsson, A.G.; Wun, C.C.; Laskey, R.; Kastelein, J.J.; Holme, I.; Pedersen, T.R. Effect of intensive lipid lowering with atorvastatin on cardiovascular outcomes in coronary heart disease patients with mild-to-moderate baseline elevations in alanine aminotransferase levels. *Int. J. Cardiol.* **2013**, *168*, 3846–3852. [CrossRef] [PubMed]

13

Non-Alcoholic Fatty Liver Disease and Extra-Hepatic Cancers

Claudia Sanna, Chiara Rosso, Milena Marietti and Elisabetta Bugianesi *

Division of Gastroenterology, Department of Medical Sciences, A.O. Città della Salute e della Scienza di Torino, University of Turin, 10126 Turin, Italy; sanna.cla@gmail.com (C.S.); chiara.rosso84@tiscali.it (C.R.); milena.marietti@gmail.com (M.M.)
* Correspondence: elisabetta.bugianesi@unito.it

Academic Editors: Amedeo Lonardo and Giovanni Targher

Abstract: Non-alcoholic fatty liver disease (NAFLD) is a leading cause of chronic liver disease but the second cause of death among NAFLD patients are attributed to malignancies at both gastrointestinal (liver, colon, esophagus, stomach, and pancreas) and extra-intestinal sites (kidney in men, and breast in women). Obesity and related metabolic abnormalities are associated with increased incidence or mortality for a number of cancers. NAFLD has an intertwined relationship with metabolic syndrome and significantly contributes to the risk of hepatocellular carcinoma (HCC), but recent evidence have fuelled concerns that NAFLD may be a new, and added, risk factor for extra-hepatic cancers, particularly in the gastrointestinal tract. In this review we critically appraise key studies on NAFLD-associated extra-hepatic cancers and speculate on how NAFLD may influence carcinogenesis at these sites.

Keywords: fatty liver; colorectal cancer; adipokines; gut microbiota

1. Introduction

Nonalcoholic fatty liver disease (NAFLD) is one of the most common causes of chronic liver disease worldwide, with an estimated global prevalence of 25% in adults and around 10% in children [1–3]. The term NAFLD includes two distinct conditions with different histologic features and prognoses: non-alcoholic fatty liver (NAFL) and non-alcoholic steatohepatitis (NASH) [4]; the presence of steatohepatitis and significant fibrosis are considered harbingers of adverse outcomes in individuals with NAFLD and are associated with an increased risk for morbidity and mortality through hepatic and non-hepatic complications [5–7]. In descending order, the majority of deaths in patients with NAFLD are, first, attributed to cardiovascular events, and, second, to malignancies at both gastrointestinal (liver, colon, esophagus, stomach, and pancreas) and extra-intestinal site (kidney in men, and breast in women), while end-stage liver disease is the third cause of death [8,9]. NAFLD is traditionally considered the hepatic manifestation of metabolic syndrome (MetS) and an impressive body of evidence indicates an increased general risk of cancer in subjects with MetS, particularly in the gastrointestinal tract. In this setting, NAFLD can either share common risk factors (*i.e.*, obesity and type 2 diabetes) or actively mediate some pathogenic mechanism, as in the case of liver cancer (hepatocellular carcinoma, HCC). Excluding the latter one, colorectal cancer (CRC) has been consistently associated with NAFLD thus far [10,11]. The mechanisms underlying the link between NAFLD and risk of neoplasms are not fully elucidated but they probably stem from the bidirectional relationship between NAFLD and MetS [12–14]. In this review we critically appraise the key studies on the association between NAFLD and extra-hepatic cancers and speculate on how NAFLD may influence carcinogenesis at these sites.

2. Nonalcoholic Fatty Liver Disease (NAFLD) and Colorectal Cancer

The association between NAFLD and CRC is the best investigated in literature (details are summarized in Table 1). Almost all of the studies showed a higher prevalence of colorectal lesions in patients with NAFLD compared to patients without. Hwang and colleagues presented the first evidence for an association of NAFLD with an increased rate of colorectal adenomatous polyps [15]. In their study, a population of 2917 participants was investigated via colonoscopy, abdominal ultrasonography, and liver tests. The prevalence of NAFLD was 41.5% in the adenomatous polyp group *versus* 30.2% in the control group; with multivariate analysis, NAFLD was associated with a three-fold increased risk of colorectal adenomas. This preliminary finding was confirmed in a large retrospective cohort study of 5.517 Korean women, where a two-fold increase in the occurrence of adenomatous polyps and a three-fold increase in the risk of colorectal cancer was found in patients with NAFLD compared to controls. However, the presence of NAFLD had no influence on the prognosis of colorectal cancer and, in particular, on the disease recurrence during follow-up [16]. Among NAFLD patients, those with histological diagnosis of NASH harbinger the most increased risk for CRC. In a cross-sectional study patients with NAFLD, diagnosed by both proton magnetic resonance spectroscopy and liver biopsy, had a significantly higher rate of colorectal adenomas (34.7% *vs.* 21.5%) and advanced neoplasms (18.6% *vs.* 5.5%) than healthy controls [17]. Almost half of NAFLD patients with advanced neoplasm had right-sided colorectal carcinoma. Importantly, CRC was more often found in patients with NASH compared to those with simple steatosis (51.0% *vs.* 25.6% and 34.7% *vs.* 14.0%). NASH remained associated with a higher risk of both adenomas (Odds Ratio (OR) 4.89) and advanced neoplasms (OR 5.34) even after adjusting for demographic and metabolic risk factor, thus, the authors concluded that screening colonoscopy should be strongly recommended in these patients [17]. In the largest study performed so far in Europe, male patients with NAFLD had significantly more colorectal adenomas and early colorectal cancers compared to those without NAFLD [18]. Multivariate regression analysis confirmed an independent association of colorectal adenomas with NAFLD (OR 1.47) [17]. Data stemming from cross-sectional studies have also been replicated longitudinally. In a prospective study where 1522 subjects underwent paired colonoscopies, while the index colonoscopy was negative in all of them, the incidence of *de novo* adenoma development was increased by 45% in those with NAFLD [19]. Lastly, a Danish cohort study evaluating the global risk of cancer in hospitalized patient showed an increased risk of CRC in those with fatty liver compared to the general population, but no difference was noticed between alcoholic and non-alcoholic fatty liver [20].

In contrast, only two studies failed to demonstrate an increased incidence of colorectal adenomas in patients with NAFLD compared to healthy controls [21,22]. The first one found a higher burden of adenomas in patients with NAFLD, but data did not reach a statistical significance, probably for the smaller sample size and the younger median age. The second one remarkably showed a lower prevalence of CRC in NAFLD patients but a higher risk for CRC in the presence of insulin resistance; however it is well known that both raised alanine aminotransferase (ALT) levels and ultrasound can underestimate the diagnosis of NAFLD.

Overall, it appears that NAFLD patients are more likely to have multiple polyps [23], more often localized more in the right and transverse segments of colon [17,23]; importantly, patients with histologic diagnosis of NASH are at higher risk for adenomatous polyps with high grade dysplasia (HGD) compared to those with simple fatty liver [17]. The relationship between NAFLD and CRC once again emphasizes the importance of a healthy lifestyle to prevent and treat the MetS and its systemic manifestations. Certainly these data suggest that NAFLD patients should undergo a closer surveillance for CRC risk according to screening guidelines [24]. If the evidence of this association will be further confirmed in larger population studies, probably these patients should be screened in advance and total colonoscopy considered as the preferred screening method, as neoplasms are more commonly found in the proximal colon [19,24].

Table 1. Principal studies on the association between nonalcoholic fatty liver disease (NAFLD) and colorectal neoplasms *.

Study	Country	Type of Study	Population Enrolled	Exclusion Criteria	NAFLD Diagnosis	Prevalence of Colorectal Lesions in Patients with NAFLD vs. Patients without NAFLD
Bhatt BD et al. [23] (2015)	USA	Retrospective	591 pts who completed LT evaluation (68 NAFLD vs. 523 non-NAFLD)	<50 years old at LT; IBD; history of multiple / recurrent adenomas; family history of CRC; known cancer-predisposing gene alteration; history of solid organ transplant; HIV pts; personal history of cancer	Biopsy + clinical criteria	Polyps prevalence: 59% vs. 40%; $p < 0.003$. OR (Odds Ratio) 2.16; $p = 0.003$. Adenomatous polyps prevalence: 32% vs. 21%; $p = 0.04$. OR 1.95; $p = 0.02$
Basyigit S et al. [22] (2015)	Turkey	Prospective observational	127 consecutive pts who underwent colonoscopy	Other causes of hepatic disease; incomplete colonoscopy; IBD; active gastrointestinal bleeding; history of colorectal surgery; history of CRC; hereditary cancer syndrome	US	Adenomas prevalence: 20% vs. 25.8%. OR 1 CRC prevalence: 4.6% vs. 24.2%. OR 1
Lin XF et al. [25] (2014)	China	Retrospective and consecutive cohort study	2315 community subjects who underwent a routine colonoscopy (263 NAFLD vs. 2052 non-NAFLD)	History of CRC, adenoma and polyp; history of other extraintestinal malignancies; contraindications to colonoscopy	US	Total colorectal lesions prevalence: 90.0% vs. 93.3% Adenomatous polyps prevalence: 44.5% vs. 55.7% CRC prevalence: 29.3% vs. 18%; $p = 0.001$. OR 1.868; 95% CI 1.360–2.567; $p < 0.05$
Wong VW-S et al. [17] (2012)	China	Cross-sectional	380 community pts + consecutive pts with biopsy proven NAFLD (in total 199 NAFLD vs. 181-non-NAFLD)	Other causes of hepatic disease; history of CRC or polyps; IBD; bowel symptoms including per rectal bleeding and altered bowel habit; prior CRC screening; contraindications to colonoscopy	Proton-magnetic resonance spectroscopy or liver biopsy	Total polyps prevalence: 52.8% vs. 38.7%; $p = 0.057$ Adenomatous polyps prevalence: 34.7% vs. 21.5%; $p = 0.043$. OR 1.61; 95% CI 0.9–2.9; $p = 0.11$ Villous polyps prevalence: 6% vs. 0.6%; $p = 0.042$ High grade dysplasia polyps prevalence: 18.1% vs. 5%; $p = 0.002$ Advance neoplasm prevalence: 18.6% vs. 5.5%; $p = 0.005$. OR 3.04; 95% CI 1.29–7.2; $p = 0.011$ CRC 1% vs. 0.6%; $p = 0.65$
Stadlmayr A et al. [18] (2011)	Austria	Cross-sectional	1211 consecutive pts who underwent screening colonoscopy (632 NAFLD vs. 597 non-NAFLD)	Incomplete colonoscopy; recent colorectal polypectomy, asymptomatic IBD; extraintestinal malignancies	US + exclusion of other causes of hepatic disease	Total colorectal lesions prevalence: 34% vs. 21.7%; $p < 0.001$ Tubular adenoma prevalence in men: 34.6% vs. 23.7%; $p = 0.006$ Rectum adenoma prevalence in men: 11% vs. 3%; $p = 0.004$ CRC prevalence in men: 1.6% vs. 0.4%; $p < 0.001$
Lee YI et al. [16] (2011)	South Korea	Retrospective cohort study	5517 women who underwent life insurance company health examinations (831 NAFLD vs. 4686 non-NAFLD)	Other causes of hepatic disease; history of receiving previous medical insurance benefits	US + exclusion of other causes of hepatic disease	Adenomatous polyps incidence: 628 vs. 185.2/10^5 person year. RR 1.94; 95% CI 1.11–3.40 CRC incidence: 233.6 vs. 27/10^5 person year. RR 3.08; 95% CI 1.02–9.34
Touzin NT et al. [21] (2011)	USA	Retrospective cohort study	233 patients who underwent screening colonoscopies (94 NAFD vs. 139 non-NAFLD)	Not available	US + liver biopsy	Adenomas prevalence: 24.4% vs. 25.1%; $p = 1$
Huang KW et al. [19] (2012)	Taiwan	Retrospective cohort study	1522 pts with two consecutive colonoscopies (216 with colorectal adenoma vs. 1306 without colorectal adenoma after negative baseline colonoscopy)	History of colorectal adenoma or CRC; adenomas during baseline colonoscopy; incomplete medical record data; alcohol consumption >20 g / day	US + exclusion of other causes of hepatic disease	NAFLD prevalence: 55.6% vs. 38.8%; $p < 0.05$. OR = 1.45; 95% CI 1.07–1.98; $p = 0.016$
Hwang ST et al. [15] (2009)	South Korea	Cross-sectional	2917 pts who underwent routine colonoscopy (556 with polyps vs. 2361 without polyps)	Incomplete colonoscopies; history of polypectomy; IBD; history of cancer; cancer detected during the study; pts with anticoagulant therapy; other causes of hepatic disease	US	NAFLD prevalence: 41.5% vs. 30.2%; $p < 0.001$. OR, 1.30; 95% CI 1.02–1.66; $p = 0.034$

* CI, confidence interval; CRC, colorectal cancer; IBD, intestinal bowel disease; LT, liver transplant; NAFLD, non-alcoholic fatty liver disease; OR, odds ratio; pts, patients; RR: relative risk; US, ultrasound.

3. NAFLD and Cancers in Other Sites

The association of NAFLD with other extra-hepatic cancers is less proven. In the previously-mentioned Danish study all-cancers risk was increased by 70% in subjects with fatty liver, either alcoholic or non-alcoholic [20]; however, those with NAFLD had a higher risk of pancreatic and kidney cancer (standardized incidence ratio (SIR) 3; 95% confidence interval (CI) 1.3–5.8 and SIR 2.7; 95% CI 1.1–5.6, respectively), malignant melanoma (SIR 2.4; 95% CI 0.8–5.6) and cancer metastases from primary unspecified sites (SIR 6.3; 95% CI 1.3–18.4), while those with alcoholic fatty liver had a higher risk for lung and breast cancer (SIR 2.2; 95% CI 1.7–2.8 and SIR 1.5; 95% CI 0.9–2.2, respectively). The latter observation contrasts with another study where a higher prevalence of breast cancers was observed in patients with ultrasound diagnosed NAFLD compared with healthy controls (63% *vs.* 48%, respectively) [26]. The burden of data available is currently too limited to draw definite conclusions about a specific role of NAFLD, as the link can be mediated by visceral obesity, which in turn is strongly associated to fatty liver in the so-called "central-axis" of obesity. A recent review summarized the well-recognized role of visceral obesity in the onset and development of various cancers [27], including CRC [28–31], esophageal [32–38] and pancreatic cancer [39], breast [40], thyroid [41], and probably prostate cancer [42]. What is currently unknown is whether both NAFLD and visceral obesity are just markers of an increased risk of cancers or also active players in this process. With this caveat in mind, we will briefly examine the association between NAFLD, visceral obesity, and cancers other than CRC.

3.1. Esophageal and Gastric Cancer

Esophageal cancer is the eighth most common form of cancer worldwide, and the World Cancer Research Fund has identified obesity as a major risk factor, able to increase the risk up to four-fold compared with lean populations [43]. Several more recent studies suggest a stronger impact of visceral fat distribution rather than body mass index (BMI) *per se* [37,44,45], but no study specifically examined hepatic fat. Strikingly, the association between visceral obesity and esophageal adenocarcinoma is independent of gastro-oesophageal reflux disease (GORD), and possibly mediated by adipose tissue insulin resistance and chronic inflammation [32,46,47]. A possible direct link between NAFLD and gastric cancer has been suggested in a recent study, performed on 1840 patients undergoing upper endoscopies over a six-month time frame; despite the limited number of gastric cancer diagnosed, the prevalence of NAFLD in subjects with gastric cancers was higher compared to the average in the Turkish population [48].

3.2. Pancreatic Cancer

In 2007 the World Cancer Research Fund/American Institute for Cancer Research (WCRF) definitively established the association between pancreatic cancer and overweight/obesity. A meta-analysis published in 2012 showed a linear increase between pancreatic cancer risk and waist circumference, with a relative risk (RR) of 1.11 (95% CI 1.05–1.18) for every 10 cm increase, and waist-to-hip ratio, with a RR of 1.19 (95% CI 1.09–1.31) for every 0.1 unit increment [39]. In a meta-analysis performed in 2012, MetS has been identified itself as a neoplastic risk factor, with a RR of 1.58 ($p < 0.0001$) for pancreatic cancer in female gender, possibly mediated by decreased physical activity, consumption of high-calorie dense foods, high dietary fat intake, low fiber intake, and oxidative stress [49]. As for esophageal cancer, NAFLD can be implicated in this association, although no direct evidence is yet available.

3.3. Renal Cancer

In addition to smoking and dietary habits, whose association with renal cancer is well established, some of the components of MetS, such as obesity and hypertension, have been recognized etiological factors and listed in specialist guidelines [50,51]. In a large study of seven European cohorts, high level of a metabolic risk score, based on the combination of BMI, blood pressure, and plasma levels of glucose, total cholesterol and triglycerides, was linearly and positively associated to higher incidence of renal cell cancer (risk increase per standard deviation of metabolic risk score increment: 43% in men and 40% in women) [52]. In patients with cT1a renal cell carcinoma visceral fat, assessed by computed tomography (CT) scan, is strongly associated with Fuhrman grade, the most frequently used neoplastic nuclear grading system for kidney, and is an independent predictor of high-grade renal cell carcinoma (RCC) [53]. In a study performed on 118 consecutive patients undergoing surgical treatment for RCC, adiponectin levels are inversely proportional to the severity of disease, with the lower levels in patients with metastatic cancer [54].

3.4. Breast Cancer

The association between breast cancer risk in postmenopausal women and components of MetS has been provided by several large studies [49,55–57]. In combined analyses of two case-control study on 3869 postmenopausal women with breast cancer and 4082 postmenopausal control cases, authors registered a higher neoplastic risk in women with MetS than those without (OR 1.75; 95% CI 1.37–2.22). In the analysis of distribution of cases and controls according to individual components of the syndrome, the resulting corresponding odds ratios were 1.33 (95% CI 1.09–1.62) for diabetes, 1.19 (95% CI 1.07–1.33) for hypertension, 1.08 (95% CI 0.95–1.22) for hyperlipidemia, 1.26 (95% CI 1.11–1.44) for BMI $\geq$ 30 kg/m^2, and 1.22 (95% CI 1.09–1.36) for waist circumference $\geq$88 cm [56]. In a study on 2092 patients, surgically treated for stage I–III invasive breast cancer in the previous five years and followed-up over 2.8 years on average, MetS appeared a major determinant of the occurrence of additional related events, such as specific mortality, presence of distant metastasis, or local recurrences and incidence of contralateral breast cancer [58]. Although each component was associated with an increased risk of cancer recurrence, the risk associated with the full syndrome was the highest, likely to be the expression of a general dysmetabolic condition rather than of a specific trait.

3.5. Prostate Cancer

The link between dysmetabolic factors, NAFLD and prostate cancer is controversial. In a systematic review and meta-regression analysis, including 31 cohort and 25 case-control, for every five kg/m^2 increment in BMI, authors described a 1.05 relative risk (95% CI 1.01–1.08), higher in patients with progressed diseases than localized diseases [59]. Two studies specifically investigated the role of NALFD. In the first one, NAFLD was found to be protective against neoplastic recurrence after radical prostatectomy for prostate cancer in 293 consecutive patients [60]. The NAFLD group showed significantly longer time-to-recurrence compared with patients without NAFLD both in the training and validation set (hazard ratio: 0.33 and 0.22; 95% CI 0.16–0.69, and 95% CI 0.11–0.43, respectively). The second one analyzed the development of malignancies and the specific site of disease in 1600 US-defined NAFLD subjects and in 1600 matched hepatitis C virus (HCV)-infected patients: prostate cancer developed in 12.6% of NAFLD compared to 3.5% in HCV patients [61], and the incidence of prostate cancer in NAFLD was higher than in the general population.

4. Putative Role of Insulin Resistance and Gut Microbiota in the Development of Extra-Hepatic Cancers in NAFLD

Although the most extensive evidence of a possible mechanistic link between NAFLD and extra-hepatic carcinogenesis currently comes from data on the pro-inflammatory and pro-carcinogenic effects of insulin resistance (IR), gut microbiota has been recently identified as a novel and intriguing player in the development of obesity, NAFLD and several types of cancer (details are summarized in Table 2). Patients with NAFLD are characterized by dysbiosis [62] and the liver stays at the cross-road of the complex interaction between changes in microbiota composition, IR, inflammation, and carcinogenesis [63,64]. Dysbiosis has been found in patients with colon cancer [65] and the possible correlation has been widely studied. Quantitative and qualitative alterations of gut microbiota lead to increased intestinal permeability through several mechanisms, including the regulation of tight junctions, such as zonulin-1, and occluding by toll like receptor 2 (TLR2) in the ileum. These alterations favor the translocation of bacterial metabolites and activation of TLRs via the recognition of microorganism-associated molecular patterns (MAMPs) and can promote tumorigenesis through the reduced release of the inflammasome-derived interleukin 18 (IL-18) and the increased IL-6 signaling which, in turn, protects normal and premalignant cells from apoptosis [11,66,67].

Table 2. Putative mechanisms linking NAFLD and extra-hepatic cancers.

Mechanism	Effects	Extra-Hepatic Site
Insulin resistance		
↑ IGF-1 axis	Proliferative and anti-apoptotic effects	Prostate/colorectal/lung/Breast cancers, Barrett's esophagus, esophageal adenocarcinoma
Dysfunctional adipose tissue		
↓ adiponectin/caspase activation ↓ adiponectin/TNF-α ↑ leptin/MAPK ↑ resistin/NF-κB	Anti-apoptotic effects Proliferation and angiogenesis Invasiveness, motility, lamellipodia formation	Gastrointestinal and extra-intestinal cancer Gastrointestinal and extra-intestinal cancer Colon/breast cancer, Barrett's esophagus, esophageal adenocarcinoma Breast/gastrointestinal and non-small cell lung cancers
Inflammation		
IL-6/JAK/STAT3 and IL-6/MAPK TNF-α/Wnt/β-catenin	Proliferation Angiogenesis, differentiation and metastasis development	Renal/gastric/colorectal cancers Colorectal cancer
Gut microbiota		
MAMPs/TLRs Inflammasome-derived IL-18	Inflammation Anti-apoptotic effects	Colon cancer Colon cancer

IGF-1, insulin growth factor-1; IL, interleukin; MAMPs, microorganism-associated molecular patterns; MAPK, mitogen-activated protein kinase; NF-κB, nuclear factor-κ B; STAT3, signal transducer and activator of transcription 3; TLRs, toll-like receptors; TNF-α, tumor necrosis factor-α.

It is well known that host diet significantly impacts on gut microbial composition. Diet-induced NAFLD may be mediated by the myeloid differentiation factor 88 (MyD88)-dependent pathway [68]. This factor is an adaptor molecule, essential for the signaling through TLRs. It is recruited after the interaction among the microorganism-associated molecular patterns (MAMPs) and TLRs (particularly TLR4) and promotes the transcription of several pro-inflammatory cytokines through the activation of NF-κB or c-Jun NH$_2$-terminal kinase (JNK) leading to the induction of IR. Loss-of-function mutation or knockout mice in TLR4 prevents IR induced by obesity underlying the important role of this receptor in the modulation of the innate immune system.

NAFLD and visceral adipose tissue are the main components of the axis of central obesity. In this setting, low-grade chronic inflammation and insulin resistance (IR) create a microenvironment suitable for cancer development through the stimulation of the insulin growth factor-1 (IGF-1) axis by hyperinsulinemia [9,69–71]. Through its proliferative and anti-apoptotic effects, this pathway can boost mutations favoring carcinogenesis [72,73]. Elevated serum levels of IGF-1 have been associated with prostate [74,75], colorectal [76], lung [77], and breast cancer [78]. Importantly, the insulin/IGF system is able to influence the risk of Barrett's esophagus and of esophageal adenocarcinoma [37,79,80], although there is no full agreement about this [81].

Several adipokines, involved in the modulation of metabolism, inflammation and fibrogenesis, can also be involved in carcinogenic processes. Adiponectin has anti-carcinogenic effects mediated by its ability to stop colon cancer cell growth through the AMPc-activated protein kinase (AMPK) and to induce a caspase-dependent pathway resulting in endothelial cell apoptosis. Adiponectin can also directly inhibit tumor necrosis factor α (TNF-α), involved in tumor cell proliferation and angiogenesis. Since NAFLD patients have reduced serum levels of adiponectin, the above described mechanisms represent an interesting link between NAFLD and cancer development at both gastrointestinal and extra-intestinal site.

The pro-carcinogenic effects of leptin, especially in the presence of low adiponectin levels, have been widely investigated. In obese animal models, leptin acts as a growth factor for CRC at early stages through the activation of signal transducer and activator of transcription 3 (STAT 3) pathway [82]. In human colon cancer cells leptin is able to promote motility and invasiveness by activation of mitogen-activated protein kinase (MAPK) pathway [83]. A case-cohort study in post-menopausal women with CRC demonstrated that high plasma concentrations of leptin were associated with an increased risk for CRC [84]. In obese subjects the combination of high leptin and low adiponectin levels may also increase the risk of Barrett's esophagus [85–90] and esophageal adenocarcinoma by enhanced cell proliferation and reduced apoptosis via extracellular signal-regulated kinase (ERK), p38 MAPK, phosphatidylinositol 3'-kinase/Akt, and Janus kinase-2 (JAK2)-dependent activation of cyclooxygenase-2 (COX-2) and prostaglandin E2 (PGE2). The association between leptin serum levels and the size of breast tumors has been summarized in a recent review [91]; higher leptin levels are related to a more aggressive disease, presence of metastasis and a lower survival rate [92] mostly in obese patients [93].

Finally, resistin can also be linked to obesity-related malignancies via activation of nuclear factor-κ B (NF-κB) pathway and amplification of the procarcinogenic effects of interleukin (IL)-1, IL-6 and TNF-α [94]. To date, a putative role of resistin has been suggested in breast cancer [94], non-small cell lung cancer [95] and in gastrointestinal tumors [96].

The low-grade chronic inflammation associated with IR also favors macrophages recruitment and massive release of several proinflammatory cytokines, such as IL-6 and TNF-α, into the systemic circulation. IL-6 induces the Janus kinase/signal transducer and activator of transcription (JAK/STAT) and MAPK pathways, stimulating cell proliferation and tumor progression, while TNF-α influences cancer angiogenesis, metastasis development and cell survival, growth, and differentiation [97–99]. Animal models have shown a relationship between TNF-α and several malignancies [100–102] including colorectal cancer [103]. Obese mice have higher TNF-α levels in the colonic mucosa, leading to β-catenin stabilization and increased transcription of the downstream Wnt pathway gene c-Myc [104]. IL-6 has been linked to renal cell carcinoma [105], gastric cancer [106], and colorectal cancer [107,108], through its modulation of several genes involved in proliferation, survival, and angiogenesis [109].

In consideration of the above described mechanisms, the increased risk of gastrointestinal cancers associated to NAFLD does not appear causal, although more extensive studies are required to demonstrate a direct link between NAFLD and cancers at various sites.

5. Conclusions

NAFLD is a complex multifactorial disease closely interrelated with obesity and type 2 diabetes, and shares with them a significant increased risk of several types of cancer. Beyond the risk of HCC, clearly mediated by NASH, substantial evidence is accumulating for a role of NAFLD as independent risk factor for cancers, particularly in the gastrointestinal tract. Once again, these preliminary, but intriguing, data convey that NAFLD patients require a multidisciplinary evaluation with a particular attention to the development of extra-hepatic complications. Further studies are necessary to better define high-risk NAFLD patients and effective screening strategies, but we encourage health care providers taking care of NAFLD patients to be vigilant for any signs and symptoms of cancer, particularly colorectal, and refer the patients for further assessment and management.

Abbreviations

AMPK	AMPc-activated protein kinase
CI	confidence interval
COX-2	cyclooxygenase 2
CRC	colorectal cancer
ERK	extracellular signal-regulated kinase
HCC	hepatocellular carcinoma
HGD	high grade dysplasia
IBD	inflammatory bowel disease
IGF	insulin growth factors
IL	interleukin
IR	insulin resistance
LT	liver transplant
MAMPs	microorganism-associated molecular patterns
MAPK	mitogen-activated protein kinase
MetS	metabolic syndrome
mTOR	mammalian target of rapamycin
NAFL	non-alcoholic fatty liver
NAFLD	non-alcoholic fatty liver disease
NASH	non-alcoholic steatohepatitis
NF-kB	nuclear factor-κ B
OR	odds ratio
PGE2	Prostaglandin E2
RR	relative risk
SIR	standardized incidence ratio
STAT3	signal transducer and activator of transcription
TNF-α	tumor necrosis factor α
US	ultrasound
JAK2	Janus kinase-2

References

1. Armstrong, M.J.; Houlihan, D.D.; Bentham, L.; Shaw, J.C.; Cramb, R.; Olliff, S.; Gill, P.S.; Neuberger, J.M.; Lilford, R.J.; Newsome, P.N. Presence and severity of non-alcoholic fatty liver disease in a large prospective primary care cohort. *J. Hepatol.* **2012**, *56*, 234–240. [CrossRef] [PubMed]
2. Younossi, Z.M.; Koenig, A.B.; Abdelatif, D.; Fazel, Y.; Henry, L.; Wymer, M. Global epidemiology of non-alcoholic fatty liver disease-meta-analytic assessment of prevalence, incidence and outcomes. *Hepatology* **2015**. [CrossRef] [PubMed]
3. Abd El-Kader, S.M.; El-Den Ashmawy, E.M.S. Non-alcoholic fatty liver disease: The diagnosis and management. *World J. Hepatol.* **2015**, *7*, 846–858. [CrossRef] [PubMed]
4. Musso, G.; Gambino, R.; Cassader, M.; Pagano, G. Meta-analysis: Natural history of non-alcoholic fatty liver disease (NAFLD) and diagnostic accuracy of non-invasive tests for liver disease severity. *Ann. Med.* **2011**, *43*, 617–649. [CrossRef] [PubMed]
5. Adams, L.A.; Lymp, J.F.; St Sauver, J.; Sanderson, S.O.; Lindor, K.D.; Feldstein, A.; Angulo, P. The natural history of nonalcoholic fatty liver disease: A population-based cohort study. *Gastroenterology* **2005**, *129*, 113–121. [CrossRef] [PubMed]
6. Ekstedt, M.; Franzén, L.E.; Mathiesen, U.L.; Thorelius, L.; Holmqvist, M.; Bodemar, G.; Kechagias, S. Long-term follow-up of patients with NAFLD and elevated liver enzymes. *Hepatology* **2006**, *44*, 865–873. [CrossRef] [PubMed]
7. Rafiq, N.; Bai, C.; Fang, Y.; Srishord, M.; McCullough, A.; Gramlich, T.; Younossi, Z.M. Long-term follow-up of patients with nonalcoholic fatty liver. *Clin. Gastroenterol. Hepatol.* **2009**, *7*, 234–238. [CrossRef] [PubMed]
8. Angulo, P. Long-term mortality in nonalcoholic fatty liver disease: Is liver histology of any prognostic significance? *Hepatology* **2010**, *51*, 373–375. [CrossRef] [PubMed]

9.   Tilg, H.; Moschen, A.R. Mechanisms behind the link between obesity and gastrointestinal cancers. *Best Pract. Res. Clin. Gastroenterol.* **2014**, *28*, 599–610. [CrossRef] [PubMed]

10. Tilg, H.; Diehl, A.M. NAFLD and extrahepatic cancers: Have a look at the colon. *Gut* **2011**, *60*, 745–746. [CrossRef] [PubMed]

11. Vanni, E.; Marengo, A.; Mezzabotta, L.; Bugianesi, E. Systemic complications of nonalcoholic fatty liver disease: When the liver is not an innocent bystander. *Semin. Liver Dis.* **2015**, *35*, 236–249. [CrossRef] [PubMed]

12. Bugianesi, E.; McCullough, A.J.; Marchesini, G. Insulin resistance: A metabolic pathway to chronic liver disease. *Hepatology* **2005**, *42*, 987–1000. [CrossRef] [PubMed]

13. Perseghin, G. Viewpoints on the way to a consensus session: Where does insulin resistance start? The liver. *Diabetes Care* **2009**, *32*, S164–S167. [CrossRef] [PubMed]

14. Scalera, A.; Tarantino, G. Could metabolic syndrome lead to hepatocarcinoma via non-alcoholic fatty liver disease? *World J. Gastroenterol.* **2014**, *20*, 9217–9228. [PubMed]

15. Hwang, S.T.; Cho, Y.K.; Park, J.H.; Kim, H.J.; Park, D.I.; Sohn, C.I.; Jeon, W.K.; Kim, B.I.; Won, K.H.; Jin, W. Relationship of non-alcoholic fatty liver disease to colorectal adenomatous polyps. *J. Gastroenterol. Hepatol.* **2010**, *25*, 562–567. [CrossRef] [PubMed]

16. Lee, Y.I.; Lim, Y.-S.; Park, H.S. Colorectal neoplasms in relation to non-alcoholic fatty liver disease in Korean women: A retrospective cohort study. *J. Gastroenterol. Hepatol.* **2012**, *27*, 91–95. [CrossRef] [PubMed]

17. Wong, V.W.-S.; Wong, G.L.-H.; Tsang, S.W.-C.; Fan, T.; Chu, W.C.; Woo, J.; Chan, A.W.; Choi, P.C.; Chim, A.M.; Lau, J.Y.; *et al.* High prevalence of colorectal neoplasm in patients with non-alcoholic steatohepatitis. *Gut* **2011**, *60*, 829–836. [CrossRef] [PubMed]

18. Stadlmayr, A.; Aigner, E.; Steger, B.; Scharinger, L.; Lederer, D.; Mayr, A.; Strasser, M.; Brunner, E.; Heuberger, A.; Hohla, F.; *et al.* Nonalcoholic fatty liver disease: An independent risk factor for colorectal neoplasia. *J. Intern. Med.* **2011**, *270*, 41–49.

19. Huang, K.-W.; Leu, H.-B.; Wang, Y.-J.; Luo, J.C.; Lin, H.C.; Lee, F.Y.; Chan, W.L.; Lin, J.K.; Chang, F.Y. Patients with nonalcoholic fatty liver disease have higher risk of colorectal adenoma after negative baseline colonoscopy. *Colorectal. Dis.* **2013**, *15*, 830–835. [CrossRef] [PubMed]

20. Sørensen, H.T.; Mellemkjaer, L.; Jepsen, P.; Thulstrup, A.M.; Baron, J.; Olsen, J.H.; Vilstrup, H. Risk of cancer in patients hospitalized with fatty liver: A Danish cohort study. *J. Clin. Gastroenterol.* **2003**, *36*, 356–359.

21. Touzin, N.T.; Bush, K.N.V.; Williams, C.D.; Harrison, S.A. Prevalence of colonic adenomas in patients with nonalcoholic fatty liver disease. *Ther. Adv. Gastroenterol.* **2011**, *4*, 169–176. [CrossRef]

22. Basyigit, S.; Uzman, M.; Kefeli, A.; Sapmaz, F.P.; Yeniova, A.O.; Nazligul, Y.; Asiltürk, Z. Absence of non-alcoholic fatty liver disease in the presence of insulin resistance is a strong predictor for colorectal carcinoma. *Int. J. Clin. Exp. Med.* **2015**, *8*, 18601–18610. [PubMed]

23. Bhatt, B.D.; Lukose, T.; Siegel, A.B.; Brown, R.S.; Verna, E.C. Increased risk of colorectal polyps in patients with non-alcoholic fatty liver disease undergoing liver transplant evaluation. *J. Gastrointest. Oncol.* **2015**, *6*, 459–468. [PubMed]

24. Wong, M.C.S.; Ching, J.Y.L.; Chan, V.C.W.; Lam, T.Y.; Luk, A.K.; Wong, S.H.; Ng, S.C.; Wong, V.W.; Ng, S.S.; Wu, J.C.; *et al.* Screening strategies for colorectal cancer among patients with nonalcoholic fatty liver disease and family history. *Int. J. Cancer* **2015**. [CrossRef]

25. Lin, X.F.; Shi, K.Q.; You, J.; Liu, W.Y.; Luo, Y.W.; Wu, F.L.; Chen, Y.P.; Wong, D.K.; Yuen, M.F.; Zheng, M.H. Increased risk of colorectal malignant neoplasm in patients with nonalcoholic fatty liver disease: A large study. *Mol. Biol. Rep.* **2014**, *41*, 2989–2997. [PubMed]

26. Bilici, A.; Ozguroglu, M.; Mihmanlı, İ.; Turna, H.; Adaletli, İ. A case—Control study of non-alcoholic fatty liver disease in breast cancer. *Med. Oncol.* **2007**, *24*, 367–371. [CrossRef]

27. Vongsuvanh, R.; George, J.; Qiao, L.; van der Poorten, D. Visceral adiposity in gastrointestinal and hepatic carcinogenesis. *Cancer Lett.* **2013**, *330*, 1–10.

28. Moore, L.L.; Bradlee, M.L.; Singer, M.R.; Splansky, G.L.; Proctor, M.H.; Ellison, R.C.; Kreger, B.E. BMI and waist circumference as predictors of lifetime colon cancer risk in Framingham Study adults. *Int. J. Obes. Relat. Metab. Disord.* **2004**, *28*, 559–567.

29. Giovannucci, E.; Ascherio, A.; Rimm, E.B.; Colditz, G.A.; Stampfer, M.J.; Willett, W.C. Physical activity, obesity, and risk for colon cancer and adenoma in men. *Ann. Intern. Med.* **1995**, *122*, 327–334. [CrossRef] [PubMed]

30. Schoen, R.E.; Tangen, C.M.; Kuller, L.H.; Burke, G.L.; Cushman, M.; Tracy, R.P.; Dobs, A.; Savage, P.J. Increased blood glucose and insulin, body size, and incident colorectal cancer. *J. Natl. Cancer Inst.* **1999**, *91*, 1147–1154. [CrossRef] [PubMed]

31. Pischon, T.; Lahmann, P.H.; Boeing, H.; Friedenreich, C.; Norat, T.; Tjønneland, A.; Halkjaer, J.; Overvad, K.; Clavel-Chapelon, F.; Boutron-Ruault, M.C.; *et al.* Body size and risk of colon and rectal cancer in the European Prospective Investigation Into Cancer and Nutrition (EPIC). *J. Natl. Cancer Inst.* **2006**, *98*, 920–931. [CrossRef] [PubMed]

32. Beddy, P.; Howard, J.; McMahon, C.; Knox, M.; de Blacam, C.; Ravi, N.; Reynolds, J.V.; Keogan, M.T. Association of visceral adiposity with oesophageal and junctional adenocarcinomas. *Br. J. Surg.* **2010**, *97*, 1028–1034. [CrossRef] [PubMed]

33. Corley, D.A.; Kubo, A.; Levin, T.R.; Block, G.; Habel, L.; Zhao, W.; Leighton, P.; Quesenberry, C.; Rumore, G.J.; Buffler, P.A. Abdominal obesity and body mass index as risk factors for Barrett's esophagus. *Gastroenterology* **2007**, *133*, 34–41. [CrossRef] [PubMed]

34. Edelstein, Z.R.; Farrow, D.C.; Bronner, M.P.; Rosen, S.N.; Vaughan, T.L. Central adiposity and risk of Barrett's esophagus. *Gastroenterology* **2007**, *133*, 403–411. [CrossRef] [PubMed]

35. El-Serag, H.B.; Kvapil, P.; Hacken-Bitar, J.; Kramer, J.R. Abdominal obesity and the risk of Barrett's esophagus. *Am. J. Gastroenterol.* **2005**, *100*, 2151–2156. [CrossRef] [PubMed]

36. Renehan, A.G.; Tyson, M.; Egger, M.; Heller, R.F.; Zwahlen, M. Body-mass index and incidence of cancer: A systematic review and meta-analysis of prospective observational studies. *Lancet* **2008**, *371*, 569–578. [CrossRef]

37. Singh, S.; Sharma, A.N.; Murad, M.H.; Buttar, N.S.; El-Serag, H.B.; Katzka, D.A.; Iyer, P.G. Central adiposity is associated with increased risk of esophageal inflammation, metaplasia, and adenocarcinoma: A systematic review and meta-analysis. *Clin. Gastroenterol. Hepatol.* **2013**, *11*, 1399–1412. [CrossRef] [PubMed]

38. Steffen, A.; Schulze, M.B.; Pischon, T.; Dietrich, T.; Molina, E.; Chirlaque, M.D.; Barricarte, A.; Amiano, P.; Quirós, J.R.; Tumino, R.; *et al.* Anthropometry and esophageal cancer risk in the European prospective investigation into cancer and nutrition. *Cancer Epidemiol. Biomark. Prev.* **2009**, *18*, 2079–2089. [CrossRef] [PubMed]

39. Aune, D.; Greenwood, D.C.; Chan, D.S.; Vieira, R.; Vieira, A.R.; Navarro Rosenblatt, D.A.; Cade, J.E.; Burley, V.J.; Norat, T. Body mass index, abdominal fatness and pancreatic cancer risk: A systematic review and non-linear dose-response meta-analysis of prospective studies. *Ann. Oncol.* **2012**, *23*, 843–852. [CrossRef] [PubMed]

40. Rose, D.P.; Vona-Davis, L. Biochemical and molecular mechanisms for the association between obesity, chronic inflammation, and breast cancer. *Biofactors* **2013**, *40*, 1–12. [CrossRef] [PubMed]

41. Schmid, D.; Ricci, C.; Behrens, G.; Leitzmann, M.F. Adiposity and risk of thyroid cancer: A systematic review and meta-analysis. *Obes. Rev.* **2015**, *16*, 1042–1054. [CrossRef] [PubMed]

42. McGrowder, D.A.; Jackson, L.A.; Crawford, T.V. Prostate cancer and metabolic syndrome: Is there a link? *Asian Pac. J. Cancer Prev.* **2012**, *13*, 1–13. [CrossRef] [PubMed]

43. Merry, A.; Schouten, L.; Goldbohm, R.; van Den Brandt, P. Body mass index, height and risk of adenocarcinoma of the oesophagus and gastric cardias: A prospective cohort study. *Gut* **2007**, *56*, 1503–1511. [CrossRef] [PubMed]

44. El-Serag, H.; Ergun, G.; Pandolfino, J.; Fitzgerald, S.; Tran, T.; Kramer, J. Obesity increases oesophageal acid exposure. *Gut* **2007**, *56*, 749–755. [CrossRef] [PubMed]

45. Kubo, A.; Cook, M.; Shaheen, N.; Vaughan, T.; Whiteman, D.; Murray, L.; Corley, D.A. Sexspecific associations between body mass index, waist circumference and the risk of Barrett's oesophagus: A pooled analysis from the international BEACON consortium. *Gut* **2013**, *62*, 1684–1691. [CrossRef] [PubMed]

46. El-Serag, H.; Hashmi, A.; Garcia, J.; Richardson, P.; Alsarraj, A.; Fitzgerald, S.; Vela, M.; Shaib, Y.; Abraham, N.S.; Velez, M.; *et al.* Visceral abdominal obesity measured by CT scan is associated with an increased risk of Barrett's oesophagus: A case-control study. *Gut* **2014**, *63*, 220–229. [CrossRef] [PubMed]

47. Garcia, J.; Splenser, A.; Kramer, J.; Alsarraj, A.; Fitzgerald, S.; Ramsey, D.; El-Serag, H.B. Circulating inflammatory cytokines and adipokines are associated with increased risk of Barrett's esophagus: A case-control study. *Clin. Gastroenterol. Hepatol.* **2014**, *12*, 229–238. [CrossRef] [PubMed]

48. Uzel, M.; Sahiner, Z.; Filik, L. Non-alcoholic fatty liver disease, metabolic syndrome and gastric cancer: Single center experience. *J. BUON* **2015**, *20*, 662. [PubMed]

49. Esposito, K.; Chiodini, P.; Colao, A.; Lenzi, A.; Giugliano, D. Metabolic syndrome and risk of cancer. *Diabetes Care* **2012**, *35*, 2402–2411. [CrossRef] [PubMed]

50. Ljungberg, B.; Bensalah, K.; Canfield, S.; Dabestani, S.; Hofmann, F.; Hora, M.; Kuczyk, M.A.; Lam, T.; Marconi, L.; Merseburger, A.S.; *et al.* EAU guidelines on renal cell carcinoma: 2014 update. *Eur. Urol.* **2015**, *67*, 913–924. [CrossRef] [PubMed]

51. Escudier, B.; Porta, C.; Schmidinger, M.; Algaba, F.; Patard, J.J.; Khoo, V.; Eisen, T.; Horwich, A. Renal cell carcinoma: ESMO clinical practice guidelines. *Ann. Oncol.* **2014**, *25*, iii49–iii56. [CrossRef] [PubMed]

52. Stocks, T.; Bjørge, T.; Ulmer, H.; Manjer, J.; Häggström, C.; Nagel, G.; Engeland, A.; Johansen, D.; Hallmans, G.; Selmer, R.; *et al.* Metabolic risk score and cancer risk: Pooled analysis of seven cohorts. *Int. J. Epidemiol.* **2015**, *44*, 1353–1363. [CrossRef] [PubMed]

53. Zhu, Y.; Wang, H.K.; Zhang, H.L.; Yao, X.D.; Zhang, S.L.; Dai, B.; Shen, Y.J.; Liu, X.H.; Zhou, L.P.; Ye, D.W. Visceral obesity and risk of high grade disease in clinical T1A renal cell carcinoma. *J. Urol.* **2013**, *189*, 447–453. [CrossRef] [PubMed]

54. Horiguchi, A.; Ito, K.; Sumitomo, M.; Kimura, F.; Asano, T.; Hayakawa, M. Decreased serum adiponectin levels in patients with metastatic renal cell carcinoma. *Jpn. J. Clin. Oncol.* **2008**, *38*, 106–111. [CrossRef] [PubMed]

55. Lawlor, D.A.; Smith, G.D.; Ebrahim, S. Hyperinsulinaemia and increased risk of breast cancer: Findings from the British Women's Heart and Health Study. *Cancer Causes Control* **2004**, *15*, 267–275. [CrossRef] [PubMed]

56. Rosato, V.; Bosetti, C.; Talamini, R.; Levi, F.; Montella, M.; Giacosa, A.; Negri, E.; La Vecchia, C. Metabolic syndrome and the risk of breast cancer in postmenopausal women. *Ann. Oncol.* **2011**, *22*, 2687–2692. [CrossRef] [PubMed]

57. Agnoli, C.; Berrino, F.; Abagnato, C.A.; Muti, P.; Panico, S.; Crosignani, P.; Krogh, V. Metabolic syndrome and postmenopausal breast cancer in the ORDET cohort: A nested case-control study. *Nutr. Metab. Cardiovasc. Dis.* **2010**, *20*, 41–48. [CrossRef] [PubMed]

58. Berrino, F.; Villarini, A.; Traina, A.; Bonanni, B.; Panico, S.; Mano, M.P.; Mercandino, A.; Galasso, R.; Barbero, M.; Simeoni, M.; *et al.* Metabolic syndrome and breast cancer prognosis. *Breast Cancer Res. Treat.* **2014**, *147*, 159–165. [CrossRef] [PubMed]

59. MacInnis, R.J.; English, D.R. Body size and composition and prostate cancer risk: Systematic review and meta-regression analysis. *Cancer Causes Control* **2006**, *17*, 989–1003. [CrossRef] [PubMed]

60. Choi, W.M.; Lee, J.H.; Yoon, J.H.; Kwak, C.; Lee, Y.J.; Cho, Y.Y.; Lee, Y.B.; Yu, S.J.; Kim, Y.J.; Kim, H.H.; *et al.* Nonalcoholic fatty liver disease is a negative risk factor for prostate cancer recurrence. *Endocr. Relat. Cancer* **2014**, *21*, 343–353. [CrossRef] [PubMed]

61. Arase, Y.; Kobayashi, M.; Suzuki, F.; Suzuki, Y.; Kawamura, Y.; Akuta, N.; Imai, N.; Kobayashi, M.; Sezaki, H.; Matsumoto, N.; *et al.* Difference in malignancies of chronic liver disease due to non-alcoholic fatty liver disease or hepatitis C in Japanese elderly patients. *Hepatol. Res.* **2012**, *42*, 264–272. [CrossRef] [PubMed]

62. Wigg, A.J.; Roberts-Thomson, I.C.; Dymock, R.B.; McCarthy, P.J.; Grose, R.H.; Cummins, A.G. The role of small intestinal bacterial overgrowth, intestinal permeability, endotoxaemia, and tumour necrosis factor α in the pathogenesis of non-alcoholic steatohepatitis. *Gut* **2001**, *48*, 206–211. [CrossRef] [PubMed]

63. Ohtani, N.; Yoshimoto, S.; Hara, E. Obesity and cancer: A gut microbial connection. *Cancer Res.* **2014**, *74*, 1885–1889. [CrossRef] [PubMed]

64. Lee, Y.Y. What is obesity doing to your gut? *Malays. J. Med. Sci.* **2015**, *22*, 1–3. [PubMed]

65. Moran, C.P.; Shanahan, F. Gut microbiota and obesity: Role in aetiology and potential therapeutic target. *Best Pract. Res. Clin. Gastroenterol.* **2014**, *28*, 585–597. [CrossRef] [PubMed]

66. Mehal, W.Z. The Gordian Knot of dysbiosis, obesity and NAFLD. *Nat. Rev. Gastroenterol. Hepatol.* **2013**, *10*, 637–644. [CrossRef] [PubMed]

67. Louis, P.; Hold, G.L.; Flint, H.J. The gut microbiota, bacterial metabolites and colorectal cancer. *Nat. Rev. Microbiol.* **2014**, *12*, 661–672. [CrossRef] [PubMed]

68. Spruss, A.; Kanuri, G.; Wagnerberger, S.; Haub, S.; Bischoff, S.C.; Bergheim, I. Toll-like receptor 4 is involved in the development of fructose-induced hepatic steatosis in mice. *Hepatology* **2009**, *50*, 1094–1104. [CrossRef] [PubMed]

69. Gilbert, C.A.; Slingerland, J.M. Cytokines, obesity, and cancer: New insights on mechanisms linking obesity to cancer risk and progression. *Annu. Rev. Med.* **2013**, *64*, 45–57. [CrossRef] [PubMed]

70. Hui, J.M.; Hodge, A.; Farrell, G.C.; Kench, J.G.; Kriketos, A.; George, J. Beyond insulin resistance in NASH: TNF-α or adiponectin? *Hepatology* **2004**, *40*, 46–54. [CrossRef] [PubMed]

71. Giovannucci, E. Nutrition, insulin, insulin-like growth factors and cancer. *Horm. Metab. Res.* **2003**, *35*, 694–704. [PubMed]

72. Pérez-Hernández, A.I.; Catalán, V.; Gómez-Ambrosi, J.; Rodríguez, A.; Frühbeck, G. Mechanisms linking excess adiposity and carcinogenesis promotion. *Front. Endocrinol.* **2014**, *5*, 65. [CrossRef]

73. Van Kruijsdijk, R.C.M.; van der Wall, E.; Visseren, F.L.J. Obesity and cancer: The role of dysfunctional adipose tissue. *Cancer Epidemiol. Biomark. Prev.* **2009**, *18*, 2569–2578. [CrossRef] [PubMed]

74. Grimberg, A.; Cohen, P. Role of insulin-like growth factors and their binding proteins in growth control and carcinogenesis. *J. Cell. Physiol.* **2000**, *183*, 1–9. [CrossRef]

75. Chan, J.M.; Stampfer, M.J.; Giovannucci, E.; Gann, P.H.; Ma, J.; Wilkinson, P.; Hennekens, C.H.; Pollak, M. Plasma insulin-like growth factor-I and prostate cancer risk: A prospective study. *Science* **1998**, *279*, 563–566. [CrossRef] [PubMed]

76. Giovannucci, E.; Pollak, M.N.; Platz, E.A.; Willett, W.C.; Stampfer, M.J.; Majeed, N.; Colditz, G.A.; Speizer, F.E.; Hankinson, S.E. A prospective study of plasma insulin-like growth factor-1 and binding protein-3 and risk of colorectal neoplasia in women. *Cancer Epidemiol. Biomark. Prev.* **2000**, *9*, 345–349.

77. Yu, H.; Spitz, M.R.; Mistry, J.; Gu, J.; Hong, W.K.; Wu, X. Plasma levels of insulin-like growth factor-I and lung cancer risk: A case-control analysis. *J. Natl. Cancer Inst.* **1999**, *91*, 151–156. [CrossRef] [PubMed]

78. Hankinson, S.E.; Willett, W.C.; Colditz, G.A.; Hunter, D.J.; Michaud, D.S.; Deroo, B.; Rosner, B.; Speizer, F.E.; Pollak, M. Circulating concentrations of insulin-like growth factor-I and risk of breast cancer. *Lancet* **1998**, *351*, 1393–1396. [CrossRef]

79. Donohoe, C.L.; O'Farrell, N.J.; Doyle, S.L.; Reynolds, J.V. The role of obesity in gastrointestinal cancer: Evidence and opinion. *Ther. Adv. Gastroenterol.* **2014**, *7*, 38–50. [CrossRef] [PubMed]

80. Doyle, S.L.; Donohoe, C.L.; Finn, S.P.; Howard, J.M.; Lithander, F.E.; Reynolds, J.V.; Pidgeon, G.P.; Lysaght, J. IGF-1 and its receptor in esophageal cancer: Association with adenocarcinoma and visceral obesity. *Am. J. Gastroenterol.* **2012**, *107*, 196–204. [CrossRef] [PubMed]

81. Siahpush, S.H.; Vaughan, T.L.; Lampe, J.N.; Freeman, R.; Lewis, S.; Odze, R.D.; Blount, P.L.; Ayub, K.; Rabinovitch, P.S.; Reid, B.J.; *et al.* Longitudinal study of insulin-like growth factor, insulin-like growth factor binding protein-3, and their polymorphisms: Risk of neoplastic progression in Barrett's esophagus. *Cancer Epidemiol. Biomark. Prev.* **2007**, *16*, 2387–2395. [CrossRef] [PubMed]

82. Endo, H.; Hosono, K.; Uchiyama, T.; Sakai, E.; Sugiyama, M.; Takahashi, H.; Nakajima, N.; Wada, K.; Takeda, K.; Nakagama, H.; *et al.* Leptin acts as a growth factor for colorectal tumours at stages subsequent to tumour initiation in murine colon carcinogenesis. *Gut* **2011**, *60*, 1363–1371. [CrossRef] [PubMed]

83. Jaffe, T.; Schwartz, B. Leptin promotes motility and invasiveness in human colon cancer cells by activating multiple signal-transduction pathways. *Int. J. Cancer* **2008**, *123*, 2543–2556. [CrossRef] [PubMed]

84. Ho, G.Y.F.; Wang, T.; Gunter, M.J.; Strickler, H.D.; Cushman, M.; Kaplan, R.C.; Wassertheil-Smoller, S.; Xue, X.; Rajpathak, S.N.; Chlebowski, R.T.; *et al.* Adipokines linking obesity with colorectal cancer risk in postmenopausal women. *Cancer Res.* **2012**, *72*, 3029–3037. [CrossRef] [PubMed]

85. Rubenstein, J.H.; Dahlkemper, A.; Kao, J.Y.; Zhang, M.; Morgenstern, H.; McMahon, L.; Inadomi, J.M. A pilot study of the association of low plasma adiponectin and Barrett's esophagus. *Am. J. Gastroenterol.* **2008**, *103*, 1358–1364. [CrossRef] [PubMed]

86. Rubenstein, J.H.; Morgenstern, H.; McConell, D.; Scheiman, J.M.; Schoenfeld, P.; Appelman, H.; McMahon, L.F., Jr.; Kao, J.Y.; Metko, V.; Zhang, M.; *et al.* Associations of diabetes mellitus, insulin, leptin, and ghrelin with gastroesophageal reflux and Barrett's esophagus. *Gastroenterology* **2013**, *145*, 1237–1244. [CrossRef] [PubMed]

87. Ryan, A.M.; Healy, L.A.; Power, D.G.; Byrne, M.; Murphy, S.; Byrne, P.J.; Kelleher, D.; Reynolds, J.V. Barrett esophagus: Prevalence of central adiposity, metabolic syndrome, and a proinflammatory state. *Ann. Surg.* **2008**, *247*, 909–915. [CrossRef] [PubMed]

88. Chandar, A.K.; Devanna, S.; Lu, C.; Singh, S.; Greer, K.; Chak, A.; Iyer, P.G. Association of serum levels of adipokines and insulin with risk of barrett's esophagus: A systematic review and meta-analysis. *Clin. Gastroenterol. Hepatol.* **2015**, *13*, 2241–2255. [CrossRef] [PubMed]

89. Francois, F.; Roper, J.; Goodman, A.J.; Pei, Z.; Ghumman, M.; Mourad, M.; de Perez, A.Z.; Perez-Perez, G.I.; Tseng, C.; Blaser, M.J. The association of gastric leptin with oesophageal inflammation and metaplasia. *Gut* **2008**, *57*, 16–24. [CrossRef] [PubMed]

90. Kendall, B.J.; Macdonald, G.A.; Hayward, N.K.; Prins, J.B.; Brown, I.; Walker, N.; Pandeya, N.; Green, A.C.; Webb, P.M.; Whiteman, D.C.; *et al.* Leptin and the risk of Barrett's oesophagus. *Gut* **2008**, *57*, 448–454. [CrossRef] [PubMed]

91. Delort, L.; Rossary, A.; Farges, M.-C.; Vasson, M.-P.; Caldefie-Chézet, F. Leptin, adipocytes and breast cancer: Focus on inflammation and anti-tumor immunity. *Life Sci.* **2015**, *140*, 37–48. [CrossRef] [PubMed]

92. Macciò, A.; Madeddu, C.; Mantovani, G. Adipose tissue as target organ in the treatment of hormone-dependent breast cancer: New therapeutic perspectives. *Obes. Rev.* **2009**, *10*, 660–670. [CrossRef] [PubMed]

93. Caldefie-Chézet, F.; Dubois, V.; Delort, L.; Rossary, A.; Vasson, M.-P. Leptin: Involvement in the pathophysiology of breast cancer. *Ann. Endocrinol.* **2013**, *74*, 90–101. [CrossRef] [PubMed]

94. Filková, M.; Haluzík, M.; Gay, S.; Senolt, L. The role of resistin as a regulator of inflammation: Implications for various human pathologies. *Clin. Immunol.* **2009**, *133*, 157–170. [CrossRef] [PubMed]

95. Karapanagiotou, E.M.; Tsochatzis, E.A.; Dilana, K.D.; Tourkantonis, I.; Gratsias, I.; Syrigos, K.N. The significance of leptin, adiponectin, and resistin serum levels in non-small cell lung cancer (NSCLC). *Lung Cancer* **2008**, *61*, 391–397. [CrossRef] [PubMed]

96. Tiaka, E.K.; Manolakis, A.C.; Kapsoritakis, A.N.; Potamianos, S.P. The implication of adiponectin and resistin in gastrointestinal diseases. *Cytokine Growth Factor Rev.* **2011**, *22*, 109–119. [CrossRef] [PubMed]

97. Codoñer-Franch, P.; Alonso-Iglesias, E. Resistin: Insulin resistance to malignancy. *Clin. Chim. Acta* **2015**, *438*, 46–54. [CrossRef] [PubMed]

98. Hursting, S.D.; Dunlap, S.M. Obesity, metabolic dysregulation, and cancer: A growing concern and an inflammatory (and microenvironmental) issue. *Ann. N. Y. Acad. Sci.* **2012**, *1271*, 82–87. [CrossRef] [PubMed]

99. Yadav, A.; Kumar, B.; Datta, J.; Teknos, T.N.; Kumar, P. IL-6 promotes head and neck tumor metastasis by inducing epithelial-mesenchymal transition via the JAK-STAT3-SNAIL signaling pathway. *Mol. Cancer Res.* **2011**, *9*, 1658–1667. [CrossRef] [PubMed]

100. Naylor, M.S.; Stamp, G.W.; Foulkes, W.D.; Eccles, D.; Balkwill, F.R. Tumor necrosis factor and its receptors in human ovarian cancer. Potential role in disease progression. *J. Clin. Investig.* **1993**, *91*, 2194–2206. [CrossRef] [PubMed]

101. Ferrajoli, A.; Keating, M.J.; Manshouri, T.; Giles, F.J.; Dey, A.; Estrov, Z.; Koller, C.A.; Kurzrock, R.; Thomas, D.A.; Faderl, S.; *et al.* The clinical significance of tumor necrosis factor-α plasma level in patients having chronic lymphocytic leukemia. *Blood* **2002**, *100*, 1215–1219. [PubMed]

102. Pikarsky, E.; Porat, R.M.; Stein, I.; Abramovitch, R.; Amit, S.; Kasem, S.; Gutkovich-Pyest, E.; Urieli-Shoval, S.; Galun, E.; Ben-Neriah, Y. NF-κB functions as a tumour promoter in inflammation-associated cancer. *Nature* **2004**, *431*, 461–466. [CrossRef] [PubMed]

103. Balkwill, F. Tumour necrosis factor and cancer. *Nat. Rev. Cancer* **2009**, *9*, 361–371. [CrossRef] [PubMed]

104. Liu, Z.; Brooks, R.S.; Ciappio, E.D.; Kim, S.J.; Crott, J.W.; Bennett, G.; Greenberg, A.S.; Mason, J.B. Diet-induced obesity elevates colonic TNF-α in mice and is accompanied by an activation of Wnt signaling: A mechanism for obesity-associated colorectal cancer. *J. Nutr. Biochem.* **2012**, *23*, 1207–1213. [CrossRef] [PubMed]

105. Angelo, L.S.; Talpaz, M.; Kurzrock, R. Autocrine interleukin-6 production in renal cell carcinoma: Evidence for the involvement of p53. *Cancer Res.* **2002**, *62*, 932–940. [PubMed]

106. Kai, H.; Kitadai, Y.; Kodama, M.; Cho, S.; Kuroda, T.; Ito, M.; Tanaka, S.; Ohmoto, Y.; Chayama, K. Involvement of proinflammatory cytokines IL-1β and IL-6 in progression of human gastric carcinoma. *Anticancer Res.* **2005**, *25*, 709–713. [PubMed]

107. Sethi, G.; Shanmugam, M.K.; Ramachandran, L.; Kumar, A.P.; Tergaonkar, V. Multifaceted link between cancer and inflammation. *Biosci. Rep.* **2012**, *32*, 1–15. [CrossRef] [PubMed]

108. Chung, Y.-C.; Chang, Y.-F. Serum interleukin-6 levels reflect the disease status of colorectal cancer. *J. Surg. Oncol.* **2003**, *83*, 222–226. [CrossRef] [PubMed]

109. Lin, W.-W.; Karin, M. A cytokine-mediated link between innate immunity, inflammation, and cancer. *J. Clin. Investig.* **2007**, *117*, 1175–1183. [CrossRef] [PubMed]

14

The Natural Course of Non-Alcoholic Fatty Liver Disease

Luis Calzadilla Bertot [1] and Leon Anton Adams [1,2,*]

[1] School of Medicine and Pharmacology, the University of Western Australia, Nedlands, WA 6009, Australia; lcbertot@gmail.com

[2] Department of Hepatology, Sir Charles Gairdner Hospital, Nedlands, WA 6009, Australia

* Correspondence: leon.adams@uwa.edu.au

Academic Editors: Amedeo Lonardo and Giovanni Targher

Abstract: Non-alcoholic fatty liver disease (NAFLD) is the most prevalent form of chronic liver disease in the world, paralleling the epidemic of obesity and Type 2 diabetes mellitus (T2DM). NAFLD exhibits a histological spectrum, ranging from "bland steatosis" to the more aggressive necro-inflammatory form, non-alcoholic steatohepatitis (NASH) which may accumulate fibrosis to result in cirrhosis. Emerging data suggests fibrosis, rather than NASH *per se*, to be the most important histological predictor of liver and non-liver related death. Nevertheless, only a small proportion of individuals develop cirrhosis, however the large proportion of the population affected by NAFLD has led to predictions that NAFLD will become a leading cause of end stage liver disease, hepatocellular carcinoma (HCC), and indication for liver transplantation. HCC may arise in non-cirrhotic liver in the setting of NAFLD and is associated with the presence of the metabolic syndrome (MetS) and male gender. The MetS and its components also play a key role in the histological progression of NAFLD, however other genetic and environmental factors may also influence the natural history. The importance of NAFLD in terms of overall survival extends beyond the liver where cardiovascular disease and malignancy represents additional important causes of death.

Keywords: nonalcoholic fatty liver; non-alcoholic steatohepatitis; fibrosis; hepatocellular carcinoma; cirrhosis; non-cirrhotic

1. Introduction

The prevalence of non-alcoholic fatty liver disease (NAFLD) parallels that of obesity, which has steadily risen throughout the world over the past thirty years [1]. The natural history of NAFLD in some individuals, is to progress to end-stage liver disease. Thus, NAFLD is projected to become the leading cause of liver related morbidity and mortality within 20 years and a leading indication for liver transplantation in the next few years [2]. Although the potential for NAFLD to progress to both cirrhosis and hepatocellular carcinoma (HCC) has been recognized for decades, more recent insights have helped define the magnitude of risk of progression and led to the understanding that NAFLD is a leading cause of cryptogenic cirrhosis [3–6]. More recently, accumulating evidence has also led to the hypotheses that even steatosis and mild inflammation can progress to fibrosis and HCC [7–9]. Nevertheless, the natural history of NAFLD remains incompletely defined, with key knowledge gaps including the lack of understanding behind the substantial inter-individual variation in disease progression and outcomes and understanding of the links between NAFLD and HCC. In this review we provide an up to date assessment of the natural history of NAFLD and emerging evidence that may impact the management of this disease in the future.

2. Histological Course of Non-Alcoholic Fatty Liver Disease (NAFLD)

Non-alcoholic fatty liver disease (NAFLD) encompasses a histological spectrum from non-alcoholic fatty liver (NAFL), which is characterized by steatosis with no or minor inflammation, to non-alcoholic steatohepatitis (NASH) where inflammation and ballooning is present, with or without fibrosis. The natural history of NASH tends to parallels the more aggressive histological picture, with prospective cohort studies demonstrating a higher rate of morbidity and mortality compared to NAFL, particularly when fibrosis is present [10,11]. Nevertheless, a limited amount of high-quality prospective data on the progression of NAFLD exists, particularly in the primary-care setting, where routine biochemical indices do not accurately reflect disease activity or progression. Paired liver biopsy studies from tertiary care cohorts provide valuable information however are limited in their generalizability due to selection bias.

At least 12 studies have analysed the progression of steatosis, steatohepatitis, and fibrosis in NAFLD cohorts by utilizing paired liver biopsies [7,9,11–20]. These studies suggest that one third of patients with NAFL and NASH have progressive fibrosis and 20% will have some regression over an average follow-up between 2.2 and 13.8 years [7,9,11–23]. The rate of fibrosis progression is characteristically slow with a recent meta-analysis determining an average progression of one stage to take 7.7 years [24]. Nevertheless, the rate of progression is twice as high in NASH subjects and a sub-group of both NASH and NAFL patients may progress rapidly from no fibrosis to advanced fibrosis over an average six year period [8,9]. In contrast to fibrosis progression over time, features of steatosis, inflammation and ballooning tend to reduce which is paralleled by reduction in amino-transaminase levels [12]. Factors that may influence the histological progression of NASH are illustrated in Table 1, Figure 1 and outlined below.

Table 1. Risk factors for fibrosis progression in non-alcoholic fatty liver disease (NAFLD): Results from paired liver biopsy studies.

Study Author, Year	n	Mean/Median (Standard Deviation or Range) Follow up in Years	Predictors of Fibrosis Progression	Odds Ratio (95% CI)
Adams (2005)	103	3.2 (±3.0)	Diabetes Fibrosis stage BMI (per kg/m^2)	1.48 0.80 1.04
Fassio (2004)	22	4.3 (3.0–14.3)	Obesity	NR
Argo (2009) *	221	5.3 (1.0–21.3)	Age Any inflammation at initial biopsy	0.98 (0.96–0.99) 2.5 (1.4–4.3)
Wong (2010)	52	3, NR	High LDL High waist circumference	2.7 (1.2 to 6.1) 1.3 (1.1 to 1.5)
Sorrentino (2010)	149	6.4	Fibronectin immunohistochemistry Hypertension HOMA-IR > 10	14.1 (6.9–32.3) 4.8 (2.7–18.2) 1.9 (1.6–12.1)
Pais (2013)	70	3.7 (±2.1)	^ steatosis grade	NR
Chan (2014)	35	6.4 (±0.8)	nil	-
McPherson (2014)	108	6.6 (1.3–22.6)	At baseline biopsy FIB 4 score At follow up biopsy FIB 4 score Diabetes	2.1 (1.1–3.9) 3.1 (1.4–6.8) 6.25 (1.88–20)
Singh (2015) **	411	NR	Hypertension Low AST:ALT ratio at baseline biopsy	1.94 (1.00–3.74) −0.08 (−0.16–0.00)

* A systematic review comprising 10 studies; ** A meta-analysis including 11 cohort studies; ^ Progression defined by progression from non-alcoholic fatty liver (NAFL) to non-alcoholic steatohepatitis (NASH), occurrence of bridging fibrosis or at least one point increase in the NAFLD activity score (NAS) score from <5 to 5, or greater; NR = Not reported; HOMA–IR = homeostasis model of assessment-insulin resistance.

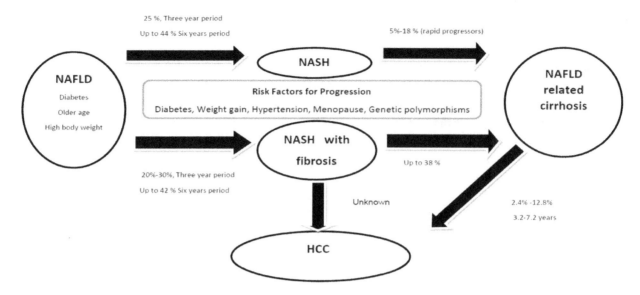

Figure 1. Progression of non-alcoholic fatty liver disease (NAFLD) to non-alcoholic steatohepatitis (NASH) with or without fibrosis, cirrhosis, and hepatocellular carcinoma. Data adapted form [7–9] and [24].

3. Predictors of Progressive Fibrosis in Non-Alcoholic Steatohepatitis (NASH)

3.1. Sex

No consistent relationship between sex and fibrosis has been found in NASH, with cross-sectional studies reporting conflicting findings [25,26]. The relationship between sex and fibrosis may be influenced by menopausal status; cross-sectional studies have found men and post-menopausal women to have a higher risk of fibrosis compared with pre-menopausal women, and early menopause and duration of menopause to be associated with a higher risk of fibrosis [27,28].

3.2. Race and Ethnicity

Hispanic patients have an increased prevalence of NAFLD compared to Caucasians; however, there appears to be no difference in degree of liver injury between these ethnic groups [29,30]. In contrast, Asian patients may be prone to more severe histological changes including ballooning, whereas African-Americans may have less severe histology, although factors such as diet may be confounding this relationship [31–33].

3.3. Genetic Polymorphisms

Polymorphisms in the *PNPLA3* and *TM6SF2* genes are common in the general population with minor allele frequencies of 20%–50% and 10%, respectively [34]. The rs738409 and rs58542926 single nucleotide polymorphisms (SNP's) of these respective genes have been identified by genome-wide association studies to be associated with an increased risk of NAFLD, as well the presence of more severe liver histology (*i.e.*, NASH and fibrosis) [34–38]. One study of over 1000 individuals with biopsy proven NAFLD, demonstrated these SNPs were associated with a 40% to 88% increased risk for advanced (F2-4) fibrosis after adjustment for age, sex, and metabolic variables [34]. Similarly, a SNP in the *IFNL4* gene, which is associated with response to interferon based treatment in chronic hepatitis C, has also been associated with fibrosis in NAFLD and has been amalgamated into a predictive score in conjunction with other clinical factors [39].

3.4. Age

Cross-sectional studies have demonstrated increasing age to be consistently associated with more severe fibrosis in NASH patients; however, this may reflect the cumulative sum of metabolic exposures and longer duration of NAFL/NASH in these populations [26,40,41]. In contrast, longitudinal studies have not consistently demonstrated age to impact the rate of fibrosis progression [24].

3.5. Metabolic Features

Diabetes and obesity have demonstrated to be predictive of a higher rate of fibrosis progression in some but not all longitudinal studies [7–9,12,22]. An increase or decrease in body mass index over time, has been associated with progression or resolution of liver fibrosis respectively in NAFLD patients and the emergence of diabetes also appears to parallel fibrosis progression, whereas improved glycemic control parallels fibrosis improvement [7–9,22]. One meta-analysis examining the full spectrum of NAFLD found hypertension to be a risk factor for fibrosis progression, however an earlier meta-analysis limited to NASH patients did not [24,42].

3.6. Histological Factors

The degree of hepatic steatosis does not appear to predict disease progression in NASH. The degree of inflammation however, has been associated with progression to advanced fibrosis in a meta-analysis, but not in any single cohort study [24].

4. Clinical Course of NAFLD

4.1. Liver Cirrhosis, Decompensation, and Liver Related Mortality

Overall, the risk of progression to cirrhosis and decompensation in NAFLD patients is low with a population based study demonstrating an incidence of 3.1% for both end-points over a mean 7.6 year follow-up [43]. Nevertheless, the risk of cirrhosis may be underestimated given the lack of systematic evaluation for its development in the community.

The risk of progression to end-stage liver disease is influenced by the severity of underlying liver histology; the majority of patients with NAFLD have simple steatosis, however, up to 30% of patients may have NASH [44] and are at greater risk. Several studies with up to 20 years follow-up, have demonstrated that the risk of progression to cirrhosis in patients with simple steatosis is between 0% and 4% [6,45,46]. In contrast, estimates of progression to cirrhosis in NASH patients varies with 10% developing decompensated liver disease over 13 years [11] and 25% developing cirrhosis over nine years [11]. The rate of progression is clearly heavily influenced by the underlying fibrosis stage, with NASH patients without fibrosis at significantly lower risk compared to those with advanced fibrosis. Progression to advanced fibrosis and cirrhosis is not uniform in all patients and metabolic factors such as presence of glucose intolerance and Type 2 diabetes mellitus (T2DM) may play a key role in this progression [47,48].

Once cirrhosis has developed, the risk of developing a major complication of portal hypertension is 17%, 23%, and 52% at one, three, and 10 years, respectively [49]. The survival of patients with NASH cirrhosis falls markedly once decompensation occurs, with a median survival of approximately two years [50]. Today, NAFLD is the second commonest etiology for listing for liver transplantation, and on the trajectory of becoming the most common cause [51–54]. Notably, the burden of NAFLD related cirrhosis may be under-estimated, as the histological signs of steatohepatitis may no longer be present at the cirrhotic stage of disease [55]. Caldwell *et al.* noted that a large proportion of patients with cryptogenic cirrhosis had been exposed to metabolic risk factors [4] and almost half of the cases of "cryptogenic" cirrhosis could ultimately be traced to the end-stage evolution of NASH [39].

Compared with individuals of the general population of the same age and gender, those with NAFLD have a lower than expected survival, at a standardized mortality ratio from 1.34 to 1.69 according to American and Swedish studies [11,12]. The increase in mortality hazard is likely in part, to be related to increased liver related mortality, with liver death the third commonest cause of death in two large cohort studies [11,12].

4.2. Non-Liver Related Death

NAFLD is associated with a significantly higher overall mortality compared to the age and sex-matched general population, which in part is likely related to excess vascular as well as liver-related death. Cross-sectional population-based studies and meta-analysis have demonstrated NAFLD to be independently associated with predictors of cardiovascular disease including endothelial dysfunction, arterial stiffness and myocardial dysfunction [56–59]. Notably, NAFLD results in hepatic insulin resistance, increased fasting glucose levels and an atherogenic lipid profile [60], and NASH is associated with increased levels of inflammatory pro-atherogenic cytokines, hyper-coagulable factors, and adhesion molecules [61].

Supporting these observations, analysis of over 11,000 participants in the NAHNES study conducted between 1989 and 2004 with median follow up of 14.5 years, demonstrated increased (69%) overall mortality in NAFLD patients with advanced fibrosis assessed by means of NAFLD fibrosis score, APRI and FIB 4. The increase in mortality in this subgroup was largely driven by cardiovascular disease (CVD) (adjusted hazard ratio 2.7 to 3.5) [62]. Other cohort studies have suggested that other sub-groups of NAFLD patients, such as those with type 2 diabetes [63] or men with an elevated gamma-glutamyl transpeptidase [57], may have an increased risk of CVD events compared to subjects without NAFLD. Thus, there may be other genetic or environmental factors that modify the association between NAFLD and CVD. Lastly, severity of liver histology may stratify risk of cardiovascular mortality with Ekstedt and colleagues demonstrating that subjects with simple steatosis did not have an increased risk of all-cause death or death related to CVD, but those with NASH were twice as likely to die from CVD compared to the reference general population (15.5% *vs.* 7.5%) over a mean follow-up period of 13.7 years [64].

5. Evolving Concepts

5.1. NAFL vs. NASH

A pioneer research published in 2006 compared the levels of serum concentrations of transforming growth factor-beta1 (TGF-β1) a marker of fibrosis, and ferritin between NAFL, and NASH patients [40]. No differences in the serum levels of TGF-β1 and ferritin were found between NAFL and NASH groups. Authors suggested that both NAFLD spectrums share common aspects regarding their progression and NAFL perhaps not so benign. Recent reports suggest NAFL may not be as benign as previously thought, with evidence of progression to advanced fibrosis, challenging the paradigm that risk of fibrosis progression is dichotomized according to the presence or absence of NASH (Table 2). Wong *et al.* [7] reported in a prospective study of paired liver biopsies taken a median three years apart, that 58% of patients with histological NAFLD activity score (NAS) <3 (*i.e.*, non-NASH) increased their activity score and 28% had fibrosis progression at three years. Fibrosis progression was seen in 20% to 30% of patients with both low and high NAS scores. Twenty-three per cent of patients with simple steatosis developed NASH in 3 years.

A retrospective study analysing a database of 70 NAFLD patients with paired biopsies showed that patients with NAFL can evolve towards well-defined steatohepatitis, and in some of them, bridging fibrosis after a follow-up of less than 5 years. The presence of mild lobular inflammation or any amount of fibrosis substantially increased the risk of histological progression in the mid-term while those with steatosis alone are at lowest risk [8]. More recently McPherson *et al.* [9] in the DELTA study included 108 patients with paired liver biopsies over a median of 6.6 years; they found overall that NAFLD had a variable natural history with 42% of patients having progression of fibrosis and 18% having regression of fibrosis. Of those with NAFL at the index liver biopsy, 44% progressed to NASH and 37% had progression of fibrosis, including 6 patients who developed stage three fibrosis.

Lastly, Singh *et al.* conducted a systematic review and meta-analysis of 11 studies involving 411 patients with paired liver biopsies [24]. Patients with both NAFL and NASH were found to develop progressive liver fibrosis, although the rate of fibrosis progression was higher in those with NASH than NAFL (one-stage progression over 7.1 years *vs.* 14.3 years, respectively). Collectively, these studies suggest that overall NAFL has a more indolent rate of progression than NASH; however, there is considerable heterogeneity, with one quarter of NAFL patients developing bridging fibrosis over a relatively short time period. Currently, reliable histological and clinical predictors of disease progression are lacking, however it appears that worsening metabolic disease (weight gain, diabetes) frequently parallels the histological progression [8,9].

Table 2. Fibrosis stage as predictor of liver related complications, death, and overall mortality.

Study Author, Year	NAFLD Patients (n)	Mean Follow up (Years)	Histological Subgroup (N)	Cirrhosis and Liver Related Complications HR	Liver Related Mortality HR	Overall Mortality HR
Ekstedt et al., 2015	229	26.4	NAS 0–8 Fibrosis stage 3–4 n = 16	10.8	3.3	3.28
Younossi et al., 2011	257	12.1	Fibrosis stage 3–4 n = NR	-	5.68	-
Angulo et al., 2015	619	12.6	Fibrosis stage			
			F1 n = 141	* 2.38	-	1.88
			F2 n = 85	* 7.51	11.2	2.89
			F3 n = 53	* 13.78	85.79	3.76
			F4 n = 18	* 47.46	-	10.9

* Results derived from a multivariate model including age, sex, race, BMI, diabetes, hypertension, statin use, site, and smoking. HR (hazard ratio).

5.2. Prognostic Significance of NASH vs. Fibrosis

The prognosis of an individual patient with NAFLD is highly variable. A greater likelihood of progressive disease was initially described in those patients with NASH, which is often defined according to the NAFLD activity score (NAS score). The NAS is the unbalanced sum of steatosis, ballooning, and lobular inflammation [10], and was originally developed as a tool for assessing efficacy in clinical trials, however has been applied more widely to define NASH and assess histological activity.

Recent evidence coming from prospective cohort studies suggest that fibrosis predicts liver and non-liver related mortality more reliably than NAS or its individual components [64–66]. A study by Younossi et al. of 209 NAFLD patients with a median follow up of 12 years found that advanced fibrosis was the only histological lesion independently associated with liver-related mortality (hazard ratio = 5.68, 95% confidence interval (1.5–21.4) [66] More recently Ekstedt and colleagues analysed a cohort of 229 biopsy proven NAFLD patients followed for a mean of 26.4 years [62]. Overall, NAFLD patients had an increased mortality compared with a matched reference population with NAFLD subjects with fibrosis stage three or four at baseline having the worst prognosis (HR 3.3, CI 2.27–4.76, $p < 0.001$). In contrast patients with a high NAS (5–8) without severe fibrosis did not have increase mortality compared with reference population. Finally, Angulo et al. conducted an international multicentre cohort study to determine the long term prognostic significance of histologic features of NAFLD [65]. This study confirmed that fibrosis stage rather than NASH, was the most important histological feature associated with overall survival and liver-related complications. Notably, even patients with mild fibrosis (stage 1) had a greater hazard for overall mortality compared to those with no fibrosis, although only those with moderate fibrosis (stage F2 and above) had a greater risk of liver related complications such as ascites, encephalopathy or varices. These studies emphasize the need to assess fibrosis routinely in all patients with NAFLD to assess their prognosis and, thus, need for monitoring and liver targeted treatment.

6. Hepatocellular Carcinoma (HCC)

6.1. HCC in NAFLD

HCC is the six most common cancer worldwide, the third most common cause of cancer related death and has a globally rising incidence [67,68]. Several studies have demonstrated an association between MetS, T2DM as well as obesity, with HCC, suggesting that NAFLD is playing a significant role in the rising incidence of HCC [67,69,70]. The potential mechanisms relating MetS, obesity, diabetes, NAFLD, and HCC, particularly in the absence of cirrhosis, are probably related to the pathogenesis of the underlying disease rather than to fibrosis alone. A fertile soil for liver carcinogenesis include insulin resistance and hepatic steatosis promoting adipose tissue-derived inflammation, hormonal changes (adipokines), oxidative stress, lipopoxicity, and stimulation of insulin-like growth factor [21,69,70]. Gut microbiome, diet, and genetics are increasingly important factors. Intestinal dysbiosis associated with obesity modify the gut microbiome and promotes the release of endotoxins [22]. High-fat diets and high fructose intake can worsen the cytokine pattern and promote lipoperoxidation [70]. Genetics contributes to increase the risk of HCC, mainly through the *PNPLA3* rs738409 variant [23].

NASH was found to be the third most common risk factor for HCC in a U.S. veterans population of 1500 with HCC diagnosed over a six year period [71]. Nevertheless, HCC remains an uncommon complication of NAFLD and heavily influenced by the presence or absence of underlying cirrhosis. For example, one Japanese study of 6508 individuals with ultrasound diagnosed NAFLD, found the HCC incidence to be only 0.2% after eight years, however subjects with advanced fibrosis determined by the AST-Platelet Ratio Index, had a 25-fold increase in risk [72]. Of concern however, are emerging reports of the development of HCC in non-cirrhotic patients; however, the magnitude of this risk remains to be defined [73–75].

6.2. HCC in NAFLD Cirrhosis

The cumulative incidence of HCC in NASH cirrhosis ranges between 2.4% and 12.8% over a 3.2–7.2 year period, and the cumulative HCC mortality in NAFLD/NASH cohorts is 0%–3% over 5.6–21 years [76]. A large series of 195 NAFLD cirrhosis patients from the Cleveland Clinic found the annual incidence of HCC to be marginally lower than a comparative population of hepatitis C cirrhosis patients (2.6% *vs.* 4.0%, *p* = 0.09) [77]. These findings have been replicated in other American and Japanese cohorts [50,78]. All these studies performs a defined protocol excluding other etiologies of HCC including Hepatitis C and Hepatitis B virus infection. Risk factors for HCC development in the NASH population included diabetes, age, any previous alcohol consumption and the presence of intra-hepatic iron [77,79]. Interestingly, the use of metformin in patients with type 2 diabetes has been associated with a reduced risk of HCC, suggesting that this risk factor may be modifiable [80].

Once HCC develops in NAFLD cirrhotic patients, survival appears to be shorter survival than patients with HCV-HCC [81]. This may be related to patients with HCC resulting from NAFLD being older, having larger tumours, and being less likely to be diagnosed by surveillance compared with HCC caused by viral hepatitis [82–84]. Nevertheless, among patients that have liver function and tumours eligible for curative HCC treatment, overall survival is similar or better that comparable patients with hepatitis C or alcohol induced cirrhosis [81,84].

6.3. HCC in NAFLD without Cirrhosis

The development of HCC in non-cirrhotic patients with NAFLD is increasingly reported with cross-sectional studies demonstrating between 15% and 50% of cases being diagnosed without cirrhosis [73,81,85,86]. Moreover, HCCs have been reported to arise in subjects without evidence of NASH or fibrosis but just simple steatosis [83]. A minority of these cases may be related to transformation of hepatic adenomas, whereas the majority appear to be related to risk factors for NAFLD, namely the MetS, obesity, and diabetes [87]. Several studies have also suggested that HCC originating in non-cirrhotic patients with NASH and/or the metabolic syndrome, are more likely to be male [85–87].

Not surprisingly, HCC associated with non-cirrhotic NAFLD is less likely to be detected during surveillance and thus is more likely to be more advanced when compared to HCC in cirrhosis patients [68,81,84]. Nevertheless, survival is equivalent or better in non-cirrhotic NAFLD patients when compared to subjects with cirrhotic-HCC, likely due to preserved liver function.

7. Conclusions

NAFLD is common in the general population, however the natural history and impact on patient morbidity and mortality is widely divergent. Metabolic factors, such as diabetes, obesity, and hypertension, as well as common genetic polymorphisms in the *PNPLA3* and *TM6SF2* genes, influence the severity of underlying liver histology and, thus, are likely to impact on risk of developing cirrhosis and HCC. Recent studies have demonstrated NAFL in addition to NASH, may lead to progressive fibrosis and have emphasized the importance of fibrosis level in determining future mortality risk. A greater understanding of the factors that alter the natural history of NAFLD will lead to better prognostication and targeting of NAFLD populations at greatest risk for specific therapies.

Acknowledgments: Luis Calzadilla Bertot has been awarded a scholarship from the Liver Foundation of Western Australia.

Author Contributions: Luis Calzadilla Bertot and Leon Anton Adams reviewed the literature and wrote the article.

Abbreviations

NAFLD	Nonalcoholic fatty liver disease
T2DM	Type 2 Diabetes mellitus
NASH	Nonalcoholic steatohepatitis
HCC	Hepatocellular carcinoma
MetS	Metabolic syndrome
NAFL	Nonalcoholic fatty liver
SNP's	Single nucleotide polymorphisms
CVD	Cardiovascular disease
NAS	NAFLD activity score
TGF-β1	Transforming growth factor-beta1

References

1. NCD-RisC. Trends in adult body mass index in 200 countries from 1975 to 2014. *Lancet* **2016**, *387*, 1377–1396.
2. Ray, K. NAFLD–The next global epidemic. *Nat. Rev. Gastroenterol. Hepatol.* **2013**, *10*, 621. [CrossRef] [PubMed]
3. Powell, E.E.; Cooksley, W.G.E.; Hanson, R.; Searle, J.; Halliday, J.W.; Powell, W. The natural history of nonalcoholic steatohepatitis: A follow-up study of forty-two patients for up to 21 years. *Hepatology* **1990**, *11*, 74–80. [CrossRef] [PubMed]
4. Caldwell, S.H.; Oelsner, D.H.; Iezzoni, J.C.; Hespenheide, E.E.; Battle, E.H.; Driscoll, C.J. Cryptogenic cirrhosis: Clinical characterization and risk factors for underlying disease. *Hepatology* **1999**, *29*, 664–669. [CrossRef] [PubMed]
5. Poonawala, A.; Nair, S.P.; Thuluvath, P.J. Prevalence of obesity and diabetes in patients with cryptogenic cirrhosis: A case-control study. *Hepatology* **2000**, *32*, 689–692. [CrossRef] [PubMed]
6. Teli, M.R.; James, O.F.; Burt, A.D.; Bennett, M.K.; Day, C.P. The natural history of nonalcoholic fatty liver: A follow-up study. *Hepatology* **1995**, *22*, 1714–1719. [CrossRef] [PubMed]
7. Wong, V.W.-S.; Wong, G.L.-H.; Choi, P.C.-L.; Chan, A.W.-H.; Li, M.K.-P.; Chan, H.-Y.; Chim, A.M.; Yu, J.; Sung, J.J.; Chan, H.L. Disease progression of non-alcoholic fatty liver disease: A prospective study with paired liver biopsies at 3 years. *Gut* **2010**, *59*, 969–974. [CrossRef] [PubMed]
8. Pais, R.; Charlotte, F.; Fedchuk, L.; Bedossa, P.; Lebray, P.; Poynard, T.; Ratziu, V.; LIDO Study Group. A systematic review of follow-up biopsies reveals disease progression in patients with non-alcoholic fatty liver. *J. Hepatol.* **2013**, *59*, 550–556. [CrossRef] [PubMed]
9. McPherson, S.; Hardy, T.; Henderson, E.; Burt, A.D.; Day, C.P.; Anstee, Q.M. Evidence of NAFLD progression from steatosis to fibrosing-steatohepatitis using paired biopsies: Implications for prognosis and clinical management. *J. Hepatol.* **2015**, *62*, 1148–1155. [CrossRef] [PubMed]

10. Angulo, P.; Hui, J.M.; Marchesini, G.; Bugianesi, E.; George, J.; Farrell, G.C.; Enders, F.; Saksena, S.; Burt, A.D.; Bida, J.P.; *et al.* The NAFLD fibrosis score: A noninvasive system that identifies liver fibrosis in patients with NAFLD. *Hepatology* **2007**, *45*, 846–854. [CrossRef] [PubMed]

11. Ekstedt, M.; Franzén, L.E.; Mathiesen, U.L.; Thorelius, L.; Holmqvist, M.; Bodemar, G.; Kechagias, S. Long-term follow-up of patients with NAFLD and elevated liver enzymes. *Hepatology* **2006**, *44*, 865–873. [CrossRef] [PubMed]

12. Adams, L.A.; Sanderson, S.; Lindor, K.D.; Angulo, P. The histological course of nonalcoholic fatty liver disease: A longitudinal study of 103 patients with sequential liver biopsies. *J. Hepatol.* **2005**, *42*, 132–138. [CrossRef] [PubMed]

13. Angulo, P.; Keach, J.C.; Batts, K.P.; Lindor, K.D. Independent predictors of liver fibrosis in patients with nonalcoholic steatohepatitis. *Hepatology* **1999**, *30*, 1356–1362. [CrossRef] [PubMed]

14. Bacon, B.R.; Farahvash, M.J.; Janney, C.G.; Neuschwander-Tetri, B.A. Nonalcoholic steatohepatitis: An expanded clinical entity. *Gastroenterol.-Orlando* **1994**, *107*, 1103–1109.

15. Evans, C.; Oien, K.; MacSween, R.; Mills, P. Non-alcoholic steatohepatitis: A common cause of progressive chronic liver injury? *J. Clin. Pathol.* **2002**, *55*, 689–692. [CrossRef] [PubMed]

16. Fassio, E.; Álvarez, E.; Domínguez, N.; Landeira, G.; Longo, C. Natural history of nonalcoholic steathepatitis: A longitudinal study of repeat liver biopsies. *Hepatology* **2004**, *40*, 820–826. [CrossRef] [PubMed]

17. Harrison, S.A.; Torgerson, S.; Hayashi, P.H. The natural history of nonalcoholic fatty liver disease: A clinical histopathological study. *Am. J. Gastroenterol.* **2003**, *98*, 2042–2047. [CrossRef] [PubMed]

18. Hui, A.; Wong, V.S.; Chan, H.Y.; Liew, C.T.; Chan, J.Y.; Chan, F.L.; Sung, J.Y. Histological progression of non-alcoholic fatty liver disease in Chinese patients. *Aliment. Pharmacol. Ther.* **2005**, *21*, 407–413. [CrossRef] [PubMed]

19. Lee, R.G. Nonalcoholic steatohepatitis: A study of 49 patients. *Hum. Pathol.* **1989**, *20*, 594–598. [CrossRef]

20. Ratziu, V.; Giral, P.; Charlotte, F.; Bruckert, E.; Thibault, V.; Theodorou, I.; Khalil, L.; Turpin, G.; Opolon, P.; Poynard, T. Liver fibrosis in overweight patients. *Gastroenterology* **2000**, *118*, 1117–1123. [CrossRef]

21. Duan, X.F.; Tang, P.; Li, Q.; Yu, Z.T. Obesity, adipokines and hepatocellular carcinoma. *Int. J. Cancer* **2013**, *133*, 1776–1783. [CrossRef] [PubMed]

22. Henao-Mejia, J.; Elinav, E.; Jin, C.; Hao, L.; Mehal, W.Z.; Strowig, T.; Thaiss, C.A.; Kau, A.L.; Eisenbarth, S.C.; Jurczak, M.J.; *et al.* Inflammasome-mediated dysbiosis regulates progression of NAFLD and obesity. *Nature* **2012**, *482*, 179–185. [CrossRef] [PubMed]

23. Oliveira, C.P.; Stefano, J.T. Genetic polymorphisms and oxidative stress in non-alcoholic steatohepatitis (NASH): A mini review. *Clin. Res. Hepatol. Gastroenterol.* **2015**, *39*, S35–S40. [CrossRef] [PubMed]

24. Singh, S.; Allen, A.M.; Wang, Z.; Prokop, L.J.; Murad, M.H.; Loomba, R. Fibrosis progression in nonalcoholic fatty liver *vs.* nonalcoholic steatohepatitis: A systematic review and meta-analysis of paired-biopsy studies. *Clin. Gastroenterol. Hepatol.* **2015**, *13*, 643–654. [CrossRef] [PubMed]

25. McPherson, S.; Stewart, S.F.; Henderson, E.; Burt, A.D.; Day, C.P. Simple non-invasive fibrosis scoring systems can reliably exclude advanced fibrosis in patients with non-alcoholic fatty liver disease. *Gut* **2010**, *59*, 1265–1269. [CrossRef] [PubMed]

26. Hossain, N.; Afendy, A.; Stepanova, M.; Nader, F.; Srishord, M.; Rafiq, N.; Goodman, Z.; Younossi, Z. Independent predictors of fibrosis in patients with nonalcoholic fatty liver disease. *Clin. Gastroenterol. Hepatol.* **2009**, *7*, 1224–1229. [CrossRef] [PubMed]

27. Yang, J.D.; Abdelmalek, M.F.; Pang, H.; Guy, C.D.; Smith, A.D.; Diehl, A.M.; Suzuki, A. Gender and menopause impact severity of fibrosis among patients with nonalcoholic steatohepatitis. *Hepatology* **2014**, *59*, 1406–1414. [CrossRef] [PubMed]

28. Klair, J.S.; Yang, J.D.; Abdelmalek, M.F.; Guy, C.D.; Gill, R.M.; Yates, K.; Unalp-Arida, A.; Lavine, J.; Clark, J.; Diehl, A.M.; *et al.* A longer duration of estrogen deficiency increases fibrosis risk among postmenopausal women with nonalcoholic fatty liver disease. *Hepatology* **2016**. [CrossRef] [PubMed]

29. Lomonaco, R.; Ortiz-Lopez, C.; Orsak, B.; Finch, J.; Webb, A.; Bril, F.; Louden, C.; Tio, F.; Cusi, K. Role of ethnicity in overweight and obese patients with nonalcoholic steatohepatitis. *Hepatology* **2011**, *54*, 837–845. [CrossRef] [PubMed]

30. Bambha, K.; Belt, P.; Abraham, M.; Wilson, L.A.; Pabst, M.; Ferrell, L.; Unalp-Arida, A.; Bass, N. Ethnicity and nonalcoholic fatty liver disease. *Hepatology* **2012**, *55*, 769–780. [CrossRef] [PubMed]

31. Mohanty, S.R.; Troy, T.N.; Huo, D.; O'Brien, B.L.; Jensen, D.M.; Hart, J. Influence of ethnicity on histological differences in non-alcoholic fatty liver disease. *J. Hepatol.* **2009**, *50*, 797–804. [CrossRef] [PubMed]

32. Solga, S.F.; Clark, J.M.; Alkhuraishi, A.R.; Torbenson, M.; Tabesh, A.; Schweitzer, M.; Diehl, A.M.; Magnuson, T.H. Race and comorbid factors predict nonalcoholic fatty liver disease histopathology in severely obese patients. *Surg. Obes. Relat. Dis.* **2005**, *1*, 6–11. [CrossRef] [PubMed]

33. Kallwitz, E.R.; Guzman, G.; TenCate, V.; Vitello, J.; Layden-Almer, J.; Berkes, J.; Patel, R.; Layden, T.J.; Cotler, S.J. The histologic spectrum of liver disease in African-American, non-Hispanic white, and Hispanic obesity surgery patients. *Am. J. Gastroenterol.* **2009**, *104*, 64–69. [CrossRef] [PubMed]

34. Liu, Y.L.; Reeves, H.L.; Burt, A.D.; Tiniakos, D.; McPherson, S.; Leathart, J.B.; Allison, M.E.; Alexander, G.J.; Piguet, A.C.; Anty, R.; *et al.* TM6SF2 rs58542926 influences hepatic fibrosis progression in patients with non-alcoholic fatty liver disease. *Nat. Commun.* **2014**, *5*, 4309. [CrossRef] [PubMed]

35. Romeo, S.; Kozlitina, J.; Xing, C.; Pertsemlidis, A.; Cox, D.; Pennacchio, L.A.; Boerwinkle, E.; Cohen, J.C.; Hobbs, H.H. Genetic variation in *PNPLA3* confers susceptibility to nonalcoholic fatty liver disease. *Nat. Genet.* **2008**, *40*, 1461–1465. [CrossRef] [PubMed]

36. Valenti, L.; Al-Serri, A.; Daly, A.K.; Galmozzi, E.; Rametta, R.; Dongiovanni, P.; Nobili, V.; Mozzi, E.; Roviaro, G.; Vanni, E.; *et al.* Homozygosity for the patatin-like phospholipase-3/adiponutrin I148M polymorphism influences liver fibrosis in patients with nonalcoholic fatty liver disease. *Hepatology* **2010**, *51*, 1209–1217. [CrossRef] [PubMed]

37. Eslam, M.; Hashem, A.M.; Romero-Gomez, M.; Berg, T.; Dore, G.J.; Mangia, A.; Chan, H.L.; Irving, W.L.; Sheridan, D.; Abate, M.L.; *et al.* FibroGENE: A gene-based model for staging liver fibrosis. *J. Hepatol.* **2016**, *64*, 390–398. [CrossRef] [PubMed]

38. Yki-Järvinen, H. Non-alcoholic fatty liver disease as a cause and a consequence of metabolic syndrome. *Lancet Diabetes Endocrinol.* **2014**, *2*, 901–910. [CrossRef]

39. Neuschwander-Tetri, B.A.; Clark, J.M.; Bass, N.M.; van Natta, M.L.; Unalp-Arida, A.; Tonascia, J.; Zein, C.O.; Brunt, E.M.; Kleiner, D.E.; McCullough, A.J.; *et al.* Clinical, laboratory and histological associations in adults with nonalcoholic fatty liver disease. *Hepatology* **2010**, *52*, 913–924. [CrossRef] [PubMed]

40. Tarantino, G.; Conca, P.; Riccio, A.; Tarantino, M.; di Minno, M.N.; Chianese, D.; Pasanisi, F.; Contaldo, F.; Scopacasa, F.; Capone, D. Enhanced serum concentrations of transforming growth factor-β1 in simple fatty liver: Is it really benign? *J. Transl. Med.* **2008**, *6*, 72. [CrossRef] [PubMed]

41. Adams, L.A.; Lymp, J.F.; Sauver, J.S.; Sanderson, S.O.; Lindor, K.D.; Feldstein, A.; Angulo, P. The natural history of nonalcoholic fatty liver disease: A population-based cohort study. *Gastroenterology* **2005**, *129*, 113–121. [CrossRef] [PubMed]

42. Williams, C.D.; Stengel, J.; Asike, M.I.; Torres, D.M.; Shaw, J.; Contreras, M.; Landt, C.L.; Harrison, S.A. Prevalence of nonalcoholic fatty liver disease and nonalcoholic steatohepatitis among a largely middle-aged population utilizing ultrasound and liver biopsy: A prospective study. *Gastroenterology* **2011**, *140*, 124–131. [CrossRef] [PubMed]

43. Dam-Larsen, S.; Becker, U.; Franzmann, M.B.; Larsen, K.; Christoffersen, P.; Bendtsen, F. Final results of a long-term, clinical follow-up in fatty liver patients. *Scand. J. Gastroenterol.* **2009**, *44*, 1236–1243. [CrossRef] [PubMed]

44. Matteoni, C.A.; Younossi, Z.M.; Gramlich, T.; Boparai, N.; Liu, Y.C.; McCullough, A.J. Nonalcoholic fatty liver disease: A spectrum of clinical and pathological severity. *Gastroenterology* **1999**, *116*, 1413–1419. [CrossRef]

45. El-serag, H.B.; Tran, T.; Everhart, J.E. Diabetes increases the risk of chronic liver disease and hepatocellular carcinoma. *Gastroenterology* **2004**, *126*, 460–468. [CrossRef] [PubMed]

46. Loomba, R.; Abraham, M.; Unalp, A.; Wilson, L.; Lavine, J.; Doo, E.; Bass, N.M. Association between diabetes, family history of diabetes, and risk of nonalcoholic steatohepatitis and fibrosis. *Hepatology* **2012**, *56*, 943–951. [CrossRef] [PubMed]

47. Hui, J.M.; Kench, J.G.; Chitturi, S.; Sud, A.; Farrell, G.C.; Byth, K.; Hall, P.; Khan, M.; George, J. Long-term outcomes of cirrhosis in nonalcoholic steatohepatitis compared with hepatitis C. *Hepatology* **2003**, *38*, 420–427. [CrossRef] [PubMed]

48. Sanyal, A.J.; Banas, C.; Sargeant, C.; Luketic, V.A.; Sterling, R.K.; Stravitz, R.T.; Shiffman, M.L.; Heuman, D.; Coterrell, A.; Fisher, R.A.; *et al.* Similarities and differences in outcomes of cirrhosis due to nonalcoholic steatohepatitis and hepatitis C. *Hepatology* **2006**, *43*, 682–689. [CrossRef] [PubMed]

49. Singal, A.K.; Guturu, P.; Hmoud, B.; Kuo, Y.-F.; Salameh, H.; Wiesner, R.H. Evolving frequency and outcomes of liver transplantation based on etiology of liver disease. *Transplantation* **2013**, *95*, 755–760. [CrossRef] [PubMed]

50. Agopian, V.G.; Kaldas, F.M.; Hong, J.C.; Whittaker, M.; Holt, C.; Rana, A.; Zarrinpar, A.; Petrowsky, H.; Farmer, D.; Yersiz, H.; et al. Liver transplantation for nonalcoholic steatohepatitis: The new epidemic. Ann. Surg. 2012, 256, 624–633. [CrossRef] [PubMed]

51. Charlton, M.R.; Burns, J.M.; Pedersen, R.A.; Watt, K.D.; Heimbach, J.K.; Dierkhising, R.A. Frequency and outcomes of liver transplantation for nonalcoholic steatohepatitis in the United States. Gastroenterology 2011, 141, 1249–1253. [CrossRef] [PubMed]

52. Wong, R.J.; Aguilar, M.; Cheung, R.; Perumpail, R.B.; Harrison, S.A.; Younossi, Z.M.; Ahmed, A. Nonalcoholic steatohepatitis is the second leading etiology of liver disease among adults awaiting liver transplantation in the United States. Gastroenterology 2015, 148, 547–555. [CrossRef] [PubMed]

53. Caldwell, S.H.; Crespo, D.M. The spectrum expanded: Cryptogenic cirrhosis and the natural history of non-alcoholic fatty liver disease. J. Hepatol. 2004, 40, 578–584. [CrossRef] [PubMed]

54. Long, M.T.; Wang, N.; Larson, M.G.; Mitchell, G.F.; Palmisano, J.; Vasan, R.S.; Hoffmann, U.; Speliotes, E.K.; Vita, J.A.; Benjamin, E.J.; et al. Nonalcoholic fatty liver disease and vascular function: Cross-sectional analysis in the Framingham heart study. Arterioscler. Thromb. Vasc. Biol. 2015, 35, 1284–1291. [CrossRef] [PubMed]

55. Huang, R.C.; Beilin, L.J.; Ayonrinde, O.; Mori, T.A.; Olynyk, J.K.; Burrows, S.; Hands, B.; Adams, L.A. Importance of cardiometabolic risk factors in the association between nonalcoholic fatty liver disease and arterial stiffness in adolescents. Hepatology 2013, 58, 1306–1314. [CrossRef] [PubMed]

56. VanWagner, L.B.; Wilcox, J.E.; Colangelo, L.A.; Lloyd-Jones, D.M.; Carr, J.J.; Lima, J.A.; Lewis, C.E.; Rinella, M.E.; Shah, S.J. Association of nonalcoholic fatty liver disease with subclinical myocardial remodeling and dysfunction: A population-based study. Hepatology 2015, 62, 773–783. [CrossRef] [PubMed]

57. Oni, E.T.; Agatston, A.S.; Blaha, M.J.; Fialkow, J.; Cury, R.; Sposito, A.; Erbel, R.; Blankstein, R.; Feldman, T.; Al-Mallah, M.H.; et al. A systematic review: Burden and severity of subclinical cardiovascular disease among those with nonalcoholic fatty liver; should we care? Atherosclerosis 2013, 230, 258–267. [CrossRef] [PubMed]

58. Anstee, Q.M.; Targher, G.; Day, C.P. Progression of NAFLD to diabetes mellitus, cardiovascular disease or cirrhosis. Nat. Rev. Gastroenterol. Hepatol. 2013, 10, 330–344. [CrossRef] [PubMed]

59. Vanni, E.; Marengo, A.; Mezzabotta, L.; Bugianesi, E. Systemic complications of nonalcoholic fatty liver disease: When the liver is not an innocent bystander. Semin. Liver Dis. 2015, 35, 236–249. [CrossRef] [PubMed]

60. Kim, D.; Kim, W.R.; Kim, H.J.; Therneau, T.M. Association between noninvasive fibrosis markers and mortality among adults with nonalcoholic fatty liver disease in the United States. Hepatology 2013, 57, 1357–1365. [CrossRef] [PubMed]

61. Haring, R.; Wallaschofski, H.; Nauck, M.; Dorr, M.; Baumeister, S.E.; Volzke, H. Ultrasonographic hepatic steatosis increases prediction of mortality risk from elevated serum gamma-glutamyl transpeptidase levels. Hepatology 2009, 50, 1403–1411. [CrossRef] [PubMed]

62. Ekstedt, M.; Hagström, H.; Nasr, P.; Fredrikson, M.; Stål, P.; Kechagias, S.; Hultcrantz, R. Fibrosis stage is the strongest predictor for disease-specific mortality in NAFLD after up to 33 years of follow-up. Hepatology 2015, 61, 1547–1554. [CrossRef] [PubMed]

63. Adams, L.A.; Ratziu, V. Non-alcoholic fatty liver—Perhaps not so benign. J. Hepatol. 2015, 62, 1002–1004. [CrossRef] [PubMed]

64. Younossi, Z.M.; Stepanova, M.; Rafiq, N.; Makhlouf, H.; Younoszai, Z.; Agrawal, R.; Goodman, Z. Pathologic criteria for nonalcoholic steatohepatitis: Interprotocol agreement and ability to predict liver-related mortality. Hepatology 2011, 53, 1874–1882. [CrossRef] [PubMed]

65. Angulo, P.; Kleiner, D.E.; Dam-Larsen, S.; Adams, L.A.; Bjornsson, E.S.; Charatcharoenwitthaya, P.; Mills, P.R.; Keach, J.C.; Lafferty, H.D.; Stahler, A.; et al. Liver fibrosis, but no other histologic features, is associated with long-term outcomes of patients with nonalcoholic fatty liver disease. Gastroenterology 2015, 149, 389–397. [CrossRef] [PubMed]

66. Bruix, J.; Gores, G.J.; Mazzaferro, V. Hepatocellular carcinoma: Clinical frontiers and perspectives. Gut 2014, 63, 844–855. [CrossRef] [PubMed]

67. Dyson, J.; Jaques, B.; Chattopadyhay, D.; Lochan, R.; Graham, J.; Das, D.; Aslam, T.; Patanwala, I.; Gaggar, S.; Cole, M.; et al. Hepatocellular cancer: The impact of obesity, type 2 diabetes and a multidisciplinary team. J. Hepatol. 2014, 60, 110–117. [CrossRef] [PubMed]

68. Baffy, G.; Brunt, E.M.; Caldwell, S.H. Hepatocellular carcinoma in non-alcoholic fatty liver disease: An emerging menace. J. Hepatol. 2012, 56, 1384–1391. [CrossRef] [PubMed]

69. Park, E.J.; Lee, J.H.; Yu, G.-Y.; He, G.; Ali, S.R.; Holzer, R.G.; Österreicher, C.H.; Takahashi, H.; Karin, M. Dietary and genetic obesity promote liver inflammation and tumorigenesis by enhancing IL-6 and TNF expression. *Cell* **2010**, *140*, 197–208. [CrossRef] [PubMed]

70. Zámbó, V.; Simon-Szabó, L.; Szelényi, P.; Kereszturi, E.; Bánhegyi, G.; Csala, M. Lipotoxicity in the liver. *World J. Hepatol.* **2013**, *5*, 550–557. [PubMed]

71. Mittal, S.; Sada, Y.H.; El-Serag, H.B.; Kanwal, F.; Duan, Z.; Temple, S.; May, S.B.; Kramer, J.R.; Richardson, P.A.; Davila, J.A. Temporal trends of nonalcoholic fatty liver disease-related hepatocellular carcinoma in the veteran affairs population. *Clin. Gastroenterol. Hepatol.* **2015**, *13*, 594–601. [CrossRef] [PubMed]

72. Kawamura, Y.; Arase, Y.; Ikeda, K.; Seko, Y.; Imai, N.; Hosaka, T.; Kobayashi, M.; Saitoh, S.; Sezaki, H.; Akuta, N.; *et al.* Large-scale long-term follow-up study of Japanese patients with non-alcoholic fatty liver disease for the onset of hepatocellular carcinoma. *Am. J. Gastroenterol.* **2012**, *107*, 253–261. [CrossRef] [PubMed]

73. Ertle, J.; Dechene, A.; Sowa, J.P.; Penndorf, V.; Herzer, K.; Kaiser, G.; Schlaak, J.F.; Gerken, G.; Syn, W.K.; Canbay, A. Non-alcoholic fatty liver disease progresses to hepatocellular carcinoma in the absence of apparent cirrhosis. *Int. J. Cancer* **2011**, *128*, 2436–2443. [CrossRef] [PubMed]

74. White, D.L.; Kanwal, F.; El-Serag, H.B. Association between nonalcoholic fatty liver disease and risk for hepatocellular cancer, based on systematic review. *Clin. Gastroenterol. Hepatol.* **2012**, *10*, 1342–1359. [CrossRef] [PubMed]

75. Ascha, M.S.; Hanouneh, I.A.; Lopez, R.; Tamimi, T.A.; Feldstein, A.F.; Zein, N.N. The incidence and risk factors of hepatocellular carcinoma in patients with nonalcoholic steatohepatitis. *Hepatology* **2010**, *51*, 1972–1978. [CrossRef] [PubMed]

76. Yatsuji, S.; Hashimoto, E.; Tobari, M.; Taniai, M.; Tokushige, K.; Shiratori, K. Clinical features and outcomes of cirrhosis due to non-alcoholic steatohepatitis compared with cirrhosis caused by chronic hepatitis C. *J. Gastroenterol. Hepatol.* **2009**, *24*, 248–254. [CrossRef] [PubMed]

77. Sorrentino, P.; D'Angelo, S.; Ferbo, U.; Micheli, P.; Bracigliano, A.; Vecchione, R. Liver iron excess in patients with hepatocellular carcinoma developed on non-alcoholic steato-hepatitis. *J. Hepatol.* **2009**, *50*, 351–357. [CrossRef] [PubMed]

78. Singh, S.; Singh, P.P.; Singh, A.G.; Murad, M.H.; Sanchez, W. Anti-diabetic medications and the risk of hepatocellular cancer: A systematic review and meta-analysis. *Am. J. Gastroenterol.* **2013**, *108*, 881–891. [CrossRef] [PubMed]

79. Piscaglia, F.; Svegliati-Baroni, G.; Barchetti, A.; Pecorelli, A.; Marinelli, S.; Tiribelli, C.; Bellentani, S.; Bolondi, L.; Zoli, M.; Malagotti, D.; *et al.* Clinical patterns of hepatocellular carcinoma (HCC) in non alcoholic fatty liver disease (NAFLD): A multicenter prospective study. *Hepatology* **2015**, *47*, e36–e37.

80. Marrero, J.A.; Fontana, R.J.; Su, G.L.; Conjeevaram, H.S.; Emick, D.M.; Lok, A.S. NAFLD may be a common underlying liver disease in patients with hepatocellular carcinoma in the United States. *Hepatology* **2002**, *36*, 1349–1354. [CrossRef] [PubMed]

81. Guzman, G.; Brunt, E.M.; Petrovic, L.M.; Chejfec, G.; Layden, T.J.; Cotler, S.J. Does nonalcoholic fatty liver disease predispose patients to hepatocellular carcinoma in the absence of cirrhosis? *Arch. Pathol. Lab. Med.* **2008**, *132*, 1761–1766. [PubMed]

82. Reddy, S.K.; Steel, J.L.; Chen, H.W.; DeMateo, D.J.; Cardinal, J.; Behari, J.; Humar, A.; Marsh, J.W.; Geller, D.A.; Tsung, A. Outcomes of curative treatment for hepatocellular cancer in nonalcoholic steatohepatitis *versus* hepatitis C and alcoholic liver disease. *Hepatology* **2012**, *55*, 1809–1819. [CrossRef] [PubMed]

83. Leung, C.; Yeoh, S.W.; Patrick, D.; Ket, S.; Marion, K.; Gow, P.; Angus, P.W. Characteristics of hepatocellular carcinoma in cirrhotic and non-cirrhotic non-alcoholic fatty liver disease. *World J. Gastroenterol.* **2015**, *21*, 1189–1196. [CrossRef] [PubMed]

84. Calle, E.E.; Rodriguez, C.; Walker-Thurmond, K.; Thun, M.J. Overweight, obesity, and mortality from cancer in a prospectively studied cohort of U.S. adults. *N. Engl. J. Med.* **2003**, *348*, 1625–1638. [CrossRef] [PubMed]

85. Paradis, V.; Zalinski, S.; Chelbi, E.; Guedj, N.; Degos, F.; Vilgrain, V.; Bedossa, P.; Belghiti, J. Hepatocellular carcinomas in patients with metabolic syndrome often develop without significant liver fibrosis: A pathological analysis. *Hepatology* **2009**, *49*, 851–859. [CrossRef] [PubMed]

86. Liu, T.C.; Vachharajani, N.; Chapman, W.C.; Brunt, E.M. Noncirrhotic hepatocellular carcinoma: Derivation from hepatocellular adenoma? Clinicopathologic analysis. *Mod. Pathol.* **2014**, *27*, 420–432. [CrossRef] [PubMed]

87. Yasui, K.; Hashimoto, E.; Komorizono, Y.; Koike, K.; Arii, S.; Imai, Y.; Shima, T.; Kanbara, Y.; Saibara, T.; Mori, T.; *et al.* Characteristics of patients with nonalcoholic steatohepatitis who develop hepatocellular carcinoma. *Clin. Gastroenterol. Hepatol.* **2011**, *9*, 428–433. [CrossRef] [PubMed]

15

The Impact of Nonalcoholic Fatty Liver Disease on Renal Function in Children with Overweight/Obesity

Lucia Pacifico [1,*], Enea Bonci [2], Gian Marco Andreoli [1], Michele Di Martino [3], Alessia Gallozzi [1], Ester De Luca [1] and Claudio Chiesa [4]

[1] Policlinico Umberto I Hospital, Sapienza University of Rome, Viale Regina Elena 324, 00161 Rome, Italy; gianmarcoandreoli@gmail.com (G.M.A.); alessia.gallozzi@gmail.com (A.G.); esterdeluca91@libero.it (E.D.L.)

[2] Department of Experimental Medicine, Sapienza University of Rome, Viale Regina Elena 324, 00161 Rome, Italy; enea.bonci@uniroma1.it

[3] Department of Radiological Sciences, Sapienza University of Rome, Viale Regina Elena 324, 00161 Rome, Italy; micdimartino@hotmail.it

[4] Institute of Translational Pharmacology, National Research Council, Via Fosso del Cavaliere 100, 00133 Rome, Italy; claudio.chiesa@ift.cnr.it

* Correspondence: lucia.pacifico@uniroma1.it

Academic Editor: Giovanni Tarantino

Abstract: The association between nonalcoholic fatty liver disease (NAFLD) and chronic kidney disease has attracted interest and attention over recent years. However, no data are available in children. We determined whether children with NAFLD show signs of renal functional alterations, as determined by estimated glomerular filtration rate (eGFR) and urinary albumin excretion. We studied 596 children with overweight/obesity, 268 with NAFLD (hepatic fat fraction $\geqslant$5% on magnetic resonance imaging) and 328 without NAFLD, and 130 healthy normal-weight controls. Decreased GFR was defined as eGFR < 90 mL/min/1.73 m^2. Abnormal albuminuria was defined as urinary excretion of $\geqslant$30 mg/24 h of albumin. A greater prevalence of eGFR < 90 mL/min/1.73 m^2 was observed in patients with NAFLD compared to those without liver involvement and healthy subjects (17.5% vs. 6.7% vs. 0.77%; $p < 0.0001$). The proportion of children with abnormal albuminuria was also higher in the NAFLD group compared to those without NAFLD, and controls (9.3% vs. 4.0% vs. 0; $p < 0.0001$). Multivariate logistic regression analysis revealed that NAFLD was associated with decreased eGFR and/or microalbuminuria (odds ratio, 2.54 (confidence interval, 1.16–5.57); $p < 0.05$) independently of anthropometric and clinical variables. Children with NAFLD are at risk for early renal dysfunction. Recognition of this abnormality in the young may help to prevent the ongoing development of the disease.

Keywords: nonalcoholic fatty liver disease; renal function; obesity; children

1. Introduction

Concurrent with the epidemic of obesity across the world, nonalcoholic fatty liver disease (NAFLD) is becoming one of the most prevalent chronic liver disorders in both adults and children. It is now known that NAFLD is not only a risk factor for hepatic failure and hepatic carcinoma, but it is also associated with a spectrum of extrahepatic diseases generally linked to metabolic syndrome (MetS) such as type 2 diabetes, and cardiovascular disease [1,2]. Recent studies in the pediatric obese population have demonstrated that the prevalence of prediabetes and MetS is significantly increased in subjects with increased hepatic fat content, and that liver steatosis, independently of visceral and intramyocellular lipid content, is a key determinant of the impairment of liver, muscle, and adipose insulin sensitivity [3,4]. Several studies have reported associations between NAFLD and subclinical atherosclerosis and between NAFLD and cardiac function alterations, independently of established risk factors [5–7]. In addition, emerging evidence suggests that subjects with NAFLD have an increased risk of chronic kidney disease (CKD), defined by a decline in the estimated glomerular filtration rate (eGFR) and/or microalbuminuria and/or overt proteinuria [8–12]. However, no data are available in children regarding a possible association between NAFLD and impaired renal function. Recognition of the influence of NAFLD on renal function in the early age would enable us to better understand the association of NAFLD and CKD, since there is less potential for confusion with adult-onset complications.

Thus, in this study we sought to determine whether children with overweight/obesity and NAFLD show signs of renal functional alterations, as assessed by eGFR and urinary albumin excretion, compared to children with overweight/obesity but without NAFLD as well as to healthy normal-weight controls.

2. Results

2.1. Clinical and Laboratory Data from the Study Population

Clinical and laboratory data from the study population are presented in Table 1. None of the enrollees had type 2 diabetes mellitus. Patients with NAFLD were on average older than those without NAFLD and healthy controls, and had higher waist circumference (WC) as well as higher values for systolic and diastolic blood pressure (BP), higher triglycerides, aspartate aminotransferase (AST), alanine aminotransferase (ALT), uric acid, fasting glucose, insulin levels and homeostasis model assessment of insulin resistance (HOMA-IR) values, and lower high-density lipoprotein-cholesterol (HDL-C) concentrations. Patients with NAFLD had significantly lower whole-body insulin sensitivity index (WBISI) than those without NAFLD. Obese children with NAFLD and obese subjects without NAFLD had significantly higher eGFR compared to healthy controls (median, 115 (interquartile range, 104–134) and 115 (96–132) vs. 108 (100–118) mL/min/1.73 m^2; $p < 0.0001$), whereas no differences were found between patients with and without NAFLD. However, a greater frequency of reduced eGFR (<90 mL/min/1.73 m^2) was observed in obese subjects with NAFLD compared to obese children without liver involvement and healthy controls (17.5% vs. 6.7% vs. 0.77%, respectively; $p < 0.0001$).

The proportion of children with microalbuminuria was also higher in the NAFLD group compared to obese children without liver involvement and healthy controls (9.3% vs. 4.0% vs. 0; $p < 0.0001$). None of the participants had eGFR < 60 mL/min/1.73 m^2 or macroalbuminuria. Compared to healthy controls, the prevalence of hyperfiltration was higher in the obese cohort, regardless of liver involvement (Table 1).

To analyze the variables associated with decreased eGFR and/or microalbuminuria, we performed a logistic regression analysis in the cohort of subjects with overweight/obesity. NAFLD (odds ratio (OR), 2.34; 95% confidence interval (CI), 1.31–4.16; $p < 0.01$) was associated with abnormal renal function independently of age, gender, and pubertal status. After further adjustment for body mass index-standard deviation (BMI-SD) score, WC, hypertension, low HDL-C values, elevated triglycerides, and glucose impairment, results did not substantially change (Table 2).

Table 1. Clinical and laboratory characteristics of the study population.

	Normal Weight	NO NAFLD	NAFLD	p Value *
No. patients	130	328	268	<0.0001
Age, years	10.6 (3.5)	10.1 (2.9)	11.2 (2.9) [d]	<0.0001
Male sex, n (%)	61 (46.9)	151 (46.0)	166 (61.9) [a,d]	<0.0001
BMI-SD score	0.17 (0.85)	1.85 (0.45) [a]	2.0 (0.45) [a,d]	<0.0001
Waist circumference, cm	65 (10)	82 (12) [a]	92 (13) [a,d]	<0.0001
Systolic BP, mmHg	102 (11)	107 (12) [b]	114 (12) [a,d]	<0.0001
Diastolic BP, mmHg	63 (7)	65 (9) [c]	69 (8) [a,d]	<0.0001
Total cholesterol, mg/dL	166 (145–186)	161 (139–187)	159 (137–181)	0.077
LDL-C	92 (72–118)	94 (76–115)	94 (74–111)	0.78
HDL-C, mg/dL	56 (50–83)	51 (44–60) [a]	46 (38–53) [a,d]	<0.0001
Triglycerides, mg/dL	62 (50–83)	70 (50–99)	89 (58–127) [a,d]	<0.0001
AST, U/L	22 (20–30)	23 (20–27) [c]	26 (21–35) [a,d]	<0.0001
ALT, U/L	16 (13–20)	18 (14–23) [b]	31 (19–54) [a,d]	<0.0001
Uric acid	0.21 (0.18–0.25)	0.25 (0.22–0.29) [a]	0.28 (0.24–0.34) [a,d]	<0.0001
Glucose, mg/dL	83 (7)	83 (7)	85 (11)	0.002
Insulin, µU/mL	7.5 (4.3–10.5)	11.1 (7.5–15.4) [a]	15.2 (10.1–23.2) [a,d]	<0.0001
HOMA-IR	1.58 (0.90–2.20)	2.30 (1.55–3.22) [a]	3.23 (2.05–5.0) [a,d]	<0.0001
WBISI	-	6.5 (4.5–9.0)	3.5 (2.4–5.6) [d]	-
eGFR, mL/min/1.73 m²	108 (100–118)	115 (104–134) [a]	115 (96–132) [a]	<0.0001
eGFR < 90 mL/min/1.73 m², n (%)	1 (0.77)	22 (6.7) [b]	47 (17.5) [a,d]	<0.0001
eGFR > 139 mL/min/1.73 m², n (%)	6 (4.6)	56 (17.0) [a]	46 (17.2) [a]	0.002
Microalbuminuria, n (%)	0	13 (4.0) [a]	25 (9.3) [a,d]	<0.0001

Results are expressed as n (%), mean (standard deviation), or median (interquartile ranges). * Anova or Kruskal-Wallis test. [a] $p < 0.0001$; [b] $p < 0.01$; [c] $p < 0.05$ vs. controls; [d] $p < 0.0001$ vs. obese children without NAFLD; NAFLD, nonalcoholic fatty liver disease; BMI-SD score, Body mass index- standard deviation score; BP, Blood pressure; LDL-C, Low density lipoprotein-cholesterol; HDL-C, High-density lipoprotein-cholesterol; AST, Aspartate aminotransferase; ALT, Alanine aminotransferase; HOMA-IR, Homeostasis model assessment of insulin resistance; WBISI, Whole-body insulin sensitivity index; eGFR, estimated glomerular filtration rate.

Table 2. Associations of NAFLD with eGFR < 90 mL/min/1.73 m² and/or microalbuminuria in children with overweight/obesity.

Variables	Odds Ratio (95% CI)	p Value
Adjusted model 1: age, gender, pubertal status	2.34 (1.31–4.16)	0.004
Adjusted model 2: model 1 plus BMI-SD score, WC, High BP, High TG, low HDL-C, and high FG	2.54 (1.16–5.57)	0.02
Adjusted model 3: model 1 plus BMI-SD score, WC, High BP, High TG, low HDL-C, and IR	2.30 (1.02–5.17)	0.04

CI, confidence interval; eGFR, estimated glomerular filtration rate; BMI-SD score, Body mass index- standard deviation score; WC, waist circumference; BP, Blood pressure; TG, triglycerides; HDL-C, High-density lipoprotein-cholesterol; FG, fasting glucose; IR, insulin resistance.

2.2. Findings in Children with Biopsy-Proven Nonalcoholic Fatty Liver Disease (NAFLD)

To investigate the association of renal dysfunction further with advanced stages of NAFLD such as steatohepatitis (NASH), we analysed the data obtained in the small subgroup of 41 patients who underwent liver biopsy. Definite-NASH was diagnosed in 26 (63.4%) children, while not-NASH in 15 (36.5%). Compared to children without NASH, those with NASH had significantly lower eGFR (median, 88 (83–107) vs. 123 (110–130) mL/min/1.73 m^2; $p < 0.01$). In addition, more children with NASH had eGFR of <90 mL/min/1.73 m^2 and/or microalbuminuria than those without NASH (17/26 (65.4%) vs. 6/15 (40.0%); $p < 0.01$).

3. Discussion

Early recognition of impaired renal function, in particular reduced GFR, is crucial to prevent serious complications [13]. Large epidemiologic studies have found a robust relationship between obesity and risk for CKD [14–16]. In a community-based sample of 2585 adult individuals with renal disease at baseline and a mean follow-up of 18.5 years, BMI was reported to determine a significant increase in the odds of developing kidney disease by 23% (OR, 1.23; 95% CI, 1.08–1.41) per standard deviation unit [14]. In 9685 adults participating to the Hypertension Detection and Follow-Up Program, free of CKD at baseline, the incidence of CKD was 28%, 31%, and 34%, respectively, in the ideal body mass index, overweight, and obese groups, after a follow-up of five years [15]. After adjustment for variables, such as age, gender, race, diabetes mellitus, mean baseline diastolic BP, and slope of diastolic BP, at baseline both overweight (OR, 1.21; 95% CI, 1.05 to 1.41) and obesity (OR, 1.40; 95% CI, 1.20 to 1.63) were associated with increased incident CKD odds at year 5 [15]. In addition, a retrospective cohort study of 320,252 adults, who were followed for 15 to 35 years, showed that a high BMI ($\geq$25.0 kg/m^2) determined who is at high risk of developing end-stage renal disease [16]. Taken together, these studies indicate that higher BMI in adults is a risk factor for the development of new onset kidney disease. Several possible pathophysiologic pathways may underlie this association. One possibility is that particular characteristics of obesity may account for the association between obesity and CKD. Indeed, obesity constitutes a complex syndrome involving metabolic traits and other factors that may interact with other environmental factors, leading to an increased risk for developing kidney disease. Clustering of these traits defines MetS, which has been reported to be consistently associated with CKD in cross-sectional studies [17,18].

NAFLD has been recently found to be an additional feature of MetS, with the main underlying cardiometabolic risk factors of the syndrome being abdominal obesity and insulin resistance [19,20]. Of note, insulin resistance is not only a metabolic determinant for the development of NAFLD but is also a predictor of incident CKD [21,22]. In addition, atherogenic dyslipidemia and type 2 diabetes are established risk factors for CKD [23,24]. As a consequence, many authors have concluded that NAFLD may have a pathogenic role in the development of CKD. The results of a recent meta-analysis have shown that (1) there is a positive relationship between NAFLD and an increased risk of CKD in adults; (2) the severity of liver disease is associated with an increased risk and severity of CKD; and (3) these relationships are maintained even after taking account of the well-known risk factors for CKD, and are independent of whole body/abdominal obesity and insulin resistance [8].

In our study, we investigated the influence of NAFLD on kidney function in a large pediatric population. This is the first study to demonstrate that overweight/obese children with NAFLD have a greater frequency of eGFR of <90 mL/min/1.73 m^2 as well as of microalbuminuria than overweight/obese children without NAFLD. Furthermore, in the small number of children with biopsy-proven NAFLD we were able to show that the decline in renal function was greater in those with NASH. It is important to point out that subjects with obesity represent a particular population in whom early renal lesion consists of hyperfiltration. In fact, in line with previous studies [25–27], one of the main findings of this study was that children with overweight/obesity compared to normal-weight subjects had a higher prevalence of hyperfiltration, regardless of liver involvement. Glomerular hyperfiltration is well-recognized as an early renal injury occurring in a number of clinical conditions, including diabetes, hypertension, and obesity [28]. Hyperfiltration is hypothesized to be a precursor of intraglomerular hypertension responsible for albuminuria. GFR then declines progressively as albuminuria increases which may cause, in the long run, end-stage renal failure [28]. Thus, in obese patients with NAFLD, we should pay attention for minor impairment on renal function, since hyperfiltration may mask a pathological decline in renal function.

The most plausible explanation for our findings is that the renal abnormalities in overweight/obese children with NAFLD may reflect the coexistence of underlying metabolic risk factors including higher BP, more dyslipidemia, and more insulin resistance compared to children without liver involvement. However, because in our study the presence of NAFLD remained significantly associated with decreased eGFR and/or microalbuminuria after taking account of traditional metabolic traits, we cannot rule out the possibility that NAFLD might at least in part contribute to the development of renal dysfunction independently of shared cardiometabolic risk factors.

The strength of our study includes a large sample size and an extensive and complete analysis of metabolic variables. Nonetheless, some limitations require consideration. First, the cross-sectional design of the study precludes the establishment of causal relationship between NAFLD and abnormal kidney function. Second, we used an estimated GFR instead of a directly measured GFR to define renal function. The gold standard technique is clearance of inulin, but practical problems limit the application of this cumbersome methodology in children because of the necessity for steady-state infusion, and a urine sampling with a bladder catheter. Other tests for determining GFR are clearance of alternative exogenous markers such as iothalamate, which are also complex and difficult to do in routine clinical practice. Recent studies in children have reported current eGFR creatinine- and/or cystatin C-based equations to be reliable methods to assess kidney function, with some variations depending on the GFR ranges and the BMI classes [29–31]. The updated Schwartz formula has been shown to be accurate for estimating GFR when compared to inulin clearance as well as to iothalamate clearance in children and adolescents, with a wide range of renal function [29,30]. Moreover, obesity has not been found to affect GFR as estimated by Schwartz formula [31]. Finally, we measured creatinine concentration by kinetic colorimetric compensated technique, whereas in the updated Schwartz formula, it was determined by an enzymatic method. The two methods, however, are highly correlated [29].

In conclusion, our present study suggests that obese children with NAFLD are at risk for early renal dysfunction. Recognition of this abnormality in the young may be important because treatment to reverse the process is most likely to be effective if applied earlier in the disease process.

4. Materials and Methods

4.1. Study Subjects

This observational cross-sectional study included 596 children and adolescents with overweight/obesity who were consecutively recruited at the outpatient Clinics (Hepatology, Lipid and Nutrition) of the Department of Pediatrics, Sapienza University of Rome, Italy, between 2007 and 2015. Two hundred and sixty eight subjects met the criteria for the diagnosis of NAFLD (i.e., hepatic fat fraction (HFF) ⩾5% on magnetic resonance imaging (MRI)) [32]. In all enrollees, hepatic virus infections (hepatitis A–E and G, cytomegalovirus, and Epstein–Barr virus), autoimmune hepatitis, metabolic liver disease, α-1-antitrypsin deficiency, cystic fibrosis, Wilson's disease, hemochromatosis, and celiac disease were excluded using appropriate tests [6,7]. In 41 of the NAFLD patients, due to persistent elevations in ALT concentrations, a liver biopsy was performed. The other 328 participants had HFF < 5% on MRI, normal levels of aminotransferases, and no evidence of chronic liver diseases (see above). Use of hepatotoxic drugs, as well as a history of type 1 or 2 diabetes, smoking and chronic alcohol intake were also exclusion criteria. None of the subjects had a history or known clinical, laboratory, and imaging signs of renal disease.

The study also included a total of 130 apparently healthy normal-weight school students drawn from four randomly selected schools in the Rome area. All students were invited to take part in a pilot study whose objective was the prevention of cardiovascular disease in childhood. Eligibility criteria included age- and gender-specific BMI; no history of renal and liver diseases as well as of alcohol consumption and smoking; normal liver ultrasound, and normal biochemical values.

All study subjects had a complete physical examination, as reported in detail elsewhere [5,6]. The degree of obesity was quantified using Cole's least mean-square method, which normalizes the skewed distribution of BMI and expresses BMI as SD score [33].

The study protocol was reviewed and approved by the Ethics Committee of Policlinico Umberto I Hospital, Rome, Italy. Written informed consent was obtained from the parents, or guardians of the children included in this study, in accordance with principles of Helsinki Declaration.

4.2. Laboratory Mmeasurements

Blood samples were taken from all study subjects, after an overnight fast, for estimation of glucose, insulin, urea nitrogen, creatinine, uric acid, total cholesterol, HDL-C, triglycerides, ALT, AST, and gamma-glutamyl transferase. An oral glucose tolerance test was performed for all overweight/obese children using 1.75 g/kg of glucose up to a maximum of 75 g. Two-hour post-load glucose and insulin were analyzed. Insulin resistance was calculated by the HOMA-IR. Insulin sensitivity was calculated by the WBISI with reduced time points according to the following formula: $10,000/\sqrt{}$ (fasting glucose × fasting insulin × 2 h post-load glucose × 2 h post-load insulin) [34].

All analyses were performed on COBAS 6000 (Roche Diagnostics, Risch-Rotkreuz, Switzerland). Creatinine concentrations were measured by the kinetic colorimetric compensated Jaffé method using the Roche platform and the CREJ2–creatinine Jaffé Gen.2 assay (Roche Diagnostics, Identification number, 0769282), which was isotope-dilution mass spectrometry standardized, traceable to National Institute of Standards and Technology creatinine standard reference material (SRM 914 and SRM 967). Urinary albumin was determined on 24 h urine collections by the turbidimetric immunoassay ALBT2 (Roche Diagnostics, Identification number, 0767433).

eGFR was calculated using the updated Schwartz formula: 0.413 × height (cm)/serum creatinine (mg/dL) [35].

4.3. Liver Ultrasound Eexamination and Magnetic Resonance Imaging

Liver ultrasound was performed by a single operator. Hepatic steatosis was diagnosed on the basis of the following features: a diffuse increase in echogenicity (a bright liver), liver to kidney contrast, deep beam attenuation, vascular blurring, and loss of definition of the diaphragm [36]. The amount of HFF was measured by MRI using the two-point Dixon method as modified by Fishbein [37], as previously described and validated [32,38].

4.4. Liver Biopsy

Liver biopsy was performed in 41 subjects because of persistent elevation in ALT. The clinical indication for biopsy was either to assess the presence of nonalcoholic steatohepatitis (NASH) or to determine the presence of other independent or competing liver diseases. The main histologic features of NAFLD were scored using the NASH Clinical Research Network criteria [39]. Biopsies were categorized into not-NASH and definite-NASH.

4.5. Definitions

Overweight and obesity were defined according to age- and gender-specific cut-off points of BMI defined by the International Obesity Task Force criteria as proposed by Cole et al. [33]. Elevated BP was defined as systolic or diastolic BP ⩾ 90th percentile for age, gender, and height [40]. Impaired fasting glucose was defined as glucose ⩾5.6 mmol/L. High waist circumference (WC), high triglycerides, and low HDL-C were defined using the cut-off proposed by Cook et al. [41]. Insulin resistance was defined by 90th percentile of HOMA-IR for age and gender in our population of healthy normal-weight children. Abnormal albuminuria was defined as a 24-h urinary albumin excretion rate $\geqslant$30 mg (i.e., microalbuminuria was diagnosed if the 24-h albumin excretion rate was 30–299 mg and macroalbuminuria if the 24-h albumin excretion rate was $\geqslant$300 mg) [42]. As recommended by Kidney Disease Improving Global Outcomes (KDIGO) guidelines, eGFR categories were classified as follows: normal or high $\geqslant$90 mL/min/1.73 m^2; mildly decreased, 60–89; mildly to moderately decreased, 45–59; moderately to severely decreased, 30–44; severely decreased, 15–29; and kidney failure <15 [42]. In the absence of an agreement in the literature, we defined glomerular hyperfiltration as eGFR > 95th percentile of that observed in our population of healthy normal-weight subjects (i.e., eGFR > 139 mL/min/1.73 m^2).

4.6. Statistical Analysis

Statistical analyses were performed using the SPSS package (version 22.0, SPSS Inc., Chicago, IL, USA). Data are reported as means and standard deviations for normally distributed variables, or as median and interquartile range for non-normally distributed variables. Differences between study groups in quantitative variables were evaluated by one-way analysis of variance (ANOVA) or Kruskal–Wallis test, as appropriate. Proportions were compared by the chi square test. Logistic regression analysis was used to assess the independent association of NAFLD with abnormal kidney function, after adjustment for age, gender, pubertal status, BMI-SD score, WC, hypertension, low HDL-C values, elevated triglycerides, and glucose impairment.

Acknowledgments: This study was supported by Sapienza University of Rome (Progetti di Ricerca Universitaria 2013/2014).

Author Contributions: Lucia Pacifico, Enea Bonci, Claudio Chiesa conceived and designed the study; Lucia Pacifico, Enea Bonci, Gian Marco Andreoli, Michele Di Martino, Alessia Gallozzi, and Ester De Luca collected and analyzed the data; Lucia Pacifico, Enea Bonci, Gian Marco Andreoli, Michele Di Martino, and Claudio Chiesa interpreted the data; Lucia Pacifico, Enea Bonci, and Claudio Chiesa wrote the manuscript. All authors read and approved the final version of the manuscript.

References

1.   Vanni, E.; Marengo, A.; Mezzabotta, L.; Bugianesi, E. Systemic complications of nonalcoholic fatty liver disease: When the liver is not an innocent bystander. *Semin. Liver Dis.* **2015**, *35*, 236–249. [CrossRef] [PubMed]
2.   Chatterjee, R.; Mitra, A. An overview of effective therapies and recent advances in biomarkers for chronic liver diseases and associated liver cancer. *Int. Immunopharmacol.* **2015**, *24*, 335–345. [CrossRef] [PubMed]
3.   Schwimmer, J.B.; Pardee, P.E.; Lavine, J.E.; Blumkin, A.K.; Cook, S. Cardiovascular risk factors and the metabolic syndrome in pediatric nonalcoholic fatty liver disease. *Circulation* **2008**, *118*, 277–283. [CrossRef] [PubMed]
4.   D'Adamo, E.; Cali, A.M.; Weiss, R.; Santoro, N.; Pierpont, B.; Northrup, V.; Caprio, S. Central role of fatty liver in the pathogenesis of insulin resistance in obese adolescents. *Diabetes Care* **2010**, *33*, 1817–1822. [CrossRef] [PubMed]
5.   Targher, G.; Day, C.P.; Bonora, E. Risk of cardiovascular disease in patients with nonalcoholic fatty liver disease. *N. Engl. J. Med.* **2010**, *363*, 1341–1350. [CrossRef] [PubMed]
6.   Pacifico, L.; Anania, C.; Martino, F.; Cantisani, V.; Pascone, R.; Marcantonio, A.; Chiesa, C. Functional and morphological vascular changes in pediatric nonalcoholic fatty liver disease. *Hepatology* **2010**, *52*, 1643–1651. [CrossRef] [PubMed]
7.   Pacifico, L.; Di Martino, M.; De Merulis, A.; Bezzi, M.; Osborn, J.F.; Catalano, C.; Chiesa, C. Left ventricular dysfunction in obese children and adolescents with nonalcoholic fatty liver disease. *Hepatology* **2014**, *59*, 461–470. [CrossRef] [PubMed]

8.   Musso, G.; Gambino, R.; Tabibian, J.H.; Ekstedt, M.; Kechagias, S.; Hamaguchi, M.; Hultcrantz, R.; Hagström, H.; Yoon, S.K.; Charatcharoenwitthaya, P.; et al. Association of non-alcoholic fatty liver disease with chronic kidney disease: A systematic review and meta-analysis. *PLoS Med.* **2014**, *11*. [CrossRef] [PubMed]

9.   Sesti, G.; Fiorentino, T.V.; Arturi, F.; Perticone, M.; Sciacqua, A.; Perticone, F. Association between noninvasive fibrosis markers and chronic kidney disease among adults with nonalcoholic fatty liver disease. *PLoS ONE* **2014**, *9*, e88569. [CrossRef] [PubMed]

10. Machado, M.V.; Gonçalves, S.; Carepa, F.; Coutinho, J.; Costa, A.; Cortez-Pinto, H. Impaired renal function in morbid obese patients with nonalcoholic fatty liver disease. *Liver Int.* **2012**, *32*, 241–248. [CrossRef] [PubMed]

11. Targher, G.; Mantovani, A.; Pichiri, I.; Mingolla, L.; Cavalieri, V.; Mantovani, W.; Pancheri, S.; Trombetta, M.; Zoppini, G.; Chonchol, M.; et al. Nonalcoholic fatty liver disease is independently associated with an increased incidence of chronic kidney disease in patients with type 1 diabetes. *Diabetes Care* **2014**, *37*, 1729–1736. [CrossRef] [PubMed]

12. Pan, L.L.; Zhang, H.J.; Huang, Z.F.; Sun, Q.; Chen, Z.; Li, Z.B.; Yang, S.Y.; Li, X.Y.; Li, X.J. Intrahepatic triglyceride content is independently associated with chronic kidney disease in obese adults: A cross-sectional study. *Metabolism* **2015**, *64*, 1077–1085. [CrossRef] [PubMed]

13. Gansevoort, R.T.; Matsushita, K.; van der Velde, M.; Astor, B.C.; Woodward, M.; Levey, A.S.; de Jong, P.E.; Coresh, J.; Chronic Kidney Disease Prognosis Consortium. Lower estimated GFR and higher albuminuria are associated with adverse kidney outcomes. A collaborative meta-analysis of general and high-risk population cohorts. *Kidney Int.* **2011**, *80*, 93–104. [CrossRef] [PubMed]

14. Fox, C.S.; Larson, M.G.; Leip, E.P.; Culleton, B.; Wilson, P.W.F.; Levy, D. Predictors of new-onset kidney disease in a community-based population. *JAMA* **2004**, *291*, 844–850. [CrossRef] [PubMed]

15. Kramer, H.; Luke, A.; Bidani, A.; Cao, G.; Cooper, R.; McGee, D. Obesity and prevalent and incident CKD: The Hypertension Detection and Follow-Up Program. *Am. J. Kidney Dis.* **2005**, *46*, 587–594. [CrossRef] [PubMed]

16. Hsu, C.Y.; McCulloch, C.E.; Iribarren, C.; Darbinian, J.; Go, A.S. Body mass index and risk for end-stage renal disease. *Ann. Intern. Med.* **2006**, *144*, 21–28. [CrossRef] [PubMed]

17. Chen, J.; Muntner, P.; Hamm, L.L.; Jones, D.W.; Batuman, V.; Fonseca, V.; Whelton, P.K.; He, J. The metabolic syndrome and chronic kidney disease in U.S. adults. *Ann. Intern. Med.* **2004**, *140*, 167–174. [CrossRef] [PubMed]

18. Hoehner, C.M.; Greenlund, K.J.; Rith-Najarian, S.; Casper, M.L.; McClellan, W.M. Association of the insulin resistance syndrome and microalbuminuria among nondiabetic native Americans. The Inter-Tribal Heart Project. *J. Am. Soc. Nephrol.* **2002**, *13*, 1626–1634. [CrossRef] [PubMed]

19. Speliotes, E.K.; Massaro, J.M.; Hoffmann, U.; Vasan, R.S.; Meigs, J.B.; Sahani, D.V.; Hirschhorn, J.N.; O'Donnell, C.J.; Fox, C.S. Fatty liver is associated with dyslipidemia and dysglycemia independent of visceral fat: The Framingham Heart Study. *Hepatology* **2010**, *51*, 1979–1987. [CrossRef] [PubMed]

20. Grundy, S.M. Metabolic syndrome pandemic. *Arterioscler. Thromb. Vasc. Biol.* **2008**, *28*, 629–636. [CrossRef] [PubMed]

21. Bugianesi, E.; Moscatiello, S.; Ciaravella, M.F.; Marchesini, G. Insulin resistance in nonalcoholic fatty liver disease. *Curr. Pharm. Des.* **2010**, *16*, 1941–1951. [CrossRef] [PubMed]

22. Cheng, H.T.; Huang, J.W.; Chiang, C.K.; Yen, C.J.; Hung, K.Y.; Wu, K.D. Metabolic syndrome and insulin resistance as risk factors for development of chronic kidney disease and rapid decline in renal function in elderly. *J. Clin. Endocrinol. Metab.* **2012**, *97*, 1268–1276. [CrossRef] [PubMed]

23. Vlagopoulos, P.T.; Sarnak, M.J. Traditional and non-traditional cardiovascular risk factors in chronic kidney disease. *Med. Clin. N. Am.* **2005**, *89*, 587–611. [CrossRef] [PubMed]

24. Athyros, V.G.; Tziomalos, K.; Katsiki, N.; Doumas, M.; Karagiannis, A.; Mikhailidis, D.P. Cardiovascular risk across the histological spectrum and the clinical manifestations of non-alcoholic fatty liver disease: An update. *World J. Gastroenterol.* **2015**, *21*, 6820–6834. [PubMed]

25. Wuerzner, G.; Pruijm, M.; Maillard, M.; Bovet, P.; Renaud, C.; Burnier, M.; Boshud, M. Marked association between obesity and glomerular hyperfiltration: A cross-sectional study in an African population. *Am. J. Kidney Dis.* **2010**, *56*, 303–312. [CrossRef] [PubMed]

26. Xiao, N.; Jenkins, T.M.; Nehus, E.; Inge, T.H.; Michalsky, M.P.; Harmon, C.M.; Helmrath, M.A.; Brandt, M.L.; Courcoulas, A.; Moxey-Mims, M.; et al. Kidney function in severely obese adolescents undergoing bariatric surgery. *Obesity* **2014**, *22*, 2319–2325. [CrossRef] [PubMed]

27. Franchini, S.; Savino, A.; Marcovecchio, M.L.; Tumini, S.; Chiarelli, F.; Mohn, A. The effect of obesity and type 1 diabetes on renal function in children and adolescents. *Pediatr. Diabetes* **2015**, *16*, 427–433. [CrossRef] [PubMed]

28. Palatini, P. Glomerular hyperfiltration: A marker of early renal damage in prediabetes and pre-hypertension. *Nephrol. Dial. Transplant.* **2012**, *27*, 1708–1714. [CrossRef] [PubMed]

29. Bacchetta, J.; Cochat, P.; Rognant, N.; Ranchin, B.; Hadj-Aissa, A.; Dubourg, L. Which creatinine and cystatin C equations can be reliably used in children? *Clin. J. Am. Soc. Nephrol.* **2011**, *6*, 552–560. [CrossRef] [PubMed]

30. Staples, A.; LeBlond, R.; Watkins, S.; Wong, C.; Brandt, J. Validation of the revised Schwartz estimating equation in a predominantly non-CKD population. *Pediatr. Nephrol.* **2010**, *25*, 2321–2326. [CrossRef] [PubMed]

31. Fadrowski, J.J.; Neu, A.M.; Schwartz, G.J.; Furth, S.L. Pediatric GFR estimating equations applied to adolescents in the general population. *Clin. J. Am. Soc. Nephrol.* **2011**, *6*, 1427–1435. [CrossRef] [PubMed]

32. Pacifico, L.; Di Martino, M.; Catalano, C.; Panebianco, V.; Bezzi, M.; Anania, C.; Chiesa, C. T1-weighted dual-echo MRI for fat quantification in pediatric nonalcoholic fatty liver disease. *World J. Gastroenterol.* **2011**, *17*, 3012–3019. [CrossRef] [PubMed]

33. Cole, T.J.; Bellizzi, M.C.; Flegal, K.M.; Dietz, W.H. Establishing a standard definition for child overweight and obesity worldwide: International survey. *BMJ* **2000**, *320*, 1240–1243. [CrossRef] [PubMed]

34. DeFronzo, R.A.; Matsuda, M. Reduced time points to calculate the composite index. *Diabetes Care* **2010**, *33*, e93. [CrossRef] [PubMed]

35. Schwartz, G.J.; Muñoz, A.; Schneider, M.F.; Mak, R.H.; Kaskel, F.; Warady, B.A.; Furth, S.L. New equations to estimate GFR in children with CKD. *J. Am. Soc. Nephrol.* **2009**, *20*, 629–637. [CrossRef] [PubMed]

36. Hamer, O.W.; Aguirre, D.A.; Casola, G.; Lavine, J.E.; Woenckhaus, M.; Sirlin, C.B. Fatty liver: Imaging patterns and pitfalls. *Radiographics* **2006**, *26*, 1637–1653. [CrossRef] [PubMed]

37. Fishbein, M.H.; Gardner, K.G.; Potter, C.J.; Schmalbrock, P.; Smith, M.A. Introduction of fast MR imaging in the assessment of hepatic steatosis. *Magn. Reson. Imaging* **1997**, *15*, 287–293. [CrossRef]

38. Pacifico, L.; Di Martino, M.; Anania, C.; Andreoli, G.M.; Bezzi, M.; Catalano, C.; Chiesa, C. Pancreatic fat and β-cell function in overweight/obese children with nonalcoholic fatty liver disease. *World J. Gastroenterol.* **2015**, *21*, 4688–4695. [PubMed]

39. Kleiner, D.E.; Brunt, E.M.; van Natta, M.; Behling, C.; Contos, M.J.; Cummings, O.W.; Ferrell, L.D.; Liu, Y.C.; Torbenson, M.S.; Unalp-Arida, A.; et al. Design and validation of a histological scoring system for nonalcoholic fatty liver disease. *Hepatology* **2005**, *41*, 1313–1321. [CrossRef] [PubMed]

40. National High Blood Pressure Education Program Working Group on High Blood Pressure in Children and Adolescents. The fourth report on the diagnosis, evaluation, and treatment of high blood pressure in children and adolescents. *Pediatrics* **2004**, *114* (Suppl. 2), 555–576.

41. Cook, S.; Auinger, P.; Huang, T.T. Growth curves for cardio-metabolic risk factors in children and adolescents. *J. Pediatr.* **2009**, *155* (Suppl. 6), e15–e26. [CrossRef] [PubMed]

42. Levey, A.S.; de Jong, P.E.; Coresh, J.; Nahas, M.E.; Astor, B.C.; Matsushita, K.; Gansevoort, R.T.; Kasiske, B.L.; Eckardt, K.U. The definition, classification, and prognosis of chronic kidney disease: A KDIGO controversities conference report. *Kidney Int.* **2011**, *80*, 17–28. [CrossRef] [PubMed]

16

Nutritional Strategies for the Individualized Treatment of Non-Alcoholic Fatty Liver Disease (NAFLD) Based on the Nutrient-Induced Insulin Output Ratio (NIOR)

Ewa Stachowska [1,*], Karina Ryterska [1], Dominika Maciejewska [1], Marcin Banaszczak [1], Piotr Milkiewicz [2,3], Małgorzata Milkiewicz [4], Izabela Gutowska [1], Piotr Ossowski [1], Małgorzata Kaczorowska [1], Dominika Jamioł-Milc [1], Anna Sabinicz [1], Małgorzata Napierała [5], Lidia Wądołowska [6] and Joanna Raszeja-Wyszomirska [3]

[1]   Department of Biochemistry and Human Nutrition, Pomeranian Medical University, Szczecin 71-460, Poland; ryterska.karina@gmail.com (K.R.); domi.maciejka@wp.pl (D.M.); banaszczak.marcin@gmail.com (M.B.); izagut@poczta.onet.pl (I.G.); zbizcz@pum.edu.pl (P.O.); szpital@szpital-zdroje.szczecin.pl (M.K.); dominikajamiol@interia.pl (D.J.-M.); kldiab@pum.edu.pl (A.S.)

[2]   Department of Clinical and Molecular Biochemistry, Pomeranian Medical University, Szczecin 70-111, Poland; p.milkiewicz@wp.pl

[3]   Liver and Internal Medicine Unit, Department of General, Transplant and Liver Surgery of the Medical University of Warsaw, Warsaw 02-097, Poland; jorasz@gmail.com

[4]   Department of Medical Biology, Pomeranian Medical University, Szczecin 70-111, Poland; milkiewm@pum.edu.pl

[5]   Department of Diabetology and Internal Diseases Pomeranian Medical University, Szczecin 72-010, Poland; malnap@sci.pum.edu.pl

[6]   Department of Human Nutrition, University of Warmia and Mazury, Olsztyn 10-718, Poland; lidia.wadolowska@wum.edu.pl

*   Correspondence: ewa.stachowska@pum.edu.pl

Academic Editors: Amedeo Lonardo and Giovanni Targher

Abstract: Nutrients play a fundamental role as regulators of the activity of enzymes involved in liver metabolism. In the general population, the action of nutrients may be affected by gene polymorphisms. Therefore, individualization of a diet for individuals with fatty liver seems to be a fundamental step in nutritional strategies. In this study, we tested the nutrient-induced insulin output ratio (NIOR), which is used to identify the correlation between the variants of genes and insulin resistance. We enrolled 171 patients, Caucasian men ($n = 104$) and women ($n = 67$), diagnosed with non-alcoholic fatty liver disease (NAFLD). From the pool of genes sensitive to nutrient content, we selected genes characterized by a strong response to the NIOR. The polymorphisms included Adrenergic receptor (*b3AR*), Tumor necrosis factor (*TNFα*), Apolipoprotein C (*Apo C III*). Uncoupling Protein type I (*UCP-1*), Peroxisome proliferator activated receptor γ2 (*PPAR-2*) and Apolipoprotein E (*APOEs*). We performed three dietary interventions: a diet consistent with the results of genotyping (NIOR (+)); typical dietary recommendations for NAFLD (Cust (+)), and a diet opposite to the genotyping results (NIOR (−) and Cust (−)). We administered the diet for six months. The most beneficial changes were observed among fat-sensitive patients who were treated with the NIOR (+) diet. These changes included improvements in body mass and insulin sensitivity and normalization of blood lipids. In people sensitive to fat, the NIOR seems to be a useful tool for determining specific strategies for the treatment of NAFLD.

Keywords: NAFLD; NAFLD diet; insulin sensitivity; NIOR; reduction of body mass; fat reduction; liver fat

1. Introduction

Non-alcoholic fatty liver disease (NAFLD) is one of the most frequently diagnosed liver diseases in the industrialized world—approximately 20%–30% of nations' populations are affected by it [1, 2]. With the increase in obesity, NAFLD has become a major risk factor for cirrhosis (and other diseases, e.g., cardiovascular diseases) [3]. Multiple trials have demonstrated that weight loss reduces histological steatosis (intrahepatic fat content) and the amount of serum enzymes [4].

One of the key causes of NAFLD is an improper diet based on caloric oversupply, the excessive intake of fats, and, at the same time, the low intake of grains, fruits, vegetables, proteins and ω-3 fatty acids [2]. This pattern of nutrition leads to the development of hyperinsulinemia, insulin resistance and obesity [2,5–7]. Therefore, on the one hand, nutrition is a major cause of NAFLD, but on the other, it presents an effective form of treatment [5,8,9].

In NAFLD, nutrition can be characterized by an appropriate choice of active nutrients that can play a regulatory role in metabolism. Nutrients regulate the activity of enzymes involved in metabolic processes, acting at the level of the proteome and metabolome and functioning as sensors that influence metabolic pathways [10–12]. Importantly, the same nutrient may have different influences on given people due to genetic polymorphisms found in the population [12]. The interactions between nutrients, genetic factors (polymorphism/mutations) and health are the subject matter of nutrigenomics [12]. This field of science aims to establish personalized nutrition strategies for the prevention and treatment of lifestyle diseases [12,13]. It can be assumed that if the action of nutrients is affected by polymorphisms, it is advisable to search for methods of individualizing a patient's nutrition. Therefore, in this study, we focused on testing a tool that could be used for the individualization of nutrition in patients with NAFLD. The specific tool used in this study was the nutrient-induced insulin output ratio (NIOR), which was selected to determine the genotype-phenotype interaction [14].

The NIOR has already been used to identify a correlation between the variants of genes (associated with the metabolism of carbohydrates and fat) and the output of insulin and the development of diet-induced insulin resistance. Using the NIOR, we identified the carriers of the alleles of gene variants characterized by a reduced tolerance to fat or carbohydrates in the diet. The pool of genes associated with NIOR includes glucose-sensitive genes, such as genes for Adrenergic receptors (*b3AR*), Tumor necrosis factor (*TNF-α*) and Apolipoprotein C (*APOC3*) [14]. The variants of these genes are described in the literature as being responsible for an increased risk of developing insulin resistance (gene *b3AR*, rs 4994) [15], the induction and development of insulin resistance and metabolic syndrome (gene *TNF-α*, rs 1800629) [16] and severe forms of hyperlipidemia (gene *APOC3*, rs 5128) [17].

Fat-sensitive genes associated with NIOR include the genes of Uncoupling Protein type I (*UCP-1*, rs 1800592), Peroxisome proliferator-activated receptor γ 2 (*PPAR-γ2*, rs 18012820) and Apolipoprotein E (*ApoE*). Selected variants of these genes are responsible for the regulation of body weight and the concentration of plasma high density lipoprotein (Type 1 uncoupling protein (*UCP1*)) [18], an increased risk of metabolic syndrome by the regulation of energy homeostasis and glucose (Peroxisome proliferator activated receptor γ2 *PPAR-γ2* gene) [19], the furthering of insulin-resistance, the development of hyperlipidemia and hypertriglyceridemia and the progression of coronary heart disease (*APOE* rs 405509, rs 7412 rs 429358) [17].

The aim of this study was to determine whether the NIOR can be useful in planning the individualized nutrition of patients with NAFLD and whether its use contributes to a more effective inhibition of NAFLD progression, defined as a reduced degree of hepatic steatosis and improved biochemical and anthropometric parameters.

2. Results

2.1. The Analysis of the Data Using Model 1

2.1.1. Changes in Anthropometric Parameters after Six Months Depending on the Type of Diet

The most beneficial changes in body composition were observed among patients treated with the NIOR (+) diet (Table 1). The body mass reduction, the reduction in waist circumference, and the reduction in fat mass were significant.

Weight reductions were also recorded in the Cust (+) group, but in comparison to NIOR (+), the reduction in fat content was less significant (-3.40 ± 6.27, $p < 0.002$ vs. -0.66 ± 3.67, $p < 0.02$) (Table 1). In Cust (+) patients, negative changes associated with the loss of lean body mass and arm circumference were also recorded (Table 1).

Slight changes in body mass, waist circumference, and hip circumference were observed in the group contrary to NIOR (−) and Cust (−) (called CONTRA in Table 1).

The analysis of changes between these groups provided interesting results. The most significant changes were observed when NIOR (+) and NIOR (−) and Cust (−) were compared (CONTRA NIOR (−) and Cust (−)). Between these groups, there were significant differences in the reduction of body mass (-6.79 ± 4.79 kg, NIOR (+) vs. -2.56 ± 2.88 kg NIOR (−), $p < 0.026$), BMI (-2.41 ± 1.73 kg/m^2 NIOR (+) vs. -0.83 ± 1.04 kg/m^2 NIOR (−), $p < 0.015$), fat mass (-5.39 ± 6.19, $p < 0.006$ NIOR (+) vs. -0.136 ± 2.97 NIOR (−), $p < 0.007$) and fat content (-2.45 ± 7.01 NIOR (+) vs. -0.88 ± 3.00 NIOR (−), $p < 0.005$) (Table 1).

Between the groups Cust (+) and NIOR (+), we observed a significant difference in the reduction of fat mass (-3.40 ± 6.27 kg Cust (+) vs. -5.39 ± 6.19 kg NIOR (+), $p < 0.04$) (Table 1).

Between the groups Cust (+) and Cust (−), we found a difference in arm circumference change (-1.45 ± 1.60 cm Cust (+) vs. 1.05 ± 3.01 cm Cust (−), $p < 0.04$) (Table 1).

2.1.2. Changes in Biochemical Parameters after Six Months in Model 1

One of the most important objectives to achieve during nutritional therapy in patients with NAFLD is a reduction in insulin resistance [20]. This effect was measured by determining. The homeostatc model assessment HOMA IR and HOMA B (used to estimate the improved β-cell "function") [21]. HOMA IR under normal physiological conditions is 1.0; higher values indicate peripheral insulin resistance or resistance of hepatic origin [22,23]. Patients in all groups were characterized by insulin resistance at the beginning (Table 1). The highest average HOMA IR value was observed for the NIOR (−) and Cust (−) groups. The reduction in HOMA IR in both of these groups reached -2.64 ± 4.57, $p < 0.05$. The initial HOMA IR in NIOR (+) patients was 3.76 ± 1.94. The recorded reduction in HOMA IR after six months was -1.34 ± 1.86, $p < 0.05$ (Table 1).

Additionally, the normalization of blood lipids (total cholesterol, triglyceride (TG), low density lipoprotein (LDL), high density lipoprotein (HDL) is an important element of nutritional therapy. Positive trends toward blood lipid normalization were observed in all types of diets (Table 1).

2.1.3. A Significant Reduction in the Degree of Fatty Liver Disease Was Observed in Patients with a Diet Selected According to NIOR

In the NIOR (+) group, the average reduction in the degree of fatty liver disease was -1.31 ± 1.01, $p < 0.002$. The difference in the reduction of fatty liver disease was significant between the NIOR (+) and NIOR (−) groups, $p < 0.04$—Mann-Whitney U test (Table 1).

Table 1. Anthropological and biochemical characteristics of the study participants' blood parameters at baseline and after six months of the diet in Model 1, with p-values of the comparison between subjects within this same intervention before and after six months. [a] $p < 0.0005$ Wilcoxon test, comparison between baseline and the fourth visit in this same group; [b] $p < 0.005$ Wilcoxon test, comparison between baseline and the fourth visit in this same group; * Mann-Whitney U test, comparison between NIOR (+) and Cust (+); # Mann-Whitney U test, comparison between NIOR (+) and contrary diets NIOR (−)/Cust (−); & Mann-Whitney U test, comparison between Cust (+) and contrary diets Cust (−) and NIOR (−). BMI: Body mass index; MUFA: monounsaturated fatty acids; PUFA: polyunsaturated fatty acids; HA: hyaluronic acid.

Parameters	Baseline			24W			p Value
	CUST (+)	NOR (+)	CONTRA CUST (−) and NOR (−)	CUST (+)	NOR (+)	CONTRA CUST (−) and NOR (−)	
Age	52.12 ± 14.74	52.80 ± 12.37	51.87 ± 12.11	52.12 ± 14.74	52.80 ± 12.37	51.87 ± 12.11	
Body mass (kg)	94.70 ± 22.55 [a]	89.01 ± 15.26 [a]	92.20 ± 19.34 [b]	87.59 ± 17.96 [a]	82.21 ± 15.35 [a,#]	89.63 ± 20.79 [b,#]	[a] $p < 0.0005$ [b] $p < 0.005$
BMI (kg/m²)	32.10 ± 4.13	30.70 ± 3.64	32.27 ± 6.59	30.01 ± 2.84	28.29 ± 15.35 [#]	28.29 ± 15.35 [#]	[#] $p < 0.015$
Arm circumference (cm)	33.30 ± 3.64 [a]	31.66 ± 2.87	32.33 ± 3.86	31.85 ± 2.56 [a,&]	30.75 ± 3.46	33.38 ± 4.53 [&]	[a] $p < 0.0005$ [&] $p < 0.04$
Waist circumference (cm)	105.14 ± 14.69 [a]	100.12 ± 11.75 [b]	106.25 ± 14.45 [b]	97.02 ± 10.63 [a]	94.00 ± 11.97 [b]	102.60 ± 16.02 [b]	[a] $p < 0.0009$ [b] $p < 0.005$
Hip circumference (cm)	105.14 ± 14.69 [a]	100.12 ± 11.75 [b]	106.25 ± 15.73 [b]	104.20 ± 14.89 [a]	94.00 ± 13.33 [b]	102.60 ± 17.04 [b]	[a] $p < 0.0009$ [b] $p < 0.005$
Fat mass (%)	34.71 ± 5.78 [b]	35.41 ± 5.67 [a]	36.02 ± 14.09	31.31 ± 5.78 [b,*]	29.74 ± 8.21 [a,#]	35.09 ± 14.94 [#]	[a] $p < 0.0006$ [b] $p < 0.002$ [#] $p < 0.007$ [*] $p < 0.04$
Fat content (%)	37.00 ± 6.63 [b]	35.61 ± 10.96 [b]	38.07 ± 7.79	36.34 ± 5.75 [b,*]	31.03 ± 13.46 [b,*,#]	38.95 ± 7.90 [#]	[b] $p < 0.005$ [#] $p < 0.005$ [*] $p < 0.04$
Lean mass (%)	60.02 ± 16.47 [b]	53.48 ± 10.96	55.94 ± 7.80 [b]	55.92 ± 14.17 [b]	51.03 ± 13.46	53.66 ± 9.28 [b]	[b] $p < 0.002$
AST (U/L)	36.10 ± 25.83 [b]	30.70 ± 13.99 [b]	32.71 ± 10.46 [b]	35.10 ± 29.60 [b]	34.20 ± 26.31 [b,#]	23.85 ± 5.21 [b,#]	[b] $p < 0.035$ [#] $p < 0.041$
ALI (U/L)	54.00 ± 36.86 [a]	46.70 ± 26.56 [a]	47.92 ± 15.85 [a]	44.40 ± 27.86 [a]	39.40 ± 33.04 [a]	32.57 ± 18.40 [a]	[a] $p < 0.0006$ [a] $p < 0.038$
Triglyceride (mg/dL)	129.30 ± 36.30 [b]	123.80 ± 52.82	238.42 ± 482.09	106.40 ± 56.24 [b]	121.80 ± 90.52	204.78 ± 319.17	[b] $p < 0.04$
HDL (mg/dL)	51.00 ± 12.22 [b]	54.40 ± 12.83	51.57 ± 15.73	54.00 ± 16.39 [b]	54.30 ± 12.82	52.14 ± 14.31	[b] $p < 0.025$
Insulin (mcU/L)	15.80 ± 9.05	14.59 ± 8.20 [b]	18.54 ± 19.69 [b]	12.07 ± 8.62	9.58 ± 6.81 [b]	9.63 ± 9.46 [b]	[b] $p < 0.05$
HOMA–IR	4.03 ± 2.31	3.76 ± 1.94 [b]	5.44 ± 6.65 [b]	3.08 ± 2.08	2.41 ± 1.74 [b]	2.80 ± 3.00 [b]	[b] $p < 0.05$
Hyaluronic acid (U/L)	54.56 ± 29.57	45.47 ± 25.82 [b]	50.23 ± 31.76	45.93 ± 22.62	32.56 ± 16.28 [b]	37.42 ± 22.21	[b] $p < 0.04$
Fatty liver Hamaguchi score	2.13 ± 0.74 [b]	2.47 ± 0.94 [b]	2.11 ± 0.98 [b]	1.2 ± 1.0 [b]	1.12 ± 1.08 [b,#]	1.11 ± 0.92 [b,#]	[b] $p < 0.01$ [#] $p < 0.04$

2.2. The Data Analysis in Model 2

Individuals from Different Groups Who Had a Similar Range of Reduction in Body Weight Obtained Different Reductions in Hepatic Steatosis and Other Parameters

Only individuals in the NIOR (+) group showed improvement in the degree of hepatic steatosis (Figure 1, Table S1).

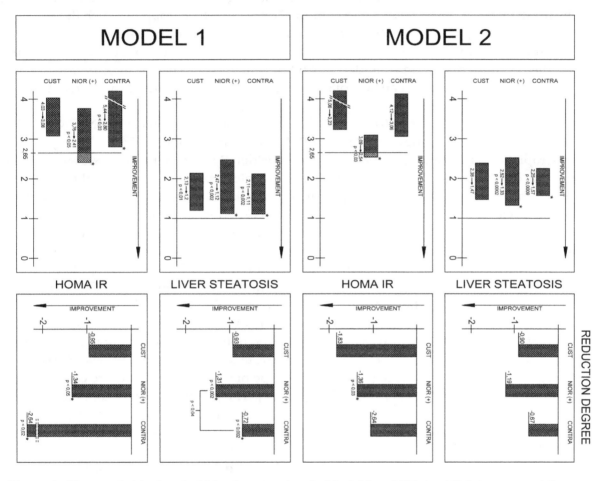

Figure 1. Changes in biochemical blood parameters in Model 1 and 2Note: All data represent the mean (standard deviation).

The analysis of the differences between the groups showed that the reduction in hepatic steatosis in the NIOR (+) group significantly differed from that observed in the NIOR (−) group (Mann-Whitney U test, $p < 0.04$). A similar significant difference between groups was observed for hyaluronic acid, with levels differing significantly between the Cust (+) and NIOR (+) groups (-26.45 ± 17.72 NIOR (+) vs. -1.94 ± 5.4 Cust (−) and NIOR (−), Mann-Whitney U test, $p < 0.005$).

3. Discussion

Obesity and insulin resistance present a considerable challenge in the nutrition plans of patients with NAFLD [24,25]. Current dietary guidelines are based on epidemiological data showing a link between diets enriched in saturated fatty acids and in fructose and the development of insulin resistance [26]. However, the response to diet differs depending on individual variations in genetic and metabolic phenotypes. Therefore, it is important to personalize patients' diets, taking into account their genetic predispositions [13,14].

One potentially interesting tool is the nutrient-induced insulin output ratio (NIOR). The NIOR makes it possible to categorize patients (gene variant carriers) into two groups: phenotypically sensitive to glucose or fat in the diet. The polymorphisms of genes associated with the NIOR have previously been associated with the severity of metabolic syndrome and susceptibility to the effects of nutrients [14–19]. In our work, we examined polymorphisms (linked with NIOR) according to their impact on the output of insulin after a meal [14]. The usefulness of NIOR as a potential tool to individualize diets was examined through the introduction of quantitative changes in nutrients (fat or simple carbohydrates), consistent with the results of genetic tests. To exclude the impact of polymorphisms themselves, some people were randomly assigned to a group in which the key nutrient contents were chosen in quantities contrary to the indications of genetic research.

The second important objective of this study was to create a nutritional plan that would be accepted by the respondents for an extended period of time. We succeeded in obtaining the results of a half-year-long diet, resulting in an acceptable reduction in the content of the tested nutrients in the diet.

We showed that a selection of nutrients consistent with the indications of the NIOR contributed to an effective reduction in hepatic steatosis in both Model 1 and Model 2. This is a very important result, as fat droplets accumulating in hepatocytes are considered the main hepatotoxic factor, inducing hepatic steatosis and fibrosis [27–29]. The reduction of lipid content in the liver, therefore, means a reduction in the intensity of fibrosis [27], which is marked by hyaluronic acid content in the blood [28,29]. Such a reduction in hyaluronic acid was recorded in all groups, but the largest decline in hyaluronic acid content was found in the NIOR (+) group, regardless of the research model (Table 1 and Figure 1).

Additionally, individual selections of nutrients based on the NIOR were intended to contribute to the reduction of fat mass (Table 1). The results seem to confirm the usefulness of NIOR for the efficient reduction in body fat mass and fat content when comparing the NIOR (+) and NIOR (−) groups. It seems that the reduction of fat mass and fat tissue was most effective in the group in which the amount of dietary fat or dietary sugar was adjusted to gene polymorphisms. Of note is that there was no significant effect of NIOR on the reduction of insulin resistance between groups. The HOMA IR ratio was effectively reduced in all groups, regardless of the type of diet (Table 1). Fats are components that play a crucial role in the progression of NAFLD [27,30–34]. The positive changes in the liver were the result of a decrease in the fat content of the diet, especially among fat-sensitive polymorphism carriers (Table 1 and Figure 1). Our study confirms the results of other authors, e.g., Marina et al. [31], who found that fat (in different contents in the diet—20% vs. 55% the total daily energy expenditure (TDEE) caused minor effects in the content of intra-abdominal fat and intrahepatic lipids. In another study (a short-term intervention), a three-week isocaloric low-fat diet (20% TDEE) decreased intrahepatic lipids by 13%, whereas a high fat diet (55% TDEE) increased the amount of lipids in the liver by up to 17% [30]. Unfortunately, both studies were limited to a short period of observation [30,31].

Though our study was longer, it suffered from a significant limitation, which was the exclusion of variants sensitive to simple sugars (after six months, only one person remained—Figure 2). This was a substantial loss because simple sugars, especially fructose (a common nutrient in western diets), is reported to be associated with an increased risk of NAFLD [35–37]. Although the consumption of fructose is high and continues to be on the rise [38], there are still no conclusive results that indicate a connection between the high intake of fructose and NAFLD [35,37]. The available evidence is not sufficiently robust to draw conclusions regarding the effects of fructose, high fructose corn syrup (HFCS) or sucrose consumption on NAFLD [37].

It seems that the lack of clear associations between the consumption of simple sugars and hepatic steatosis can result from yet another important variable, i.e., gender. Research from 2014 shows that the severity of hepatic steatosis may be significantly influenced by feeding patterns associated with gender [27]. Unfortunately, our study cannot be included in the discussion in this area. Slightly more severe hepatic steatosis was shown in our analysis of diets before the initiation of the prescribed diet. The analysis of the FFQ results indicates a lack of a relationship between the consumption of products containing large amounts of sugars and the degree of hepatic steatosis among our respondents, regardless of gender (unpublished results). Understanding the specific interaction between nutrients and dietary needs and maintaining this balance is extremely important in providing treatment for NAFLD [39,40].

4. Materials and Methods

4.1. Patients

A group of 171 eligible participants, Caucasian men (n = 104) and women (n = 67) diagnosed with NAFLD, were prospectively enrolled in the study (Figure 2). Of the 171 total recruited patients, only 166 confirmed patients with NAFLD met the inclusion criteria. We conducted the measurements at the beginning of the study and at check points conducted at the first visit, after the first month, the second month and after six months—the final check point (Figure 2).

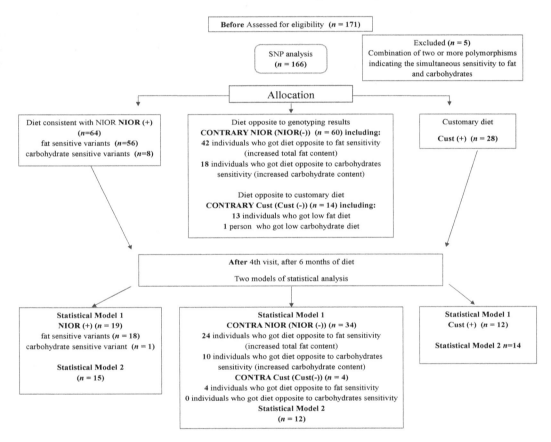

Figure 2. Flowchart for the selection of individuals from the nutrient-induced insulin output ratio (NIOR) cohort. Participants entering subsequent phases of the study as well as dropouts out are indicated in the total. NIOR (+) represents individuals consuming a diet consistent with the results of genotyping; Cust (+), individuals consuming a diet comprising the typical dietary recommendations for non-alcoholic fatty liver disease (NAFLD); NIOR (−) and Cust (−), individuals consuming a diet contrary to the genotyping results.

The exclusion criteria included the following: diabetes mellitus (DMII); infection with either HBV (Hepatitis B Virus) or HCV (Hepatitis C Virus); obesity (body mass index (BMI) >30 kg/m^2); high levels of physical activity (>3000 kcal/week in leisure-time physical activity); changes in physical activity during the dietary intervention; use of statins; any condition that could limit the mobility of the participant; not being able to attend control visits; vegetarianism or a need for other special diets; the excessive consumption of alcohol (≥20 g in women and ≥30 g in men, per day); and other drug addiction.

Physical activity was assessed during the first visit and in subsequent appointments using the International Physical Activity Questionnaire (IPAQ) [41]. In this study we recommended moderate activity and we advised our patients not to change physical activity during the time of intervention. The degree of fatty liver disease was assessed by a trained physician according to the Hamaguchi score [42], using a high-resolution B-mode abdominal ultrasound scanner (Acuson X300, Simens, San Jose, CA, USA).

The study protocol was approved by the ethics committee of the Pomeranian Medical University (Szczecin, Poland, 25 01 2010 KB-0012/09/10) and conformed to the ethical guidelines of the 1975 Declaration of Helsinki. The volunteers provided written informed consent before the study.

4.2. The Anthropometric Data

Anthropometric assessments were performed routinely during each of the four visits. The study included measurements of height (m), body weight (kg), skinfold thickness (mm), arm circumference (cm), waist circumference (cm) and hip circumference (cm). The measurements of body weight and height were obtained by means of medical scales with a stadiometer. Body mass index was calculated according to these measurements (BMI = body weight (kg)/square of height (m)) [24,43]. Using a medical tape measure, waist circumference was measured (midway between the bottom edge of the ribs and the iliac crest) as was hip circumference. Based on these measurements, WHR was calculated (WHR = waist circumference (cm)/hip circumference (cm)) [24]. A caliper was used to measure skinfold thicknesses: biceps, triceps, subscapular and abdominal skinfolds. In addition, in each subject, body composition was measured with a multifrequency bioimpedance meter, BIA-101 (Akern, Bioresearch SRL, PONASSIEVE, Florence, Italy).

4.3. Methods and Experimental Design

A randomized parallel controlled clinical trial with three dietary interventions was performed:

1. A diet consistent with the results of genotyping, called NIOR (+);
2. A diet with typical dietary recommendations for NAFLD, called Cust (+) [8];
3. A diet opposite to genotyping results, called (NIOR (−) and Cust (−) (CONTRA NIOR and Cust) (Figure 3).

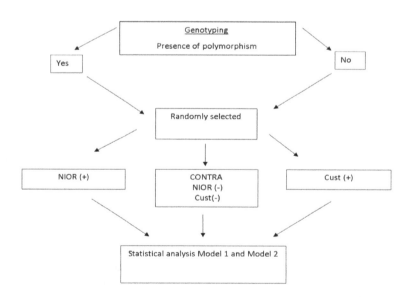

Figure 3. Baseline treatment characteristics. NIOR (+) represents individuals consuming a diet consistent with the results of genotyping; Cust (+), individuals consuming a diet comprising the typical dietary recommendations for NAFLD; NIOR (−) and Cust (−), individuals consuming a diet contrary to the genotyping results.

4.4. Allocation to Groups

The patients were randomly assigned to the NIOR (+) group. They represented:

(a) a single polymorphism indicative of sensitivity to carbohydrates or fats
(b) more than one polymorphism indicative of sensitivity to carbohydrates or to fats (e.g., two polymorphisms indicative of sensitivity to fat)

Only eight patients from the NIOR (+) group had polymorphisms indicative of sensitivity to carbohydrates. Unfortunately, these people dropped out of the study at various stages of the study. Only one carrier of sensitivity to carbohydrates completed the study (19 patients remained in the group).

Persons with a combination of two or more polymorphisms indicating simultaneous sensitivity to fat and carbohydrates were excluded from the study.

4.5. Dietary Intervention

4.5.1. General Recommendation

The diet was calculated individually according to the patient's caloric needs. Individuals with a BMI indicating that they were overweight or obese received a reduced caloric diet of 500 kcal/day. People with a BMI within the normal range were given a normocaloric diet that allowed them to maintain their current body weight.

The total daily energy expenditure (TDEE) was calculated using the direct measurement of resting metabolic rate (RMR). RMR was measured during the first visit and in subsequent follow-up visits with a Fitmate apparatus (Pro, COSMED). The activity factor (AF) was determined in accordance with the generally accepted norm (TDEE = AF $\times$ RMR). The caloric content of the diet was adjusted during visits to the changing values of the patient's TDEE.

All patients received weekly menus and guidelines on the timing of meals throughout the day, their composition and the size of the portions. Menus were prepared in the form of a daily plan for the seven days of the week and included guidance on the timing during the day of the five meal times.

The recommended sources of fat included vegetable fats, with a predominance of rapeseed oil and olive oil. It was permissible to use butter and margarine. Animal fats such as lard were excluded.

The recommended sources of carbohydrates included products with a low and medium glycemic index (GI). These included whole wheat bread, whole wheat pasta, cereal and brown rice. Sweets were excluded from the diet.

The recommended protein sources comprised poultry, fish (oily fish three times a week), fermented dairy products (two times a day), eggs (four to five times a week), lean cottage cheese, and cheese with a reduced fat content. Pork fat and offal products were excluded from the diet. The amount of fruit and vegetables recommended in the diets included three portions of vegetables and two portions of fruit. The amount of fluid intake was calculated to be 35 mL/kg of actual body weight.

4.5.2. Recommendations Based on the Nutrient-Induced Insulin Output Ratio (NIOR)

(a) NIOR (+) patients received dietary recommendations with a reduced fat content (20% TDEE when NIOR polymorphisms showed sensitivity to fat) or reduced carbohydrate content (55% of TDEE, including <5% of sugars, when the polymorphisms showed sensitivity to simple carbohydrates).
(b) Cust (+) patients received dietary advice with the following nutrient content: fat content at 30% of TDEE and carbohydrates at 55% of TDEE (including 10% of simple carbohydrates).
(c) NIOR (−) patients, when they had "fat-sensitive" gene variants, received dietary recommendations that increased total fat content up to 30% of TDEE.

When participants had sugar-sensitive variants of genes, they received an increased amount of carbohydrates (10% simple carbohydrates).

Cust (−) patients were randomly assigned to groups with a reduced fat content or lower carbohydrate content.

4.5.3. Dietary Control

Nutrition patterns were analyzed with a Food Frequency Questionnaire (FFQ) and a 72 h food diary (including two working days and one day free of work) during the first visit. At all check points, the patients brought their completed 72 h food diary. The amounts consumed were recorded in household units, by volume or by measuring with a ruler. The dietary records were validated by a nutritionist according to a corresponding food table and nutrient database (Table 2).

4.6. Laboratory Analyses

After overnight fasting, venous blood was collected into tubes containing anticoagulant Ethylenediaminetetraacetic acid (EDTA).

Blood samples were centrifuged at 3500 rpm for 10 min at 4 °C within 2 h of collection. Standard blood biochemical analyses were carried out at the University Hospital Laboratory (Szczecin, Poland). Hyaluronic acid was determined with an ELISA kit (Wuhan EIAab Science, A1710 Guangguguoji, Wuhan, China).

4.7. Genotyping

From the pool of genes sensitive to nutrient content, we selected genes that were characterized by a strong response to the oral glucose tolerance test after 75 g of glucose or after a high-fat meal. These included the b3-adrenergic receptor (b3AR), tumor necrosis factor (TNF-α) and apolipoprotein C III (apo CIII) [14].

From the pool of carbohydrate-sensitive genes, we selected Type 1 uncoupling protein (UCP-1), peroxisome proliferator-activated receptor γ 2 (PPAR-Y2) and apolipoprotein E (ApoE).

DNA from mononuclear peripheral blood was isolated using a DNeasy Blood and Tissue kit (Qiagen, Valencia, CA, USA). Genotypes were determined by the real-time polymerase chain reaction using TaqMan® Genotyping 36 g Assays for polymorphisms, including b3AR rs4994 (Applied Biosystems Assay ID C___2215549_20); TNF-rs1800629 (C___7514879_10); Apo C III-rs5128 (C___8907537_1); Ucp-1-rs1800592 (C___8866368_20); PPAR-2-rs 1801282 (C___1129864_10); APOE-rs 405509 (C____905013_10); APOE-rs7412 (C_904973_10); and APOE-rs429358 (C___3084793_20). Fluorescence data were analyzed with allelic discrimination—7500 Software v 2.0.2 (Foster City, CA, USA).

4.8. Statistical Analysis

Statistica 7.1 software (Statsoft, Poznań, Poland) was used for the statistical analysis, and all results are expressed as the mean ± standard deviation. As the distribution, in most cases, deviated from normal (Shapiro-Wilk's test), non-parametric tests were used: Wilcoxon tests were used for comparisons among groups and Mann-Whitney U tests were used for comparisons between groups. A $p < 0.05$ was considered significant.

Two Models of Statistical Analysis

Model 1 included the analysis of the results of the anthropometric and biochemical measurements with the criterion of the dietary recommendations that were adopted by the patients throughout the study (six months). The caloric value of the patients' menus was estimated during checkups, which took place after one, two and six months, based on their 72 h diaries. The patients who were included in the statistical analysis followed the diet carefully (which was estimated based on menus in relation to the recommended caloric content ±200 kcal/day). Patients who exceeded that value at any stage of the study were excluded from the statistical analysis in Model 1.

Table 2. Characteristics of dietary interventions. Nutrient-induced insulin output ratio (NIOR) (+) represents individuals consuming a diet consistent with the results of genotyping; Cust (+), individuals consuming a diet comprising the typical dietary recommendations for non-alcoholic fatty liver disease (NAFLD); NIOR (−) and Cust (−), individuals consuming a diet contrary to the genotyping results. * Group with a lower amount of carbohydrate (CHO) or fat.

Content of Diet	NIOR (+) Variant Sensitive for Fat	NIOR (+) Variant Sensitive for Carbohydrate	Cust (+)	CONTRA NIOR NIOR (−) If Variant Was Sensitive for Fat	CONTRA NIOR NIOR (−) If Variant Was Sensitive for Carbohydrate	CONTRA Cust Cust (−) Randomly Selected to Group with Lower Amount of Fat of CHO *
Energy	Calculated individually	Calculated individually	Calculated individually	Calculated individually	Calculated individually	Calculated individually
Fat percent of total caloric in %	20	30	30	30	20	20 or 30 *
Carbohydrates in %	65	55	55	55	65	65 or 55 *
Simple carbohydrate in %	≥10	<5	≥10	<5	≥10	≥10 or <5 *
Protein (%)	15	15	15	15	15	15
Fiber (g/day)	30–35	30–35	30–35	30–35	30–35	30–35
Fluid (mL/kg)	35	35	35	35	35	35

Model 2 included the analysis of the anthropometric and biochemical results with the criterion of weight loss in the range of 8–10 kg over six months. We excluded patients who were characterized by normal weight at the beginning of the experiment from this analysis.

5. Conclusions

It seems that by introducing an individual nutrition and genotyping plan that takes into account the normal supply of calories, nutrients, proteins, and micro- and macronutrients, we are able to prevent problems that result from the progression of disease. Therefore, individualization, understood as the work of a dietitian with the patient, seems to be a therapeutic necessity, and the nutrient-induced insulin output ratio in people sensitive to fat seems to be n useful tool for determining specific strategies for patients with NAFLD.

Acknowledgments: Supported by a grant from the Narodowe Centrum Nauki (NCN), Nr N404 150539.

Author Contributions: Ewa Stachowska conceived and designed the experiments, wrote the paper; Karina Ryterska performed the experiments; Dominika Maciejewska performed the experiments (biochemistry); Marcin Banaszczak performed the experiments (biochemistry); Piotr Milkiewicz conceived and designed the experiments (medical support); Małgorzata Milkiewicz performed the experiments (biochemistry-PCR); Izabela Gutowska analyzed the data; Piotr Ossowski performed the experiments (biochemistry); Małgorzata Kaczorowska performed the experiments (nutrition); Dominika Jamioł-Milc performed the; experiments (nutrition); Anna Sabinicz performed the experiments (nutrition); Małgorzata Napierała performed the experiments (nutrition); Lidia Wądołowska contributed reagents/materials/analysis tools (nutritional analysis); Raszeja-Wyszomirska Joanna analyzed the data (medical support).

References

1. Vernon, G.; Baranova, A.; Younossi, Z.M. Systematic review: The epidemiology and natural history of non-alcoholic fatty liver disease and non-alcoholic steatohepatitis in adults. *Aliment. Pharmacol. Ther.* **2011**, *34*, 274–285. [CrossRef] [PubMed]

2. Argo, C.K.; Northup, P.G.; Al-Osaimi, A.M.; Caldwell, S.H. Systematic review of risk factors for fibrosis progression in non-alcoholic steatohepatitis. *J. Hepatol.* **2009**, *51*, 371–379. [CrossRef] [PubMed]

3. Targher, G.; Day, C.P.; Bonora, E. Risk of cardiovascular disease in patients with nonalcoholic fatty liver disease. *N. Engl. J. Med.* **2010**, *363*, 1341–1350. [CrossRef] [PubMed]

4. Promrat, K.; Kleiner, D.E.; Niemeier, H.M.; Jackvony, E.; Kearns, M.; Wands, JR.; Fava, J.L.; Wing, R.R. Randomized controlled trial testing the effects of weight loss on nonalcoholic steatohepatitis. *Hepatology* **2010**, *51*, 121–129. [CrossRef] [PubMed]

5. Yoon, H.J.; Cha, B.S. Pathogenesis and therapeutic approaches for non-alcoholic fatty liver disease. *World J. Hepatol.* **2014**, *6*, 800–811. [CrossRef] [PubMed]

6. Hassan, K.; Bhalla, V.; El Regal, M.E.; A-Kader, H.H. Nonalcoholic fatty liver disease: A comprehensive review of a growing epidemic. *World J. Gastroenterol.* **2014**, *20*, 12082–120101. [CrossRef] [PubMed]

7. Weiß, J.; Rau, M.; Geier, A. Non-alcoholic fatty liver disease: Epidemiology, clinical course, investigation, and treatment. *Dtsch. Ärzteblatt Int.* **2014**, *111*, 447–452.

8. Kargulewicz, A.; Stankowiak-Kulpa, H.; Grzymisławski, M. Dietary recommendations for patients with nonalcoholic fatty liver disease. *Prz. Gastroenterol.* **2014**, *9*, 18–23. [CrossRef] [PubMed]

9. Barrera, F.; George, J. The role of diet and nutritional intervention for the management of patients with NAFLD. *Clin. Liver. Dis.* **2014**, *18*, 91–112. [CrossRef] [PubMed]

10. Keijer, J.; Hoevenaars, F.P.; Nieuwenhuizen, A.; van Schothorst, E.M. Nutrigenomics of body weight regulation: A rationale for careful dissection of individual contributors. *Nutrients* **2014**, *6*, 4531–4551. [CrossRef] [PubMed]

11. Arslan, N. Obesity, fatty liver disease and intestinal microbiota. *World J. Gastroenterol.* **2014**, *20*, 16452–16463. [CrossRef] [PubMed]

12. Hesketh, J.; Wybranska, I.; Dommels, Y.; King, M.; Elliott, R.; Pico, C.; Keijer, J. Nutrient-gene interactions in benefit-risk analysis. *Br. J. Nutr.* **2006**, *95*, 1232–1239. [CrossRef] [PubMed]

13. Kang, J.X. The coming of age of nutrigenetics and nutrigenomics. *J. Nutr. Nutr.* **2012**, *5*. [CrossRef] [PubMed]

14. Wybranska, I.; Malczewska-Malec, M.; Partyka, L.; Kiec-Wilk, B.; Kosno, K.; Leszczynska-Golabek, I.; Zdzienicka, A.; Gruca, A.; Kwasniak, M.; Dembinska-Kiec, A. Evaluation of genetic predisposition to insulin resistance by nutrient-induced insulin output ratio (NIOR). *Clin. Chem. Lab. Med.* **2007**, *45*, 1124–1132. [CrossRef] [PubMed]

15. Zafarmand, M.H.; van der Schouw, Y.T.; Grobbee, D.E.; de Leeuw, P.W.; Bots, M.L. T64A polymorphism in β3-adrenergic receptor gene (*ADRB3*) and coronary heart disease: A case-cohort study and meta-analysis. *J. Intern. Med.* **2008**, *263*, 79–89. [CrossRef] [PubMed]

16. Miranda, J.L.; Perez-Martinez, P.P.; Marin, C.F.; Fuentes, F.; Delgado, J.; Pérez-Jiménez, F. Dietary fat, genes, and insulin sensitivity. *J. Mol. Med.* **2007**, *85*, 213–226. [CrossRef] [PubMed]

17. Henneman, P.; van der Sman-de Beer, F.; Moghaddam, P.H.; Huijts, P.; Stalenhoef, AF.; Kastelein, J.J.; van Duijn, C.M.; Havekes, L.M.; Frants, R.R.; van Dijk, K.W.; et al. The expression of type III hyperlipoproteinemia: Involvement of lipolysis genes. *Eur. J. Hum. Genet.* **2009**, *54*, 3043–3048. [CrossRef] [PubMed]

18. Hamada, T.; Kotani, K.; Nagai, N. Low-calorie diet-induced reduction in serum HDL cholesterol is ameliorated in obese women with the −3826 G allele in the uncoupling protein-1 gene. *Tohoku J. Exp. Med.* **2009**, *219*, 337–342. [CrossRef] [PubMed]

19. Meirhaeghem, A.; Cottel, D.; Amouyel, P.; Dallongeville, J. Association between peroxisome proliferator-activated receptor γ haplotypes and the metabolic syndrome in French men and women. *Diabetes* **2005**, *54*, 3043–3048. [CrossRef]

20. Marchesini, G.; Pagotto, U.; Bugianesi, E.; De Iasio, R.; Manini, R.; Vanni, E.; Pasquali, R.; Melchionda, N.; Rizzetto, M. Low ghrelin concentrations in nonalcoholic fatty liver disease are related to insulin resistance. *J. Clin. Endocrinol. Metab.* **2003**, *88*, 5674–5679. [CrossRef] [PubMed]

21. Pfützner, A.; Derwahl, M.; Jacob, S.; Hohberg, C.; Blümner, E.; Lehmann, U.; Fuchs, W.; Forst, T. Limitations of the HOMA-B score for assessment of β-cell functionality in interventional trials-results from the PIOglim study. *Diabetes. Technol. Ther.* **2010**, *12*, 599–604.

22. Haffner, S.M.; Kennedy, E.; Gonzalez, C.; Stern, M.P.; Miettinen, H. A prospective analysis of the HOMA model. The Mexico City Diabetes Study. *Diabetes Care* **1996**, *19*, 1138–1141. [CrossRef] [PubMed]

23. Eslamparast, T.; Eghtesad, S.; Poustchi, H.; Hekmatdoost, A. Recent advances in dietary supplementation, in treating non-alcoholic fatty liver disease. *World J. Hepatol.* **2015**, *7*, 204–212. [CrossRef] [PubMed]

24. Zheng, R.D.; Chen, Z.R.; Chen, J.N.; Lu, Y.H.; Chen, J. Role of body mass index, waist-to-height and waist-to-hip ratio in prediction of nonalcoholic fatty liver disease. *Gastroenterol. Res. Pract.* **2012**, *2012*, 362147. [CrossRef] [PubMed]

25. Dudekula, A.; Rachakonda, V.; Shaik, B.; Behari, J. Weight loss in nonalcoholic Fatty liver disease patients in an ambulatory care setting is largely unsuccessful but correlates with frequency of clinic visits. *PLoS ONE* **2014**, *9*, e111808. [CrossRef]

26. Deer, J.; Koska, J.; Ozias, M.; Reaven, P. Dietary models of insulin resistance. *Metabolism* **2015**, *64*, 163–171. [CrossRef] [PubMed]

27. Jia, Q.; Xia, Y.; Zhang, Q.; Wu, H.; Du, H.; Liu, L.; Wang, C.; Shi, H.; Guo, X.; Liu, X.; et al. Dietary patterns are associated with prevalence of fatty liver disease in adults. *Eur. J. Clin. Nutr.* **2015**, *69*, 914–921. [CrossRef] [PubMed]

28. Adams, L.A. Biomarkers of liver fibrosis. *J. Gastroenterol. Hepatol.* **2011**, *26*, 802–809. [CrossRef] [PubMed]

29. Rossi, E.; Adams, L.A.; Ching, H.L.; Bulsara, M.; MacQuillan, G.C.; Jeffrey, G.P. High biological variation of serum hyaluronic acid and Hepascore, a biochemical marker model for the prediction of liver fibrosis. *Clin. Chem. Lab. Med.* **2013**, *51*, 1107–1114. [CrossRef] [PubMed]

30. Van Herpen, N.A.; Schrauwen-Hinderling, V.; Schaart, G.; Mensink, R.P.; Schrauwen, P. Three weeks on a high-fat diet increases intrahepatic lipid accumulation and decreases metabolic flexibility in healthy overweight men. *JCEM* **2011**, *96*, E691–E695. [CrossRef] [PubMed]

31. Marina, A.; von Frankenberg, A.D.; Suvag, S.; Callahan, H.S.; Kratz, M.; Richards, T.L.; Utzschneider, K.M. Effects of dietary fat and saturated fat content on liver fat and markers of oxidative stress in overweight/obese men and women under weight-stable conditions. *Nutrients* **2014** *6*, 4678–4690. [CrossRef] [PubMed]

32. Westerbacka, J.; Lammi, K.; Hakkinen, A.M.; Rissanen, A.; Salminen, I.; Aro, A.; Yki-Järvinen, H. Dietary fat content modifies liver fat in overweight nondiabetic subjects. *J. Clin. Endocrinol. Metab.* **2005**, *90*, 2804–2809. [CrossRef] [PubMed]

33. Moore, J.B.; Gunn, P.J.; Fielding, B.A. The role of dietary sugars and de novo lipogenesis in non-alcoholic fatty liver disease. *Nutrients* **2014**, *6*, 5679–5703. [CrossRef] [PubMed]
34. Bémeur, C.; Butterworth, R.F. Nutrition in the management of cirrhosis and its neurological complications. *J. Clin. Exp. Hepatol.* **2014**, *4*, 141–150. [CrossRef] [PubMed]
35. Jin, R.; Welsh, J.A.; Le, N.A.; Holzberg, J.; Sharma, P.; Martin, D.R.; Vos, M.B. Dietary fructose reduction improves markers of cardiovascular disease risk in Hispanic-American adolescents with NAFLD. *Nutrients* **2014**, *6*, 3187–3201. [CrossRef] [PubMed]
36. Chiu, S.; Sievenpiper, J.L.; de Souza, R.J.; Cozma, A.I.; Mirrahimi, A.; Carleton, A.J.; Ha, V.; di Buono, M.; Jenkins, A.L.; Leiter, L.A.; et al. Effect of fructose on markers of non-alcoholic fatty liver disease (NAFLD): A systematic review and meta-analysis of controlled feeding trials. *Eur. J. Clin. Nutr.* **2014**, *68*, 416–423. [CrossRef] [PubMed]
37. Chung, M.; Ma, J.; Patel, K.; Berger, S.; Lau, J.; Lichtenstein, A.H. Fructose, high-fructose corn syrup, sucrose, and nonalcoholic fatty liver disease or indexes of liver health: A systematic review and meta-analysis. *Am. J. Clin. Nutr.* **2014**, *100*, 833–849. [CrossRef] [PubMed]
38. Sluik, D.; Engelen, A.I.; Feskens, E.J. Fructose consumption in the Netherlands: The Dutch National Food Consumption Survey 2007–2010. *Eur. J. Clin. Nutr.* **2015**, *69*, 475–481. [CrossRef] [PubMed]
39. Veena, J.; Muragundla, A.; Sidgiddi, S.; Subramaniam, S. Non-alcoholic fatty liver disease: Need for a balanced nutritional source. *Br. J. Nutr.* **2014**, *112*, 1858–1872. [CrossRef] [PubMed]
40. Rinella, M.E.; Sanyal, A.J. Management of NAFLD: A stage-based approach. *Nat. Rev. Gastroenterol. Hepatol.* **2016**, *13*, 196–205. [CrossRef] [PubMed]
41. Hagströmer, M.; Oja, P.; Sjöström, M. The International Physical Activity Questionnaire (IPAQ): A study of concurrent and construct validity. *Public Health Nutr.* **2006**, *9*, 755–762. [CrossRef] [PubMed]
42. Hamaguchi, M.; Kojima, T.; Itoh, Y.; Harano, Y.; Fujii, K.; Nakajima, T.; Kato, T.; Takeda, N.; Okuda, J.; Ida, K.; et al. The severity of ultrasonographic findings in nonalcoholic fatty liver disease reflects the metabolic syndrome and visceral fat accumulation. *Am. J. Gastroenterol.* **2007**, *102*, 2708–2715. [CrossRef] [PubMed]
43. Wells, J.C. Commentary: The paradox of body mass index in obesity assessment: Not a good index of adiposity, but not a bad index of cardio-metabolic risk. *Int. J. Epidemiol.* **2014**, *43*, 672–674. [CrossRef] [PubMed]

17

The Dipeptidyl Peptidase-4 Inhibitor Teneligliptin Attenuates Hepatic Lipogenesis via AMPK Activation in Non-Alcoholic Fatty Liver Disease Model Mice

Takayasu Ideta [1], Yohei Shirakami [1,2,*], Tsuneyuki Miyazaki [1], Takahiro Kochi [1], Hiroyasu Sakai [1], Hisataka Moriwaki [1] and Masahito Shimizu [1]

[1] Department of Gastroenterology, Internal Medicine, Gifu University Graduate School of Medicine, 1-1 Yanagido, Gifu 501-1194, Japan; taka.mailbox.789@gmail.com (T.I.); tsunemiyazaking@yahoo.co.jp (T.M.); kottii924@yahoo.co.jp (T.K.); sakaih03@gifu-u.ac.jp (H.S.); hmori@gifu-u.ac.jp (H.M.); shimim-gif@umin.ac.jp (M.S.)

[2] Informative Clinical Medicine, Gifu University Graduate School of Medicine, 1-1 Yanagido, Gifu 501-1194, Japan

* Correspondence: ys2443@gifu-u.ac.jp

Academic Editor: Amedeo Lonardo

Abstract: Non-alcoholic fatty liver disease (NAFLD), which is strongly associated with metabolic syndrome, is increasingly a major cause of hepatic disorder. Dipeptidyl peptidase (DPP)-4 inhibitors, anti-diabetic agents, are expected to be effective for the treatment of NAFLD. In the present study, we established a novel NAFLD model mouse using monosodium glutamate (MSG) and a high-fat diet (HFD) and investigated the effects of a DPP-4 inhibitor, teneligliptin, on the progression of NAFLD. Male MSG/HFD-treated mice were divided into two groups, one of which received teneligliptin in drinking water. Administration of MSG and HFD caused mice to develop severe fatty changes in the liver, but teneligliptin treatment improved hepatic steatosis and inflammation, as evaluated by the NAFLD activity score. Serum alanine aminotransferase and intrahepatic triglyceride levels were significantly decreased in teneligliptin-treated mice ($p < 0.05$). Hepatic mRNA levels of the genes involved in *de novo* lipogenesis were significantly downregulated by teneligliptin ($p < 0.05$). Moreover, teneligliptin increased hepatic expression levels of phosphorylated AMP-activated protein kinase (AMPK) protein. These findings suggest that teneligliptin attenuates lipogenesis in the liver by activating AMPK and downregulating the expression of genes involved in lipogenesis. DPP-4 inhibitors may be effective for the treatment of NAFLD and may be able to prevent its progression to non-alcoholic steatohepatitis.

Keywords: AMPK; DPP-4 inhibitor; lipogenesis; non-alcoholic fatty liver disease; NAFLD; SREBP1c; teneligliptin

1. Introduction

Obesity is considered to be a serious health problem, as it frequently causes various medical concerns, including type 2 diabetes mellitus (T2DM), cardiovascular diseases, dyslipidemia and many types of cancer [1]. Non-alcoholic fatty liver disease (NAFLD), which is strongly associated with obesity, has become one of the most common causes of chronic liver disease in developed countries. The clinical importance of NAFLD is illustrated by its high prevalence (6.3%–33%, with a median of 20%) in the general population [2]. NAFLD is defined as a chronic hepatic status with fat accumulation in the liver after the exclusion of secondary causes of hepatic fat accumulation, such as remarkable alcohol consumption, autoimmune or viral hepatitis and certain medications [3]. Some patients with

NAFLD develop a more serious disease condition, non-alcoholic steatohepatitis (NASH), and 10%–15% of patients with NASH develop liver cirrhosis, leading to hepatocellular carcinoma (HCC) [4–6]. The incidence of HCC due to NASH is almost the same as that due to chronic hepatitis C virus [7], which suggests that chronic liver damage or liver carcinogenesis associated with NAFLD/NASH are critical healthcare problems that should be resolved.

NAFLD is strongly associated with several aspects of metabolic syndrome, *i.e.*, obesity, dyslipidemia (primarily increased triglycerides), insulin resistance and concomitant glucose intolerance, including T2DM [6,8,9]. Therefore, improvement of these medical conditions may be beneficial to ameliorate NAFLD. For instance, pitavastatin, a drug used for the treatment of dyslipidemia, improved liver steatosis and decreased serum levels of free fatty acid (FFA) and alanine aminotransferase (ALT) in obese and diabetic *db/db* mice [10]. In the same strain of mice, treatment with green tea catechins, which have characteristics facilitating the prevention of metabolic syndrome, attenuated liver steatosis and suppressed chronic inflammation in the liver [11]. In addition, metformin, an anti-diabetic agent, markedly improve insulin resistance and inhibited obesity-related liver tumorigenesis in *db/db* mice [12]. Recently, it was reported that NAFLD is a strong determinant for the development of metabolic syndrome [13,14], suggesting that interventions purposing to ameliorate NAFLD are appropriate for the prevention and treatment of metabolic syndrome and related diseases.

Intestinal hormone incretins, such as glucagon-like peptide-1 (GLP1), regulate blood glucose levels by promoting insulin secretion in pancreatic β cells, as well as decreasing glucagon secretion in pancreatic α cells. Following their secretion from the intestines, incretins are rapidly decomposed by dipeptidyl peptidase (DPP)-4. DPP-4 inhibitors prevent GLP1 from decomposing, and this leads to appropriate secretion of insulin and glucagon from the pancreas. Therefore, DPP-4 inhibitors are commonly used in practice as medicinal agents for T2DM [15,16]. Recently, incretins have been reported to have various bioactivities, not only in pancreas cells, but also outside the pancreas [17]. Moreover, several studies have revealed the potential roles of incretin-based therapies, including DPP-4 inhibitors and GLP-1 receptor agonists, in the treatment of NAFLD [18,19]. DPP-4 inhibitors may be able to attenuate the pathology of NASH, because patients with NAFLD/NASH have increased DPP-4 activity, which correlates with the histological severity of NASH [20–22].

Monosodium glutamate (MSG)-treated animals exhibit obesity and metabolic dysfunction [23–25]. In the present study, we established a novel mouse model of NAFLD by injecting them with MSG and then feeding them a high-fat diet (HFD); these mice display obesity and severe fatty changes in the liver with an early onset. Using this model, we evaluated the preventive and therapeutic efficacy of teneligliptin, a DPP-4 inhibitor, on NAFLD and investigated the underlying mechanisms.

2. Results and Discussion

2.1. Results

2.1.1. General Observations

At the end of the experiment, there were no significant differences in body weight or relative weight of organs, including the liver and white adipose tissue (periorchis and retroperitoneum), between the two groups (Table 1). No significant difference was seen in the amount of food ingested by the two groups during the experiment. No clinical symptoms of adverse event by teneligliptin were observed throughout the experiment. Histopathological examination also displayed no toxicity due to teneligliptin treatment in important organs, including the liver, kidney and spleen (data not shown).

Table 1. Body, liver and fat weights of the experimental mice.

Measurement Item	Control	Teneligliptin
Body weight (g)	83.4 ± 7.1 [a]	80.7 ± 8.3
Liver weight (g)	5.5 ± 1.4	5.1 ± 0.8
Liver-to-body weight ratio	0.066 ± 0.013	0.063 ± 0.016
White adipose tissue [b] (g)	2.8 ± 0.7	2.8 ± 1.1

[a] Mean ± SD; [b] white adipose tissue of the periorchis and retroperitoneum.

2.1.2. Effects of Teneligliptin on the Histopathology of the Experimental Mouse Liver

The hematoxylin and eosin (H&E)-stained liver sections showed fatty degeneration, inflammation and hepatocellular ballooning in both groups. Macrovesicular fat deposits and glycogen storage were observed in the livers of both groups, but teneligliptin treatment attenuated fat accumulation in the experimental mice (Figure 1A). Liver sections were histologically evaluated using the NAFLD activity score (NAS) system [26]. The total NAS in Group 2 was significantly decreased compared to that in Group 1 (Figure 1B). When comparing each scoring factor in the NAS system, hepatic steatosis and inflammation were significantly attenuated in Group 2 compared to those in Group 1 at this experimental time point (14 weeks of age) (Figure 1C). Liver fibrosis was not detected in either group.

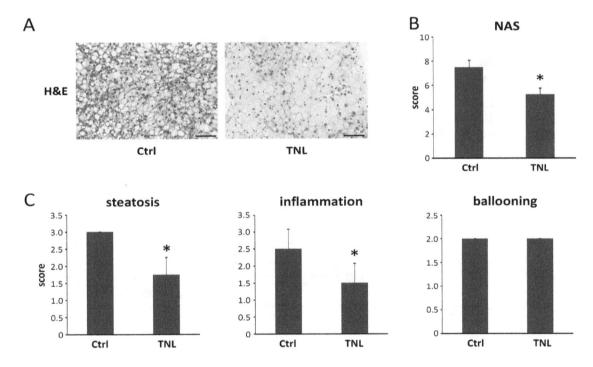

Figure 1. Effects of teneligliptin on hepatic histopathology in experimental mice. (**A**) Hematoxylin and eosin (H&E) staining of liver sections from experimental mice. Representative photomicrographs of the liver sections of MSG/high-fat diet (HFD)-administered mice treated with or without teneligliptin. Bar, 100 μm; (**B,C**) The NAFLD activity score (NAS) was determined based on histopathological analysis (steatosis, inflammation and ballooning). Ctrl, control. TNL, teneligliptin. The values are expressed as the mean ± SD. * $p < 0.05$ *versus* the control group.

2.1.3. Effects of Teneligliptin on the Intrahepatic Triglyceride Levels and the Activation of AMP-Activated Protein Kinase in the Livers of Experimental Mice

Triglyceride levels in the liver were significantly decreased in the teneligliptin-treated group (Figure 2A). This was consistent with histological findings of attenuated hepatic steatosis in the livers of mice in the group treated with teneligliptin, as evaluated by Oil Red O-stained liver sections

(Figure 2B). Moreover, teneligliptin administration significantly increased the hepatic expression levels of phosphorylated (*i.e.*, activated) AMPK (p-AMPK) protein (Figure 2C), which may be associated with the improvement of liver steatosis [27].

2.1.4. Effects of Teneligliptin on the Expression Levels of Acetyl-CoA Carboxylase, Fatty Acid Synthetase, Sterol Regulatory Element-Binding Protein 1c and Elongation of Very Long Chain Fatty Acid-Like Family Member 6 mRNA in the Livers of Experimental Mice

We determined the mRNA expression levels of *Acc*, *Fas*, *Srebp1c* and *Elovl6* to elucidate the effects of teneligliptin on lipid metabolism in the livers of experimental mice. As shown in Figure 3, the expression levels of *Acc*, *Fas* and *Srebp1c*, which regulate lipogenesis [28,29], were significantly decreased in the mice treated with teneligliptin when compared to those without teneligliptin. In addition, teneligliptin administration also decreased the hepatic expression levels of *Elovl6*, which is also one of the key molecules controlling fatty acid metabolism and lipotoxicity [28].

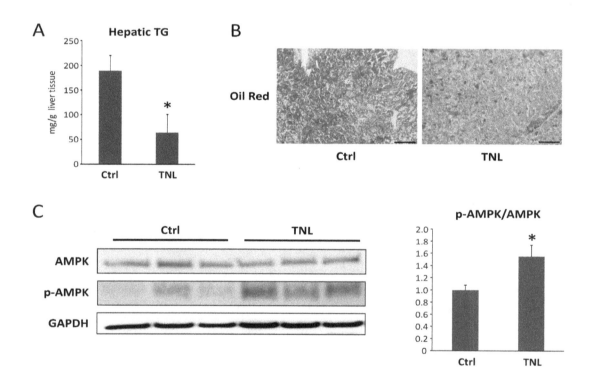

Figure 2. Effects of teneligliptin on hepatic steatosis and the levels of AMPK and p-AMPK in the livers of experimental mice. (**A**) Hepatic lipids were extracted from liver samples, and intrahepatic triglyceride (TG) levels were measured ($n = 6$); (**B**) steatosis in frozen liver sections from experimental mice treated with or without teneligliptin was analyzed with Oil Red O staining. Bar, 100 μm; (**C**) Total proteins were extracted from the livers of experimental mice, and the expression levels of AMPK and p-AMPK proteins were examined by Western blot analysis using the respective antibodies. GAPDH served as a loading control (**left** panel). Band intensities were quantified using densitometry. After the average of band intensity ratios of p-AMPK to GAPDH and AMPK to GAPDH were calculated in each sample, the ratios of these calculated values, which was expressed as p-AMPK/AMPK, were determined (**right** panel). Similar results were obtained in repeat experiments. The values are expressed as the mean ± SD. * $p < 0.05$ *versus* the control group.

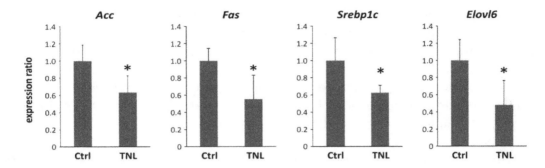

Figure 3. Effects of teneligliptin on the expression levels of genes related to lipogenesis in the livers of experimental mice. Total RNA was isolated from the livers of the experimental mice ($n = 6$), and the expression levels of *Acc*, *Fas*, *Srebp1c* and *Elovl6* mRNAs were examined using quantitative real-time RT-PCR with specific primers. The values are expressed as the mean ± SD. * $p < 0.05$ *versus* the control group.

2.1.5. Effects of Teneligliptin on Biochemical Parameters

Blood samples were collected from the inferior vena cava at sacrifice after six hours of fasting for chemical analyses. The levels of serum ALT were significantly reduced by teneligliptin administration. On the other hand, other parameters, including FFA, glucose, insulin and triglyceride, were not significantly different between the groups (Table 2).

Table 2. Serum parameters in serum of the experimental mice. FFA, free fatty acid.

Measurement Item	Control	Teneligliptin
FFA (μEQ/mL)	2091.0 ± 328.9 [a]	1550.4 ± 267.5
Glucose (mg/dL)	295.2 ± 108.2	528.0 ± 102.0
Insulin (ng/mL)	2.3 ± 0.9	2.14 ± 1.8
ALT (IU/L)	239.8 ± 20.4	162.0 ± 16.5 [b]
Triglyceride (mg/mL)	56.4 ± 32.2	65.2 ± 9.3

[a] Mean ± SD; [b] significantly different from the control group by the Welch *t*-test.

2.2. Discussion

The incidence of NAFLD/NASH is expected to continue to increase because of the global obesity epidemic. Therefore, efficacious therapeutic medications and preventive strategies for NAFLD/NASH are required. The novel animal model used in our present study is considered to reflect the pathological conditions in human NAFLD/NASH characterized by macrovesicular steatosis and chronic liver inflammation and is thought to be a practical and feasible model for investigating NAFLD and for testing preventive and therapeutic modalities that can suppress the progression of simple hepatic steatosis into NASH. In addition, this mouse model has the advantage of developing NAFLD with earlier onset compared to other animal models reported previously [11,23,30]. Although NAFLD/NASH has been considered as a hepatic manifestation of metabolic syndrome, it was recently found that NAFLD appears to be a precursor and a strong risk factor for the future development of metabolic syndrome [13,14]. A previous report by Misu *et al.* [31] suggested this reciprocal causality by demonstrating that the serum level of selenoprotein P, which is a liver-derived secretory protein and which is higher in subjects with NAFLD [32], causes insulin resistance. From this point of view, it is considered an appropriate action to intervene in ameliorating NAFLD by various medications, including the DPP-4 inhibitors, for the prevention and treatment of metabolic syndrome and related diseases.

DPP-4 inhibitors are commonly used in practice as medical agents for T2DM [15,16]. The present study clearly demonstrated that teneligliptin, a DPP-4 inhibitor, suppresses lipogenesis and steatosis in the liver of NAFLD model mice generated by administering MSG and HFD, whereas body weight and white adipose tissue weight were not reduced by this condition. We consider that the positive effect of teneligliptin on hepatic steatosis is associated, at least in part, with the suppression of the expression of specific genes, including *Srebp1c*, *Acc* and *Fas*, which play a key role in *de novo* lipogenesis [29]. *Srebp1c* is a key lipogenic transcription factor abundantly present in the mammalian liver [33]. It has been reported that hepatic gene expression of *Srebp1c* is increased in subjects with NAFLD as compared to those without [34]. In addition, treatment with linagliptin, the other DPP-4 inhibitor, also decreased liver expression of *Srebp1c* and *Fas* and, thus, improved steatosis in a mouse model of diet-induced obesity [35]. These reports may suggest that targeting lipogenic molecules, such as *Srebp1c* and *Fas*, with a DPP-4 inhibitor is a promising strategy for improving hepatic steatosis.

Among various agents investigated and thought to be candidates targeting NAFLD, the effects on fibrosis, ballooning degeneration, steatosis and lobular inflammation are analyzed in a recent publication comparing vitamin E, thiazolidinediones (TZDs), pentoxifylline and obeticholic acid (OCA) [36]. The effects of these agents are different; pentoxifylline, TZDs and OCA have ameliorating effects on lobular inflammation, but vitamin E has no effect on that compared to placebo. Furthermore, only pentoxifylline shows no effect on ballooning [36]. According to the results in our present study displaying the effects of teneligliptin on histopathology in the liver, teneligliptin could ameliorate hepatic steatosis and inflammation, but not ballooning in the NAS system (Figure 1). This might be because the major effect of teneligliptin as well as pentoxifylline [37] on NAFLD is inhibition of lipogenesis in the liver.

In the present study, the teneligliptin-treated group showed the tendency of a higher serum glucose level. This is assumed to be due possibly to the effect of fasting before sacrifice. In the feeding state, the serum glucose level must be lower than that in the control group, because the effect of this medicine on the serum glucose level has already been proven in experiments in the drug development process, as well as in clinical practice. Furthermore, in the feeding state, serum incretin levels appear to be higher in the teneligliptin-treated group, and it can be suspected that serum glucose metabolism was relatively dependent on the functions of incretins, including the functions that induce insulin secretion from the pancreas and enhance the insulin signaling pathway in the hepatocyte [17], due to the continuous influence of the DPP-4 inhibitor. Then, in the fasting state at sacrifice, intestines did not secrete incretins, leading probably to the relatively higher glucose levels shown in teneligliptin-treated mice. Although the serum levels of incretins and insulin, as well as glucose in the feeding state were not measured in our study, the levels of these might be able to let us interpret those unexpected data.

AMPK is a key regulator of energy balance and nutrient metabolism [38]. In the liver, AMPK has been demonstrated to inhibit cholesterol and triglyceride biosynthesis by reducing the activities of *Srebp1c* and *Fas* [27]. AMPK activation also promotes fatty acid β-oxidation by inactivation of ACC activity [39]. Moreover, GLP-1 suppresses hepatic lipogenesis through the activation of the AMPK pathway [40]. Other studies reported by Svegliati-Baroni *et al.* [41] and Lee *et al.* [42] also demonstrate that enhanced AMPK signaling due to GLP-1 activation can lead to inhibiting hepatic steatosis. Therefore, AMPK is considered to be a therapeutic target for NAFLD/NASH associated with metabolic syndrome [27]. In the present study, teneligliptin treatment significantly increased the levels of phosphorylated AMPK in the livers of NAFLD model mice (Figure 2C). These findings suggest that teneligliptin may attenuate lipogenesis in hepatocytes through the activation of AMPK and, subsequently, downregulation of *Srebp1c* and *Fas* (Figure 3). These findings are also consistent with the results of a previous report showing that AMPK inhibition resulted in elevated cleavage and transcription of hepatic *Srebp1c* in insulin-resistant mice [27]. In our study, it can be considered that teneligliptin elevated the level of GLP-1 due to attenuating the effect of the DDP-4 inhibitor and then enhanced AMPK in hepatocytes through the GLP-1 receptor (GLP-1R). The levels of GLP-1 and other incretins, however, were not determined in this study, as mentioned above. In addition, it is still controversial whether GLP-1R is present or responsible for the GLP-1 signal in the hepatocyte [43]. Moreover, there may be direct effects of DPP-4 inhibitors on hepatic steatosis through AMPK activation or other signaling pathways. Further investigations are required in order to clarify the effect of DPP-4 inhibitors and incretins on lipid metabolism in the hepatocyte.

One of the key mechanisms of incretin-based therapies, including DPP-4 inhibitors, for improving liver steatosis is the reduction of FFA [44] and improvement of glucose metabolism [15,16]. Therefore, we initially expected that teneligliptin would attenuate liver steatosis in the MSG/HFD-treated mice by improving these metabolic abnormalities. However, serum levels of FFA, glucose, insulin and triglycerides were not decreased by treatment with teneligliptin in the present study. We speculated that this was likely due to the study protocols, because MSG plus HFD treatment induced very severe obesity and steatosis within a short period of time. The present experimental condition (10 weeks of treatment with teneligliptin) may have been insufficient to obtain anti-diabetic effects, which is one of the limitations of the present study. Another limitation is that plasma levels of GLP-1 were not measured, and therefore, inhibition of DPP-4 by teneligliptin was not evaluated. We also did not assay the plasma DPP-4 activity or concentration. Therefore, future long-term studies should be conducted to confirm that teneligliptin improves liver steatosis by decreasing serum levels of FFA and improving glucose metabolism, focusing on the serum levels of GLP-1 and the activity of DPP-4 in several animal models.

3. Experimental Section

3.1. Animals and Chemicals

ICR mice were obtained from Charles River Japan (Kanagawa, Japan), and their newborns were employed in the study. MSG was purchased from Wako Pure Chemical (Osaka, Japan). CRF-1, a basal diet and HFD were from Oriental Yeast (Tokyo, Japan). Teneligliptin (Tenelia™) was kindly provided by Mitsubishi Tanabe Pharma Corporation (Tokyo, Japan). We fully complied with the Guidelines Concerning Experimental Animals issued by the Japanese Association for Laboratory Animal Science [45] and exercised due consideration to minimize pain and suffering.

3.2. Experimental Procedure

MSG was administered into the neonatal ICR mice at birth as a single-dose subcutaneous injection (4 mg/g body weight). Among these mice, males were divided into two groups at 4 weeks of age: the MSG/HFD group ($n = 6$, Group 1) and the MSG/HFD/teneligliptin-treated group ($n = 6$, Group 2). The mice in Group 2 were administered teneligliptin (30 mg/kg per day) in the drinking water from 4 weeks of age. The treatment dose of teneligliptin was determined according to the data from the animal experiments in the drug development process. Although the dose was relatively higher than that for humans in clinical practice, no notable adverse effect was observed in the treatment with the dose for the experimental animal in the process. Both groups were fed HFD from 4–14 weeks of age. At the termination of the experiment (14 weeks of age), all animals were sacrificed by CO_2 asphyxiation to analyze hepatic histopathology.

3.3. Histopathological Examination

Maximum sagittal sections of three hepatic sublobes were used for histopathological examination. For all experimental mice, 4 μm-thick sections of formalin-fixed and paraffin-embedded livers were stained with H&E for conventional histopathology. The histological features of the liver were evaluated using the NAS system [26].

3.4. Clinical Chemistry

Blood samples were collected from the inferior vena cava at sacrifice after 6 h of fasting for chemical analyses. Unfortunately, one blood sample could not be taken properly in the sampling procedure in each group; therefore, 5 blood samples in each were used to analyze. The serum concentrations of glucose (BioVision Research Products, Mountain View, CA, USA), triglycerides (Wako Pure Chemical), FFAs (Wako Pure Chemical) and insulin (Shibayagi, Gunma, Japan) were measured as previously reported [46]. ALT was measured using a standard clinical automatic analyzer (Type 7180; Hitachi, Tokyo, Japan).

3.5. RNA Extraction and Quantitative Real-Time Reverse Transcription-PCR Analysis

Total RNA was extracted from the mice livers using the RNeasy Mini Kit (QIAGEN, Venlo, The Netherlands). cDNA was synthesized from 0.2 µg of total RNA with the High Capacity cDNA Reverse Transcription Kit (Applied Biosystems, Foster City, CA, USA). A quantitative real-time reverse transcription-PCR (RT-PCR) analysis was applied using a LightCycler Nano (Roche Diagnostics, Indianapolis, IN, USA) and FastStart Essential DNA Green Master (Roche Diagnostics). The sequences of specific primers for amplifying eElovl6, Fas, Acc, Srebp1c and 18S genes were obtained by Primer-BLAST [47] (Table 3). The expression level of each gene was normalized to that of 18S.

Table 3. Primer sequences.

Genes	5′-Primer	3′-Primer
Acc	GGCTCAAACTGCAGGTATCC	TTGCCAATCCACTCGAAGA
Elovl6	CAGCAAAGCACCCGAACTA	AGGAGCACAGTGATGTGGTG
Fas	GCTGCTGTTGGAAGTCAGC	AGTGTTCGTTCCTCGGAGTG
Srebp1c	CTGGAGCTGCGTGGTTT	GCCTCATGTAGGAATACCCTCCTCATA
18s	CCATCCAATCGGTAGTAGCG	GTAACCCGTTGAACCCCATT

3.6. Hepatic Lipid Analysis

Approximately 200 mg of frozen liver samples were homogenized, and lipids were extracted using Folch's method [48]. The triglyceride levels in the liver were measured with the Triglyceride E-test Kit (Wako Pure Chemical), as previously reported [49]. To visualize the intrahepatic lipids, Oil Red O staining was performed based on the standard protocol for frozen liver sections.

3.7. Protein Extraction and Western Blot Analysis

Total protein was extracted from the mice livers, and equivalent amounts of proteins (10 µg/lane) were examined by Western blot analysis [11]. Primary antibodies were obtained from Cell Signaling Technology (Beverly, MA, USA), including AMPK (#2603), p-AMPK (#2535) and GAPDH (#2118). The antibody for p-AMPK was used to detect the phosphorylation site at Thr172 in the activation loop. GAPDH served as the loading control. The intensities of the bands were quantified with NIH Image software ver. 1.62 (Bethesda, MD, USA). After the average of band intensity ratios of p-AMPK to GAPDH and AMPK to GAPDH was calculated in each sample, the ratio of these calculated values, which was expressed as p-AMPK/AMPK, were determined.

3.8. Statistical Analysis

The results are presented as the means $\pm$ SD and were analyzed using JMP software Version 10 (SAS Institute, Cary, NC, USA). Differences among the two groups were analyzed by Welch's t-test. The differences were considered significant at p-values of less than 0.05.

4. Conclusions

Teneligliptin, the DPP4 inhibitor, improved the histopathological appearance of the liver and decreased intrahepatic triglyceride levels in an NAFLD model mouse, which was associated with downregulation of hepatic lipogenesis-related genes due to AMPK activation. Interestingly, the hepatic Dpp-4 mRNA expression level is significantly higher in patients with NAFLD compared to healthy subjects [50]. The results of the present study, together with those of previous reports [19,21,22], have prompted us to conduct a clinical trial to determine the effectiveness of DPP-4 inhibitors for the prevention and treatment of NAFLD.

Acknowledgments: This work was supported in part by Grants-in-Aid from the Ministry of Education, Science, Sports, and Culture of Japan (Nos. 22790638, 25460988 and 26860498).

Author Contributions: Takayasu Ideta, Yohei Shirakami and Masahito Shimizu conceived of and designed the experiments. Tsuneyuki Miyazaki, Takahiro Kochi and Hiroyasu Sakai performed the experiments. Takayasu Ideta, Yohei Shirakami analyzed the data. Takayasu Ideta, Yohei Shirakami, Hisataka Moriwaki and Masahito Shimizu wrote the paper.

References

1. Calle, E.E.; Rodriguez, C.; Walker-Thurmond, K.; Thun, M.J. Overweight, obesity, and mortality from cancer in a prospectively studied cohort of U.S. adults. *N. Engl. J. Med.* **2003**, *348*, 1625–1638. [CrossRef] [PubMed]

2. Chalasani, N.; Younossi, Z.; Lavine, J.E.; Diehl, A.M.; Brunt, E.M.; Cusi, K.; Charlton, M.; Sanyal, A.J. The diagnosis and management of non-alcoholic fatty liver disease: Practice guideline by the american association for the study of liver diseases, american college of gastroenterology, and the american gastroenterological association. *Hepatology* **2012**, *55*, 2005–2023. [CrossRef] [PubMed]

3. Sass, D.A.; Chang, P.; Chopra, K.B. Nonalcoholic fatty liver disease: A clinical review. *Dig. Dis. Sci.* **2005**, *50*, 171–180. [CrossRef] [PubMed]

4. Bacon, B.R.; Farahvash, M.J.; Janney, C.G.; Neuschwander-Tetri, B.A. Nonalcoholic steatohepatitis: An expanded clinical entity. *Gastroenterology* **1994**, *107*, 1103–1109. [PubMed]

5. Kim, C.H.; Younossi, Z.M. Nonalcoholic fatty liver disease: A manifestation of the metabolic syndrome. *Clevel. Clin. J. Med.* **2008**, *75*, 721–728.

6. Vanni, E.; Bugianesi, E.; Kotronen, A.; De Minicis, S.; Yki-Jarvinen, H.; Svegliati-Baroni, G. From the metabolic syndrome to NAFLD or vice versa? *Dig. Liver Dis.* **2010**, *42*, 320–330. [CrossRef] [PubMed]

7. Ascha, M.S.; Hanouneh, I.A.; Lopez, R.; Tamimi, T.A.; Feldstein, A.F.; Zein, N.N. The incidence and risk factors of hepatocellular carcinoma in patients with nonalcoholic steatohepatitis. *Hepatology* **2010**, *51*, 1972–1978. [CrossRef] [PubMed]

8. Marchesini, G.; Brizi, M.; Morselli-Labate, A.M.; Bianchi, G.; Bugianesi, E.; McCullough, A.J.; Forlani, G.; Melchionda, N. Association of nonalcoholic fatty liver disease with insulin resistance. *Am. J. Med.* **1999**, *107*, 450–455. [CrossRef]

9. Sanyal, A.J.; American Gastroenterological, A. Aga technical review on nonalcoholic fatty liver disease. *Gastroenterology* **2002**, *123*, 1705–1725. [CrossRef] [PubMed]

10. Shimizu, M.; Yasuda, Y.; Sakai, H.; Kubota, M.; Terakura, D.; Baba, A.; Ohno, T.; Kochi, T.; Tsurumi, H.; Tanaka, T.; *et al.* Pitavastatin suppresses diethylnitrosamine-induced liver preneoplasms in male C57BL/KsJ-*db/db* obese mice. *BMC Cancer* **2011**, *11*, 281. [CrossRef] [PubMed]

11. Shimizu, M.; Sakai, H.; Shirakami, Y.; Yasuda, Y.; Kubota, M.; Terakura, D.; Baba, A.; Ohno, T.; Hara, Y.; Tanaka, T.; *et al.* Preventive effects of (−)-epigallocatechin gallate on diethylnitrosamine-induced liver tumorigenesis in obese and diabetic C57BL/KsJ-*db/db* mice. *Cancer Prev. Res.* **2011**, *4*, 396–403. [CrossRef] [PubMed]

12. Ohno, T.; Shimizu, M.; Shirakami, Y.; Baba, A.; Kochi, T.; Kubota, M.; Tsurumi, H.; Tanaka, T.; Moriwaki, H. Metformin suppresses diethylnitrosamine-induced liver tumorigenesis in obese and diabetic C57BL/KsJ-+Lepr*db*/+Lepr*db* mice. *PLoS ONE* **2015**, *10*, e0124081. [CrossRef] [PubMed]

13. Lonardo, A.; Ballestri, S.; Marchesini, G.; Angulo, P.; Loria, P. Nonalcoholic fatty liver disease: A precursor of the metabolic syndrome. *Dig. Liver Dis.* **2015**, *47*, 181–190. [CrossRef] [PubMed]

14. Zhang, Y.; Zhang, T.; Zhang, C.; Tang, F.; Zhong, N.; Li, H.; Song, X.; Lin, H.; Liu, Y.; Xue, F. Identification of reciprocal causality between non-alcoholic fatty liver disease and metabolic syndrome by a simplified bayesian network in a chinese population. *BMJ Open* **2015**, *5*, e008204. [CrossRef] [PubMed]

15. Aschner, P.; Kipnes, M.S.; Lunceford, J.K.; Sanchez, M.; Mickel, C.; Williams-Herman, D.E.; Sitagliptin Study, G. Effect of the dipeptidyl peptidase-4 inhibitor sitagliptin as monotherapy on glycemic control in patients with type 2 diabetes. *Diabetes Care* **2006**, *29*, 2632–2637. [CrossRef] [PubMed]

16. Pi-Sunyer, F.X.; Schweizer, A.; Mills, D.; Dejager, S. Efficacy and tolerability of vildagliptin monotherapy in drug-naive patients with type 2 diabetes. *Diabetes Res. Clin. Pract.* **2007**, *76*, 132–138. [CrossRef] [PubMed]

17. Gupta, N.A.; Mells, J.; Dunham, R.M.; Grakoui, A.; Handy, J.; Saxena, N.K.; Anania, F.A. Glucagon-like peptide-1 receptor is present on human hepatocytes and has a direct role in decreasing hepatic steatosis *in vitro* by modulating elements of the insulin signaling pathway. *Hepatology* **2010**, *51*, 1584–1592. [CrossRef] [PubMed]

18. Trevaskis, J.L.; Griffin, P.S.; Wittmer, C.; Neuschwander-Tetri, B.A.; Brunt, E.M.; Dolman, C.S.; Erickson, M.R.; Napora, J.; Parkes, D.G.; Roth, J.D. Glucagon-like peptide-1 receptor agonism improves metabolic, biochemical, and histopathological indices of nonalcoholic steatohepatitis in mice. *Am. J. Physiol. Gastrointest. Liver Physiol.* **2012**, *302*, G762–G772. [CrossRef] [PubMed]

19. Klein, T.; Fujii, M.; Sandel, J.; Shibazaki, Y.; Wakamatsu, K.; Mark, M.; Yoneyama, H. Linagliptin alleviates hepatic steatosis and inflammation in a mouse model of non-alcoholic steatohepatitis. *Med. Mol. Morphol.* **2014**, *47*, 137–149. [CrossRef] [PubMed]

20. Balaban, Y.H.; Korkusuz, P.; Simsek, H.; Gokcan, H.; Gedikoglu, G.; Pinar, A.; Hascelik, G.; Asan, E.; Hamaloglu, E.; Tatar, G. Dipeptidyl peptidase IV (DDP IV) in nash patients. *Ann. Hepatol.* **2007**, *6*, 242–250. [PubMed]

21. Schuppan, D.; Gorrell, M.D.; Klein, T.; Mark, M.; Afdhal, N.H. The challenge of developing novel pharmacological therapies for non-alcoholic steatohepatitis. *Liver Int.* **2010**, *30*, 795–808. [CrossRef] [PubMed]

22. Yilmaz, Y.; Atug, O.; Yonal, O.; Duman, D.; Ozdogan, O.; Imeryuz, N.; Kalayci, C. Dipeptidyl peptidase IV inhibitors: Therapeutic potential in nonalcoholic fatty liver disease. *Med. Sci. Res.* **2009**, *15*, HY1-5. [CrossRef]

23. Collison, K.S.; Makhoul, N.J.; Zaidi, M.Z.; Al-Rabiah, R.; Inglis, A.; Andres, B.L.; Ubungen, R.; Shoukri, M.; Al-Mohanna, F.A. Interactive effects of neonatal exposure to monosodium glutamate and aspartame on glucose homeostasis. *Nutr. Metabol.* **2012**, *9*, 58. [CrossRef] [PubMed]

24. Nagata, M.; Suzuki, W.; Iizuka, S.; Tabuchi, M.; Maruyama, H.; Takeda, S.; Aburada, M.; Miyamoto, K. Type 2 diabetes mellitus in obese mouse model induced by monosodium glutamate. *Exp. Anim. Jpn. Assoc. Lab. Anim. Sci.* **2006**, *55*, 109–115. [CrossRef]

25. Roman-Ramos, R.; Almanza-Perez, J.C.; Garcia-Macedo, R.; Blancas-Flores, G.; Fortis-Barrera, A.; Jasso, E.I.; Garcia-Lorenzana, M.; Campos-Sepulveda, A.E.; Cruz, M.; Alarcon-Aguilar, F.J. Monosodium glutamate neonatal intoxication associated with obesity in adult stage is characterized by chronic inflammation and increased mRNA expression of peroxisome proliferator-activated receptors in mice. *Basic Clin. Pharmacol. Toxicol.* **2011**, *108*, 406–413. [CrossRef] [PubMed]

26. Kleiner, D.E.; Brunt, E.M.; Van Natta, M.; Behling, C.; Contos, M.J.; Cummings, O.W.; Ferrell, L.D.; Liu, Y.C.; Torbenson, M.S.; Unalp-Arida, A.; *et al.* Design and validation of a histological scoring system for nonalcoholic fatty liver disease. *Hepatology* **2005**, *41*, 1313–1321. [CrossRef] [PubMed]

27. Li, Y.; Xu, S.; Mihaylova, M.M.; Zheng, B.; Hou, X.; Jiang, B.; Park, O.; Luo, Z.; Lefai, E.; Shyy, J.Y.; *et al.* AMPK phosphorylates and inhibits *Srebp* activity to attenuate hepatic steatosis and atherosclerosis in diet-induced insulin-resistant mice. *Cell Metabol.* **2011**, *13*, 376–388. [CrossRef] [PubMed]

28. Serviddio, G.; Bellanti, F.; Vendemiale, G. Free radical biology for medicine: Learning from nonalcoholic fatty liver disease. *Free Radic. Biol. Med.* **2013**, *65*, 952–968. [CrossRef] [PubMed]

29. Blaslov, K.; Bulum, T.; Zibar, K.; Duvnjak, L. Incretin based therapies: A novel treatment approach for non-alcoholic fatty liver disease. *World J. Gastroenterol.* **2014**, *20*, 7356–7365. [CrossRef] [PubMed]

30. Shimizu, M.; Sakai, H.; Shirakami, Y.; Iwasa, J.; Yasuda, Y.; Kubota, M.; Takai, K.; Tsurumi, H.; Tanaka, T.; Moriwaki, H. Acyclic retinoid inhibits diethylnitrosamine-induced liver tumorigenesis in obese and diabetic C57BLKS/J- +lepr^{db}/+lepr^{db} mice. *Cancer Prev. Res.* **2011**, *4*, 128–136. [CrossRef] [PubMed]

31. Misu, H.; Takamura, T.; Takayama, H.; Hayashi, H.; Matsuzawa-Nagata, N.; Kurita, S.; Ishikura, K.; Ando, H.; Takeshita, Y.; Ota, T.; *et al.* A liver-derived secretory protein, selenoprotein *p*, causes insulin resistance. *Cell Metabol.* **2010**, *12*, 483–495. [CrossRef] [PubMed]

32. Choi, H.Y.; Hwang, S.Y.; Lee, C.H.; Hong, H.C.; Yang, S.J.; Yoo, H.J.; Seo, J.A.; Kim, S.G.; Kim, N.H.; Baik, S.H.; *et al.* Increased selenoprotein *p* levels in subjects with visceral obesity and nonalcoholic fatty liver disease. *Diabetes Metabol. J.* **2013**, *37*, 63–71. [CrossRef] [PubMed]

33. Musso, G.; Gambino, R.; Cassader, M. Recent insights into hepatic lipid metabolism in non-alcoholic fatty liver disease (NAFLD). *Progress Lipid Res.* **2009**, *48*, 1–26. [CrossRef] [PubMed]

34. Higuchi, N.; Kato, M.; Shundo, Y.; Tajiri, H.; Tanaka, M.; Yamashita, N.; Kohjima, M.; Kotoh, K.; Nakamuta, M.; Takayanagi, R.; *et al.* Liver X receptor in cooperation with *Srebp*-1c is a major lipid synthesis regulator in nonalcoholic fatty liver disease. *Hepatol. Res.* **2008**, *38*, 1122–1129. [CrossRef] [PubMed]

35. Kern, M.; Kloting, N.; Niessen, H.G.; Thomas, L.; Stiller, D.; Mark, M.; Klein, T.; Bluher, M. Linagliptin improves insulin sensitivity and hepatic steatosis in diet-induced obesity. *PLoS ONE* **2012**, *7*, e38744. [CrossRef] [PubMed]

36. Singh, S.; Khera, R.; Allen, A.M.; Murad, M.H.; Loomba, R. Comparative effectiveness of pharmacological interventions for nonalcoholic steatohepatitis: A systematic review and network meta-analysis. *Hepatology* **2015**, *62*, 1417–1432. [CrossRef] [PubMed]

37. Shirakami, Y.; Shimizu, M.; Kubota, M.; Ohno, T.; Kochi, T.; Nakamura, N.; Sumi, T.; Tanaka, T.; Moriwaki, H.; Seishima, M. Pentoxifylline prevents nonalcoholic steatohepatitis-related liver pre-neoplasms by inhibiting hepatic inflammation and lipogenesis. *Eur. J. Cancer Prev.* **2015**. [CrossRef] [PubMed]

38. Hardie, D.G.; Ross, F.A.; Hawley, S.A. Ampk: A nutrient and energy sensor that maintains energy homeostasis. *Nat. Rev. Mol. Cell Biol.* **2012**, *13*, 251–262. [CrossRef] [PubMed]

39. Viollet, B.; Mounier, R.; Leclerc, J.; Yazigi, A.; Foretz, M.; Andreelli, F. Targeting AMP-activated protein kinase as a novel therapeutic approach for the treatment of metabolic disorders. *Diabetes Metab.* **2007**, *33*, 395–402. [CrossRef] [PubMed]

40. Ben-Shlomo, S.; Zvibel, I.; Shnell, M.; Shlomai, A.; Chepurko, E.; Halpern, Z.; Barzilai, N.; Oren, R.; Fishman, S. Glucagon-like peptide-1 reduces hepatic lipogenesis via activation of AMP-activated protein kinase. *J. Hepatol.* **2011**, *54*, 1214–1223. [CrossRef] [PubMed]

41. Svegliati-Baroni, G.; Saccomanno, S.; Rychlicki, C.; Agostinelli, L.; de Minicis, S.; Candelaresi, C.; Faraci, G.; Pacetti, D.; Vivarelli, M.; Nicolini, D.; *et al.* Glucagon-like peptide-1 receptor activation stimulates hepatic lipid oxidation and restores hepatic signalling alteration induced by a high-fat diet in nonalcoholic steatohepatitis. *Liver Int.* **2011**, *31*, 1285–1297. [CrossRef] [PubMed]

42. Lee, J.; Hong, S.W.; Chae, S.W.; Kim, D.H.; Choi, J.H.; Bae, J.C.; Park, S.E.; Rhee, E.J.; Park, C.Y.; Oh, K.W.; *et al.* Exendin-4 improves steatohepatitis by increasing Sirt1 expression in high-fat diet-induced obese C57BL/6J mice. *PLoS ONE* **2012**, *7*, e31394. [CrossRef] [PubMed]

43. Samson, S.L.; Bajaj, M. Potential of incretin-based therapies for non-alcoholic fatty liver disease. *J. Diabetes Complicat.* **2013**, *27*, 401–406. [CrossRef] [PubMed]

44. Boschmann, M.; Engeli, S.; Dobberstein, K.; Budziarek, P.; Strauss, A.; Boehnke, J.; Sweep, F.C.; Luft, F.C.; He, Y.; Foley, J.E.; *et al.* Dipeptidyl-peptidase-IV inhibition augments postprandial lipid mobilization and oxidation in type 2 diabetic patients. *J. Clin. Endocrinol. Metab.* **2009**, *94*, 846–852. [CrossRef] [PubMed]

45. The Japanese Association for Laboratory Animal Science (JALAS). Available online: http://www.jalas.jp/english/en_about_jalas.html (accessed on 26 July 2013).

46. Shimizu, M.; Shirakami, Y.; Iwasa, J.; Shiraki, M.; Yasuda, Y.; Hata, K.; Hirose, Y.; Tsurumi, H.; Tanaka, T.; Moriwaki, H. Supplementation with branched-chain amino acids inhibits azoxymethane-induced colonic preneoplastic lesions in male C57BL/KsJ-*db/db* mice. *Clin. Cancer Res.* **2009**, *15*, 3068–3075. [CrossRef] [PubMed]

47. Primer Blast. Available online: http://www.ncbi.nlm.nih.gov/tools/primer-blast/ (accessed on 26 July 2013).

48. Folch, J.; Lees, M.; Sloane Stanley, G.H. A simple method for the isolation and purification of total lipides from animal tissues. *J. Biol. Chem.* **1957**, *226*, 497–509. [PubMed]

49. Iwasa, J.; Shimizu, M.; Shiraki, M.; Shirakami, Y.; Sakai, H.; Terakura, Y.; Takai, K.; Tsurumi, H.; Tanaka, T.; Moriwaki, H. Dietary supplementation with branched-chain amino acids suppresses diethylnitrosamine-induced liver tumorigenesis in obese and diabetic C57BL/KsJ-*db/db* mice. *Cancer Sci.* **2010**, *101*, 460–467. [CrossRef] [PubMed]

50. Miyazaki, M.; Kato, M.; Tanaka, K.; Tanaka, M.; Kohjima, M.; Nakamura, K.; Enjoji, M.; Nakamuta, M.; Kotoh, K.; Takayanagi, R. Increased hepatic expression of dipeptidyl peptidase-4 in non-alcoholic fatty liver disease and its association with insulin resistance and glucose metabolism. *Mol. Med. Rep.* **2012**, *5*, 729–733. [CrossRef] [PubMed]

Permissions

List of Contributors

Simone Leonetti and Domenico Tricò
Department of Surgical, Medical and Molecular Pathology and Critical Care Medicine, University of Pisa, 56126 Pisa, Italy

Raimund I. Herzog
Department of Internal Medicine, Section of Endocrinology, Yale University School of Medicine, New Haven, CT 06510, USA

Sonia Caprio
Department of Pediatrics, Yale University School of Medicine, New Haven, CT 06510, USA

Nicola Santoro
Department of Pediatrics, Yale University School of Medicine, New Haven, CT 06510, USA
Department of Medicine and Health Sciences, "V.Tiberio" University of Molise, 86100 Campobasso, Italy

Yvonne Oligschlaeger and Ronit Shiri-Sverdlov
Department of Molecular Genetics, School of Nutrition and Translational Research in Metabolism (NUTRIM), Maastricht University, Universiteitssingel 50, 6229 ER, Maastricht, The Netherlands

Martina Colognesi, Daniela Gabbia and Sara De Martin
Department of Pharmaceutical and Pharmacological Sciences, University of Padova, L.go Meneghetti 2, 35131 Padova, Italy

Silvia Fargion
Department of Pathophysiology and Transplantation, IRCCS "Ca' Granda" IRCCS Foundation, Poiliclinico Hospital, University of Milan, Centro delle Malattie Metaboliche del Fegato, Milan 20122, Italy

Francesco Baratta, Daniele Pastori and Licia Polimeni
Department of Internal Medicine and Medical Specialities and Department of Anatomical, Histological, Forensic Medicine and Orthopedics Sciences-Sapienza University, Rome 00185, Italy

Giulia Tozzi
Unit for Neuromuscular and Neurodegenerative Diseases, Children's Hospital and Research Institute "Bambino Gesù", Rome 00165, Italy

Francesco Violi and Maria Del Ben
Department of Internal Medicine and Medical Specialities, Sapienza University, Rome 00185, Italy

Francesco Angelico
Department of Public Health and Infectious Diseases, Sapienza University, Policlinico Umberto I, I Clinica Medica, Viale del Policlinico 155, Rome 00161, Italy

Elizabeth M. Brunt
Department of Pathology and Immunology, Washington University School of Medicine, St. Louis, MO 63110, USA

Natalia Nuño-Lámbarri and Varenka J. Barbero-Becerra
Traslational Research Unit, Médica Sur Clinic & Foundation, Mexico City 14050, Mexico

Misael Uribe
Obesity and Digestive Diseases Unit, Médica Sur Clinic & Foundation, Mexico City 14050, Mexico

Norberto C. Chávez-Tapia
Traslational Research Unit, Médica Sur Clinic & Foundation, Mexico City 14050, Mexico
Obesity and Digestive Diseases Unit, Médica Sur Clinic & Foundation, Mexico City 14050, Mexico

Mariana Verdelho Machado and Helena Cortez-Pinto
Departamento de Gastrenterologia, Hospital de Santa Maria, Centro Hospitalar Lisboa Norte (CHLN), 1649-035 Lisbon, Portugal
Laboratório de Nutrição, Faculdade de Medicina de Lisboa, Universidade de Lisboa, Alameda da Universidade, 1649-004 Lisboa, Portugal

Giuseppina Pisano and Rosa Lombardi
Department of Pathophysiology and Transplantation, Ca' Granda IRCCS Foundation, Policlinico Hospital, University of Milan, Centre of the Study of Metabolic and Liver Diseases, Via Francesco Sforza 35, 20122 Milan, Italy

Michael France
Department of Clinical Biochemistry, Cobbett House, Central Manchester Foundation Trust, Oxford Road, Manchester M13 9WL, UK

See Kwok
Cardiovascular Trials Unit, The Old St Mary's Hospital, Hathersage Road, Oxford Road, Manchester M13 9WL, UK

Handrean Soran and Jan Hoong Ho
Department of Medicine, Central Manchester Foundation Trust, Oxford Road, Manchester M13 9WL, UK

Anna Ludovica Fracanzani
Department of Imaging Science, University of Manchester, Oxford Road, Manchester M13 9PT, UK
Department of Pathophysiology and Transplantation, Ca' Granda IRCCS Foundation, Policlinico Hospital, University of Milan, Centre of the Study of Metabolic and Liver Diseases, Via Francesco Sforza 35, 20122 Milan, Italy

Safwaan Adam
Department of Imaging Science, University of Manchester, Oxford Road, Manchester M13 9PT, UK

Dexter Canoy
Cancer Epidemiology Unit, University of Oxford, Richard Doll Building, Roosevelt Drive, Oxford OX3 7LF, UK

Yifen Liu and Paul N. Durrington
School of Biomedicine, 3rd floor, Core Technology Facility, 46 Grafton Street, Manchester M13 9NT, UK

Patrick Wainwright
Clinical Biochemistry, University Hospital Southampton, Tremona Road, Southampton SO16 6YD, UK

Christopher D. Byrne
Nutrition and Metabolism, Faculty of Medicine, University of Southampton, Tremona Road, Southampton SO16 6YD, UK
Southampton National Institute for Health Research Biomedical Research Centre, University Hospital Southampton, Tremona Road, Southampton SO16 6YD, UK

Morgan Marcuccilli
Division of Renal Diseases and Hypertension, University of Colorado Hospital, Aurora, CO 80045, USA

Michel Chonchol
Division of Renal Diseases and Hypertension, University of Colorado Denver, 13199 East Montview Boulevard, Suite 495, Aurora, CO 80045, USA

Claudia Sanna, Chiara Rosso, Milena Marietti and Elisabetta Bugianesi
Division of Gastroenterology, Department of Medical Sciences, A.O. Città della Salute e della Scienza di Torino, University of Turin, 10126 Turin, Italy

Leon Anton Adams
School of Medicine and Pharmacology, the University of Western Australia, Nedlands, WA 6009, Australia
Department of Hepatology, Sir Charles Gairdner Hospital, Nedlands, WA 6009, Australia

Luis Calzadilla Bertot
School of Medicine and Pharmacology, the University of Western Australia, Nedlands, WA 6009, Australia

Lucia Pacifico, Alessia Gallozzi, Ester De Luca and Gian Marco Andreoli
Policlinico Umberto I Hospital, Sapienza University of Rome, Viale Regina Elena 324, 00161 Rome, Italy

Enea Bonci
Department of Experimental Medicine, Sapienza University of Rome, Viale Regina Elena 324, 00161 Rome, Italy

Michele Di Martino
Department of Radiological Sciences, Sapienza University of Rome, Viale Regina Elena 324, 00161 Rome, Italy

Claudio Chiesa
Institute of Translational Pharmacology, National Research Council, Via Fosso del Cavaliere 100, 00133 Rome, Italy

Ewa Stachowska, Karina Ryterska, Dominika Maciejewska, Marcin Banaszczak, Izabela Gutowska, Piotr Ossowski, Małgorzata Kaczorowska, Dominika Jamioł-Milc and Anna Sabinicz
Department of Biochemistry and Human Nutrition, Pomeranian Medical University, Szczecin 71-460, Poland

Piotr Milkiewicz
Department of Clinical and Molecular Biochemistry, Pomeranian Medical University, Szczecin 70-111, Poland
Liver and Internal Medicine Unit, Department of General, Transplant and Liver Surgery of the Medical University of Warsaw, Warsaw 02-097, Poland

Małgorzata Milkiewicz
Department of Medical Biology, Pomeranian Medical University, Szczecin 70-111, Poland

Małgorzata Napierała
Department of Diabetology and Internal Diseases
Pomeranian Medical University, Szczecin 72-010,
Poland

Lidia Wądołowska
Department of Human Nutrition, University of
Warmia and Mazury, Olsztyn 10-718, Poland

Joanna Raszeja-Wyszomirska
Liver and Internal Medicine Unit, Department of
General, Transplant and Liver Surgery of the Medical
University of Warsaw, Warsaw 02-097, Poland

**Takayasu Ideta, Tsuneyuki Miyazaki, Takahiro
Kochi, Hiroyasu Sakai, Hisataka Moriwaki and
Masahito Shimizu**
Department of Gastroenterology, Internal Medicine,
Gifu University Graduate School of Medicine, 1-1
Yanagido, Gifu 501-1194, Japan

Yohei Shirakami
Department of Gastroenterology, Internal Medicine,
Gifu University Graduate School of Medicine, 1-1
Yanagido, Gifu 501-1194, Japan
Informative Clinical Medicine, Gifu University Graduate
School of Medicine, 1-1 Yanagido, Gifu 501-1194, Japan

Index

Printed in the USA
CPSIA information can be obtained
at www.ICGtesting.com
JSHW061537161023
50268JS00005B/54